Being a doctor

Understanding medical practice

Hamish Wilson & Wayne Cunningham

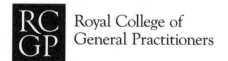
Royal College of
General Practitioners

Published by the Royal College of General Practitioners, 2014
30 Euston Square, London NW1 2FB
www.rcgp.org.uk

First published 2013 by Otago University Press, Dunedin, New Zealand
Copyright © Hamish Wilson and Wayne Cunningham 2013
ISBN 978-0-85084-365-1

Cover image: Gretchen Albrecht, *Violet Surge*, 2012, Oil and acrylic on Belgian linen, 85 x 150 cm, Collection of the artist

Cover and type design by Fiona Moffat
Printed by Hobbs the Printers Ltd

Text acknowledgements
The authors and publisher gratefully acknowledge the permission granted to reproduce the copyright material in this book. Every effort has been made to trace copyright holders and to obtain their permission for the use of copyright material. The publisher apologises for any errors or omissions in the below list and would be grateful if notified of any corrections that should be incorporated in future reprints or editions of this book.

Figure 1.1 (p.18), Figure 1.2 (p.19), Table 6.1 (p.113): adapted from Hutchinson TA, Mount BM, Kearney M, 'The healing journey'. In: Hutchinson T, ed., *Whole person care: a new paradigm for the 21st century*, pp.23–30. Copyright © 2011. Reprinted with kind permission of Springer Science+Business Media.

Figure 3.1 (p.56): adapted from *The American Journal of Psychiatry* 137(5), Engel G, 'The clinical application of the bio-psychosocial model', 535–544. Copyright © 1980. Reprinted with kind permission of the American Psychiatric Association.

Figure 4.1 (p.73): adapted from *Patient Education and Counseling* 85(3), Jagosh J, Boudreau J, Steinert Y, MacDonald M, Ingram L, 'The importance of physician listening from the patients' perspective: enhancing diagnosis, healing and the doctor-patient relationship', 369–374. Copyright © 2011. Reprinted with kind permission of Elsevier.

Figure 4.2 (p.74): adapted from *Patient Education and Counseling* 74(3), Street Jr RL, Makoul G, Arora NK, Epstein RM, 'How does communication heal? Pathways linking clinician-patient communication to health outcomes', 295–301. Copyright © 2009. Reprinted with kind permission of Elsevier.

Figure 6.2 (p.102), Box 6.1 (p.103), Figure 6.3 (p.104): adapted from Stewart M, Belle Brown J, Weston W, McWhinney I, McWilliam C, Freeman T, *Patient-centered medicine: transforming the clinical method*. 2nd edn. Copyright © 2003. Reprinted with kind permission of Radcliffe Publishing.

Figure 6.2 (p.102), Box 6.2 (p.106), Figure 6.4 (p.108), Figure 6.5 (p.109), Table 7.1 (p.128): adapted from Silverman J, Kurtz S, Draper J, *Skills for communicating with patients*. 2nd edn. Copyright © 2003. Reprinted with kind permission of Radcliffe Publishing.

Figure 6.6 (p.111), Figure 6.7 (p.112): adapted from Hutchinson T, Brawer J, 'The challenge of medical dichotomies and the congruent physician–patient relationship in medicine'. In: Hutchinson T, ed., *Whole person care: a new paradigm for the 21st century*, pp. 31–44. Copyright © 2011. Reprinted with kind permission of Springer Science+Business Media.

Table 7.2 (p.130): from Meador CK, *Symptoms of unknown origin: a medical odyssey*. Copyright © 2005. Reprinted with kind permission of Vanderbilt University Press.

Figure 8.2 (p.151): from *The Lancet* 374(9702), Wallace JE, Lemaire JB, Ghali WA, 'Physician wellness: A missing quality indicator', 1714–21. Copyright © 2009. Reprinted with kind permission of Elsevier.

Figure 12.1 (p.229): from *The New England Journal of Medicine* 344(26), Green LA, Fryer Jr GE, Yawn BP, Lanier D, Dovey SM, 'The ecology of medical care revisited', 2021–5. Copyright © 2001. Reprinted with kind permission of Massachusetts Medical Society.

Figure 12.2 (p.233): adapted from Howden-Chapman P, Tobias M, eds., *Social Inequalities in Health: New Zealand 1999*. Copyright © 2000. Reprinted with kind permission of New Zealand Ministry of Health.

Contents

Acknowledgements

This book arises from many years of discussion with our postgraduate students. We are indebted to them for their contribution to these emerging ideas and their generosity in providing so many rich examples of clinical practice.

We are particularly grateful for the helpful critique and advice from members of the Department of General Practice and Rural Health, Dunedin School of Medicine, especially Associate Professor Jim Reid, Professor Susan Dovey and Dr Katharine Wallis. Drs Katherine Glover and Roz McKechnie provided excellent editorial comments.

We also consulted more widely, sending early drafts of chapters to a range of colleagues. We received invaluable comments from Dr Alison Begg, Professor Peter Crampton, Dr Mark Davis, Dr Tom Egnew (Washington State University), Dr Sue Hawken and Dr Peter Huggard (University of Auckland), Professor Jane Lemaire (University of Calgary), Dr Brett Mann, Dr Lucy O'Hagan, Richard O'Neill-Dean and George Sweet.

Special thanks to Dr Glenn Colquhoun for his encouragement of our conceptual ideas and his insightful foreword.

Finally, our heartfelt thanks go to our families for their continued love and support: Annette Rose and Flavia Wilson; Joanne, Renee, Andrew and Courtney Cunningham.

Dedication

Being a Doctor is dedicated to the memory of Dr Pat Farry: mentor, colleague and friend.

Foreword to the UK edition

The cabaret trio Fascinating Aïda perform a song that opens with a dismal litany of the stresses, threats and false ideologies currently contaminating the Western world. Then the music swells optimistically as the comediennes imagine a simpler, purer, nobler life in the Antipodes. 'Suddenly New Zealand,' they sing, 'is attractively remote.'

I suspect that many British readers of this book, struggling in a torrent of targets, diktats and reorganisations, will nod approvingly, knowing just how they feel.

Hamish Wilson and Wayne Cunningham come from the School of Medicine in Dunedin, in the far south of New Zealand's South Island, which, geographically, is about as far as it's possible to get from the UK. But their book – perceptive, inspirational, and in its way more nutritious even than the lamb or butter of their native land – locates them, philosophically, as close as it's possible to get to the heart of what general practice is (or ought to be) about.

Being a Doctor is born of a long-running disconnect between medicine as applied biomedical science on the one hand and, on the other, as a conduit of consolation from one human being to another in distress. Wilson and Cunningham rightly denounce this as a false schism, and seek to help doctors at every career stage bridge the gap between the personal and the impersonal. In elegant, easy-to-read prose they lead us on a comprehensive journey through general practice's landmark concepts, explaining and illustrating as they go. Disease, they remind us, can be understood through the methods of science; but to understand the felt experience of illness calls in addition for narrative competency and emotional intelligence on the part of the doctor. The relationship between doctor and patient is both the setting for healing and a powerful tool for achieving it, and requires to be managed no less expertly than the physical pathologies our patients present. To this end, doctors need to be attentive to their own health and well-being, and to cultivate the habit of reflective practice as part of their professionalism.

Many GPs of my generation, and maybe the one after, will recall nostalgically the genuine thrill of discovering how such insights could illuminate our clinical work. The days of my professional youth were the heydays of the Balint movement and the 'long last appointment', a period when notions like patient-centredness and consultation models were intriguingly new. They were also less pressured, more contemplative times. It felt then as if reflecting on the process and psychodynamics of our consultations enhanced rather than impeded our ability to get through the day's work. But for today's rising generation of GPs – preoccupied first with passing the MRCGP exam, then coping with mounting demands in the teeth of a gale of information and regulation, trying the while to build a career on constantly shifting bureaucratic sands – the philosophising of my youth might seem at best a luxury, at worst an irrelevance and a distraction. I could understand how, to some of my younger colleagues, the New Zealand of *Being a Doctor* might at first appear remote, and not necessarily attractively so.

And now a further complication has arisen. The dichotomous nature of our profession – 'medicine as a science' or 'medicine as a humanity' – has been rendered three-tailed by the emergence of a new persona – 'medicine as a state institution'. It was inevitable, as populations age, health-care costs escalate and electorates become more articulate, that general practice would become a societal enterprise with impact and implications more far-reaching than the sum of its individual constituent doctor–patient consultations. Inevitable too, therefore, that we would find ourselves a focus of attention for all the familiar apparatchiks of a national organisation: the managers and accountants, the commissioners and regulators, the economists and statisticians, the drafters of contracts and guidelines, the political naggers and snipers. Overwhelmed by all this attention, we risk succumbing to the common fallacy that to be a doctor nowadays is to be little more than a distributor of a commercial commodity called 'health care'. Suddenly New Zealand …

Stephen Karpman, a transactional analysis therapist, described in a classic paper what can happen when three parties get themselves entwined in a 'drama triangle' of interdependent relationships. One of them takes the role of 'Victim' to another's 'Persecutor', while the third becomes the 'Rescuer'. An everyday example is a patient who falls victim to a disease (persecutor), which the doctor/rescuer is expected to cure. Other common triangles are patient/GP/specialist, or medical profession/public/politicians. In Karpman's analysis the roles are not fixed, and can rotate endlessly. A familiar variant of the patient/disease/doctor scenario is when it becomes the patient who persecutes the doctor/victim with medically unexplained symptoms, from which predicament the doctor can be rescued by the chance finding of an abnormal pathology result, providing a pseudo-disease to pursue. Equally common, and probably more damaging, is the interminable *pas de trois* in which profession, public and politicians squabble over who is the good guy, who the bad guy and who the fall guy in the long-running drama that is our National Health Service.

Medicine's three identities – science, humanity and institution – all too readily form drama triangles, in which one sneers at another, who calls on the third to intercede in support. 'Doctor–patient relationship?' scoffs hard-nosed science. 'Eyewash and window-dressing!' 'Ah, but it's very popular window-dressing,' say the institutions of state, 'and it doesn't do to alienate the voters – sorry, the patients.' Or, 'Give us more money!' high-tech medicine demands of the government. 'Here, let us help,' says general practice. 'We would make much better use of resources.' Or, 'You erode the personal element in medicine at your peril,' humanity warns the latest political new broom. Science is invoked: 'Where's the evidence for that?' it demands. 'We need more research.'

And so on and – never-endingly and addictively – on. Whole medical, academic and political careers can be wasted in such cyclical in-fighting, in which nobody stays a winner for long and patients seem always to lose.

The only escape from a drama triangle is not to play the game at all – to eschew stereotyping, misrepresentation and name-calling, and make a determined stand for balanced rationality. Wilson and Cunningham have managed this beautifully. Being a doctor their way is to compromise neither the science of medicine nor its humanity. They manage to keep things simple without being naïve. They show us complexity without making it impenetrable. They integrate medicine's disparate strands and roles into coherence without loss of identity. To have succeeded in this task is an act of healing on a grand – a global – scale. The lessons they teach and the vision they vouchsafe are every bit as relevant to us in the UK as in their own homeland. So you see, Fascinating Aïda, half the world away is no distance at all.

Roger Neighbour OBE DSc MA FRCP FRCGP FRACGP
Past President, Royal College of General Practitioners
Bedmond, Hertfordshire
April 2014

Foreword to the NZ edition

Dark matters

The last time I worked in a hospital I flew in a helicopter. I was based at an intensive care unit that served a large area of the country. My patients were unconscious and I carried a pocket full of syringes to keep it that way. The views were glorious. Patients had something wrong with them. Medicine had medicines. The world was a Google map. Then I entered general practice and became lost. In general practice I am pressed so close to what I am looking at that most of the time I cannot see it at all. On days when I am able to follow the thread of an illness through the body it often disappears in front of me, leaving me grasping, as though what is wrong with someone might really be wrong in some imaginary part of them or in a web of connections around them. Sometimes diseases simply change shape. Here they are diseases and here they aren't, now you see them, now you don't, like particles blinking in and out of existence. I think I am dumb all the time.

It has taken some time to realise that it is supposed to be this way. Diseases have to begin somewhere. It can take a while to see them sticking out against the background. When is unhappiness too much unhappiness? When is too much drinking too much drinking? Then there are the treatments: those that should work but don't, those that shouldn't work but do, those we are sorry we ever used in the first place and, most frustrating of all, those that work but taste bad. Still, I stay. The view might be distorted and involving but it is no less beautiful. In general practice I am in the paint, dripping. I am forced to see the world street-first. Joy and sorrow change like lights at a busy intersection.

Last Wednesday morning I saw a young woman with eczema. I saw a man who wanted to stop smoking. I read letters about a patient who had had his gallbladder removed and another whose heart was dancing. I saw a young woman for a repeat prescription. Her story was so large I knew not to ask about it in the morning when the day is fragile with need. I received the results of a blood test that told me a man I saw last week with a twisted knee probably has diabetes. A woman is no longer anaemic. Another man's blood is neither too thick nor too thin. A teenager has no bugs in her urine. I read an insurance report. It told me the prolonged sexual abuse of my patient has caused her post-traumatic stress but not her depression. They will treat her for one but not the other. People are made of per cents and they are able to account for them. I saw an old woman for no good reason other than she wanted to say hello to me. We talked about knitting and I made her laugh. I saw another old woman who is running out of puff and has a sore neck. Her sticks click as she walks. We smile. I get a text from a patient who needs her pills. I get another from a woman who has been fighting with the man she loves and fears. I promise to talk to him but I haven't yet. I want to but I fear him too. Most gratifying of all, I finish on time. Life has come along in the right-sized bundles and I have ignored it when it hasn't.

Doctors sit in rooms with patients. Their conversations usually begin innocuously, with courtesies, rituals of meeting, ways of putting each other at ease. After this they move on to the business of the day. What is it you have come for? What is it that can be done? Transactions are conducted. At some point, no matter how straightforward the interaction, there will be a moment, a change in pitch, a thing unsaid. The room will not be empty. If you look around you will see the doctor and the patient and the desk and the chair but that will not be the sum total of the room. There will also be a weight. Dark matter is present. And dark matter does what dark matter does. It distorts. It bends us around it. It creates a gravity that cannot be explained and draws us together. It makes no difference whether you ignore it or not, it is there. It is a sort of death, a lovely death, a thing beyond, a very full kind of emptiness.

Patients have taught me that this gap between people is jam-packed, that the pauses between us can lead to a question someone wants to ask or to a burden they want to share and that in this exchange human beings are medicine to human beings. People drink each other like shy deer at pools. At these points the greatest tenderness possible is simply not to scare each other. We can send satellites to space, we can smash matter together inside superconductors, but talk to someone, listen to them, be with them when they doubt or are in pain and you will see all the dark matter you need. It is no surprise at all. Medicine is full of it.

Wednesday afternoon things change. Nothing is the right size at all. I visit a young man with cystic fibrosis. His older brother died of the same disease a few years ago and he and his mother are tired. I try to encourage them but they know better. I see a young woman who was abused as a child. She is clever, speaks three languages and loves literature. Anxieties float around her like butterflies. We try to separate what is real from what is real. The next patient wants me to sign a piece of paper. While my pen is scratching she tells me she is in dispute with her partner. He is leaving her for someone else. He is trying to evict her from her home and their case is to be heard shortly. I try to write faster so that the story will stop before it reaches its inevitable conclusion but I am too late. As she speaks her resolve falters and melts. The paper sits on the desk like a small patterned tablecloth at a picnic. Great grey tears splotch on top of it.

I linger over the body of my next patient looking for a reason why she could feel so tired. I know it is unlikely I will find one but I need to try. It gives me permission to ask how she is sleeping and to wonder what else is going on in her life. She unravels and weeps: relationships, money and work come flooding out. The last patient of the day is frustrated and alone and wants me to listen and pay somehow. She is tired. She grew up in care. Her family is in care and she is angry. She wants to hit out and cling on and sob all at the same time. In a strange way she likes me. In a strange way I like her too. But not right now. I am tired. The afternoon has barely been in control. Its lives have been threatening to run amok into mine. I try to articulate hope every way I can but that is only making things worse. She provokes me. It is a gift. She wants me to feel what she feels but instead I tell her to leave. Not like that. Not in so many words. I do it in a doctor way so that it is covered up and respectable but she is clever enough by half to know what I am saying. She has hurt me. I only sleep half the night. Our conversation plays over and over in my head and I don't know what it means except that it means something. It feels like love and I wonder why that is.

Doctors have edges. At best I am only ever temporarily reasonable. If pushed I can be condescending and rude and petty and stubborn. On any given day I see only a fraction of what makes up a human life and make a series of judgements based on that. Sometimes they are accurate and often they aren't. I am constantly humbled when I find out who my patients really are at home or in the community and by what they really see in me. One of the distinctions of general practice is that it sees its patients over time. It is to our great advantage as doctors that this time allows people to emerge bit by bit out of the conditions they come to see us with. Time after time these people have taken me by the hand, checked my pulse and calmed me down. They have taught me that human beings come in layers. What is important to them may not be immediately obvious and may not be what they first point towards. If doctors can be trusted with one layer they might be trusted with the next. At times there may be a layer a patient will feel the presence of but cannot name or a layer they are unaware they want to reveal. If you are prepared to wait long enough they might do so. This sort of waiting can save a lot of time.

More than anything else, my patients have taught me that we die. Even when they come to me with something that medicine is able to treat, once it is treated they return to dying. It may be a month later, a year later, a lifetime later. However long it takes, the body will return a little the worse for wear. All medicine fails in the end. My handiwork comes back to me less polished, unravelling, the laces undone. My patients and I both know it and if we are lucky we get to talk about it at times. Perhaps this is the most splendid view general practice offers. Those that have been my best teachers have carried the dead with them, have hinted at the arrogance of the living thinking they are the only ones who know what is going on. They chuckle. There is a sense that everything will be accounted for in the end. We are all rolled back into a context greater than ourselves, whatever that may be. Perhaps this is dark matter after all. I don't know. Such a view forces a sort of spirituality and that spirituality has power because it gives connection to something beyond our extinction as individuals. What we believe is always at least as important as what we know, however inconvenient. The imagination is the most powerful medicine of all.

On Sunday I get a call from an elderly patient. Her husband is dying of bowel cancer. He cannot sleep. I started him on a sleeping pill to help a month ago. Recently she has seen a programme on television about how people who take sleeping pills die earlier than those that don't and so she has stopped it and her husband is up half the night again which means she is as well. I promise to visit but I wonder why I am, 'Heck, he's dying. Why not sleep well?' When I get to the door I knock three times but no one hears me. I go back to the car and call my patient to say I am there. She lets me in and we talk for a long time about randomised controlled trials and what can be inferred and the inevitability of her husband's illness. She encourages and nods and nods and encourages until I remember she is deaf on the side I am talking to. She is not sure what I am saying but she thinks it is her husband's own fault he doesn't sleep because he stays up to watch rugby and she says to lie down and close his eyes and think of God and what do I think? I smile and say it is ok to take the pill. She says that's good then.

And this is my life outside the helicopter: no one opens the door, people cannot hear properly, medicines taste bad, something is on television, husbands ignore their wives and God is always interfering. What little medicine I have left must thread its way through all of these. Perhaps this is medicine itself. Maybe. It is a different view to the one from the mountain top but no less spectacular for all that.

This is a book about that view. General practice is not about anything grand like brains or kidneys or livers or hearts. General practitioners do what no one else will do, the little things, the bits in between. They bear witness. But it is in that bearing witness that they see over time a real living human being lift out of a collection of symptoms and body parts and startle. As much as anything else, general practice is a point of view, a way of looking. This book made me feel less lonely about medicine when I read it. Sometimes I wanted to punch the air. Sometimes I sagged with the feeling that someone had put into words what I didn't know I already knew. It felt like I was with those who see what is beautiful about our ordinariness, who love people, who see how remarkably complex an everyday life is and how the dead are always with us. It is about dark matter. Read it and go outside. The world will click and buzz and wink. It is good medicine.

Glenn Colquhoun
January 2013

Introduction

Early in my training in general practice, I attended a patient with poorly controlled asthma. Trying to improve her condition, I reviewed her clinical notes, hospital admissions, respiratory clinic letters, and changed her medications. Yet despite my efforts, she remained unwell. Feeling quite impotent in the face of her ongoing asthma, I asked my family medicine teacher what I should do.

In reply, he posed a question: 'Are you there to cure disease or to help people with their lives?' I found the stark choice he was offering at that time very challenging. Who was I to try and help someone with their life? Was I also supposed to be a counsellor, a psychologist or even a priest?

Just doing the 'disease stuff' seemed hard enough to me. I was frustrated by his question, wanting a simple answer that would lead to a cure. Although the question could have been phrased differently, his insight into what I needed to learn was quite accurate. It suggested I had to choose between one goal or another. However, with my disease-focused training failing me, I also lacked skills that would address any wider perspectives. A better question might have been 'How can you both manage her disease and help her with this illness?' Either way, his question stayed in my mind for many years and I now appreciate the wisdom behind it. In retrospect, he started me on a pathway of learning about what being a doctor really means.[1]

Since the mid-1990s, we have led a postgraduate course for doctors called 'The Nature of Medical Practice' at the University of Otago. This course is quite different in style from most other postgraduate education. Instead of solely providing theory, the modules of learning are based on the combined clinical experience of these mature general practitioners. By setting their knowledge of practice against theory, we provide them with opportunities to explore and critique their assumptions and goals.

Over time, we have considerably refined and developed the course. After years of participating in many fascinating discussions about clinical practice, we gradually realised we were also exploring what it *means* to be a doctor. This is more than having sufficient knowledge and skills, or being generally competent. Being a doctor starts with a complex socialisation process, where professional identity is shaped and moulded. Doctors learn to conform to the prevailing medical norms, while also grappling with aspects of medical culture that can be at odds with their own values.

Similarly, these GPs also noted how their predominantly hospital-based training was poor preparation for family medicine or general practice. While their knowledge of disease was usually adequate, they were struck by the different spectrum of disease in the community, where the influence of the person of the patient was more obvious and significant. Their feeling of disquiet about the mismatch between training and practice has been labelled as dissonance: it comes from the often substantial gap between theory and real-life clinical experience.

---

1   This particular story is from Wayne Cunningham's personal experience.

This book arises from these iterative discussions about what it is like to be a doctor. We also hope to resolve some of the dissonance between 'received theory' and the reality of modern medicine.

Dissonance can be felt in hospital practice as well as in community settings. In the emergency department and in outpatient work, many patients continue to bewilder the most competent of doctors. Such difficulties arise from two main sources. First, there can be a mismatch between biomedical theory and the problems that patients present to us. This mismatch was never discussed in our own training, where biomedical knowledge was deemed sufficient. Some doctors internalise this dissonance as a personal lack of knowledge or competence. Sometimes the patient is ridiculed or demonised instead. A better approach is to become more objective about biomedicine as the predominant model of clinical practice, exploring both its strengths and weaknesses.

Second, in our training we were provided with little awareness of the importance of the doctor–patient relationship. Somehow the doctor was considered to be separate or detached from the patient. The problem here is that that relationship includes oneself. Critiquing the doctor–patient relationship and its effect on outcomes of care implies a quite different set of assumptions about the nature of medicine and the role of the doctor. The profession needs to be more scientific about this relationship, looking at it in the same way as any other component of patient care. In this book, we explore these issues carefully, building the case that relationship is a core aspect of medicine as a healing profession.

We are academic general practitioners who have been immersed in clinical practice and in teaching for many decades. Although we are writing from a general practice perspective, this book is sufficiently generic to be helpful for everyone. Our hope is that doctors in all specialties can use these ideas to reflect on their approach to clinical work.

We would like this book to inform medical teachers, especially family medicine teachers or GP preceptors who host vocational trainees. It will be particularly relevant for trainee doctors who are making the transition from hospital practice into community settings. For undergraduate students, the concepts here may bridge their learning about disease and their early clinical experiences. While undergraduate education has changed considerably, there is still a long way to go before future graduates are fully prepared for clinical practice. Ideally, this book will reduce the gaps between theory, training and clinical work.

This book, then, is about the current practice of medicine. It aims to improve patient care by helping doctors to understand and achieve their tasks, especially when faced with the difficulties that our work often presents. We believe each doctor, as a person, is inseparable from the task of delivering medical care. Enhancing our ability to deliver that care is essential for patients, communities and society. Just as patients need 'whole person' care, the profession needs 'whole person' doctors. Being a doctor, and deriving meaning from clinical experience, are at the heart of this book.

The following brief introduction to each chapter will illustrate how we have developed our approach to whole person care and to whole person doctoring.

We begin by considering the role of the healer, challenging the reader to explore their own roles and goals in medicine. In Chapter 2, we explore the patient's illness experience in depth. We introduce the idea of narrative and how the doctor can help shape that narrative, illustrating how suffering and healing are linked.

To 'be' a doctor involves understanding the philosophy of medicine and how that philosophy underpins clinical practice. Both teaching and practice rest on assumptions that are seldom recognised or made explicit. In Chapter 3, we define and critique the modern biomedical paradigm, identifying what are known as 'anomalies'. The 'placebo effect' and somatisation are particularly interesting clinical situations, where theory does not match with clinical experience.

Doctor and patient are always in a relationship of one sort or another: the doctor–patient relationship (Chapter 4) is the channel through which we deliver medical care. The book explores the various components of this relationship, what goes well, what does not go so well, and why that could be so. Chapter 5 looks at particular challenges in relationship. While there has been an emerging thread of discussion about 'heartsink' or 'difficult' patients, we prefer the term 'heartsink' *experience*, as the issues usually lie within the doctor's experience of that particular patient.

In Chapter 6, we review various models or frameworks of the consultation. These models provide insight into the moment-to-moment consultation process. By being explicit about current models of practice, our hope is that doctors can better reflect on their consulting style. This leads to recognising which strategies or approaches are most effective and what can be modified or avoided. Linking back to somatisation in Chapter 3, we also propose a revised approach to the patient where no disease can be found (Chapter 7).

The next three chapters focus on the person of the doctor. The health and well-being of practitioners are crucial to the effective delivery of medical care. If doctors are not well, struggling to cope, traumatised, or heading towards burnout, their ability to care for patients will be compromised. In Chapter 8, we review this difficult area of professional practice, offering suggestions for how doctors can maintain and improve their resilience. Similarly, in Chapter 9, we explore the ways in which the culture of medicine impacts on doctors. Medical culture is a complex subject, experienced by all practitioners, but rarely discussed. Tools to define and critique that culture are offered. We also explore the complex socialisation process through which novice students develop their professional identities.

Reflective practice (Chapter 10) is the key to effective experiential learning. Reflection used to lie outside the culture of medicine, perhaps because the traditional or 'scientific' approach would have us believe that doctors are independent observers. Once the barriers to reflection have been identified, various methods can be used to reflect constructively on clinical practice. Balint work is particularly interesting as a form of reflective practice, illustrating many of the key themes in this book. This method is outlined in detail in the Appendix.

The culture of medicine is also integral to the increasing problem of adverse outcomes of clinical care and the emerging concept of patient safety (Chapter 11). This chapter outlines the profession's rather curious delay in responding to these unexpected consequences of health care. We look to the future and consider how such events can be both expected and prevented. The focus here is largely on hospital practice, as patient safety is still an emerging concept in primary care. However, the issues are once again generic.

Doctors working in primary care are often challenged by patients' living circumstances that are influencing their health. The penultimate chapter considers how primary medical care is located within primary health care, as well as the interface with secondary care. This is an important chapter for doctors making the transition to general practice or starting in family medicine training. Adjusting to differences in the scope of practice can take some time.

We conclude in Chapter 13 by considering what is needed to educate and train the doctor of the future. By incorporating the strengths of biomedicine with models of clinical practice such as whole person care, we believe doctors can adopt a more coherent and effective approach. Whole person care brings the patient, the doctor and the disease together in a framework that helps answer the challenging question of how to practise medicine and how to be a doctor.

This book is not a list of updates or latest therapies. It is assumed that the reader is a competent doctor, or at least is in the process of becoming one. We refer to medical conditions, treatments and clinical behaviour without further explanation. Similarly, this book does not cover financial structures of practice or private to public health service arrangements, as these vary from country to country. Instead, this book explores the underlying philosophy of modern medicine and so will help competent doctors to better understand their practice, regardless of local context. It will also help them to grapple more effectively with the complexities and challenges of day-to-day work.

In several chapters we have drawn on our own clinical experience and used stories or 'vignettes' to illustrate particular ideas. Where appropriate, vignettes have been edited by the patients themselves, and in all cases names and particulars have been altered to preserve confidentiality. These vignettes are not exemplars of perfect practice. We hope that readers will imagine themselves in these situations and reflect on their own experiences. Some chapters include a list of 'further reading', relevant books we have found useful.

While the chapters build progressively on ideas, readers may 'lift' each one out if it meets their learning or teaching needs. For pronouns, we have avoided the repetitive use of 's/he' and 'they', preferring instead to use 'she' and 'he' in different vignettes.

Our hope is that this book will help inform doctors about the nature of their work, help them face and resolve some of their daily challenges, and make them more effective in their practice. Being a doctor is much more than simply providing medical care: our overall aim is to increase the resilience and wellness of doctors. This helps the profession to provide better care for patients, through a deep and thoughtful approach to clinical work.

Hamish Wilson and Wayne Cunningham
January 2013

Chapter 1

Medicine, Suffering and Healing

CONTENTS

Introduction

The practice of medicine is usually quite straightforward: this or that abdominal pain may have a surgical cause; a broken leg can be set; diabetes can be managed. Routine practice, regardless of context, does not usually ask questions of meaning or professional identity. Yet now and again there is a sense that a straightforward approach is not enough. We encounter patients who challenge our ideas about medicine and what we hope to achieve: the more complex, even 'difficult' patients. Underlying issues now need to be addressed.

We start this chapter, then, with two questions: 'Is medicine a healing profession?' and 'Are doctors healers?' While these questions are challenging and provocative, they are a useful start for thinking about the aims of clinical practice. If doctors are not involved in healing, regardless of specialty, then what is their purpose?

We will explore suffering and healing as separate from cure, as well as the concept of doctors as healers. We will then draw these ideas together, identifying an apparent contradiction as doctors learn to use themselves as the healing agent.

While our observations of clinical practice are located in primary care, these ideas about doctoring are generic and apply to doctors in all specialties. Making the transition from hospital to general practice can simply make these issues more apparent.

We start with a short vignette about a patient with an acute illness. While the setting is the emergency department, this patient might just as easily present herself in general practice or be referred to a gastroenterology clinic for review. The vignette illustrates some of the major themes in this chapter. The doctor's perspective will be discussed later.

VIGNETTE 1.1 HOLDING IT ALL IN

A 20-year-old woman came to the emergency department with four hours of severe dry-retching every 10 to 15 minutes. This had happened a few times previously and she usually required an injection for the bouts to stop. She initially attributed this episode to last night's meal of chicken, although others who ate a similar meal were unaffected. She looked anxious, but her examination was unremarkable. BP and pulse were normal, no evidence of dehydration, abdomen soft. She had a friend with her.

Over the next two hours she had two anti-emetic injections that made no difference at all.

A second doctor came on duty and was asked to take over this patient's care. He took the history a little further. She outlined a story of previous bouts of such vomiting over the past seven years, occurring about once per year. Exploration of her family history revealed that her mother had problems with undiagnosed headaches and that her father was physically well. Her only sibling, an older sister, had died some years before in a tragic accident. She said this was an ongoing issue for her, although she had a reputation of 'coping well'.

On further enquiry about her life, she said she was studying for a degree but had yet to apply for the one she really wanted. She was also ambivalent about whether or not to hold her 21st birthday party in the next few months, aware that her father's life plans had changed dramatically since the death of her sibling. She was fearful that a 21st celebration would cause her family even more pain. The change in family dynamics after her sister's death had been very difficult. She had not really discussed these issues with anyone (including her friend who was present), as they might see her as not coping so well.

This second consultation took about 15 minutes. At this stage, she appeared calm and relaxed, and the dry retching had completely stopped. She thanked the doctor and made arrangements to leave.

What was going on here? Why did the patient suddenly improve? What did the doctor actually achieve, and how?

Rather than presenting this vignette as a 'diagnostic puzzle' to be solved, the story is intended to stimulate thought about possible links between acute illness and suffering, and how we might consider the doctor's role. First, though, we will consider the central concept of 'suffering'. What is it, and how does it relate to our work as doctors?

Suffering and healing

Dr Eric Cassell is a physician from New York who has written extensively on suffering. His 1982 article 'The nature of suffering and the goals of medicine', in the *New England*

Journal of Medicine, has been widely quoted,(1) and his later book of the same title is one of the classic modern texts on this subject.(2)

Cassell helpfully distinguishes between pain and suffering. Patients with their first bout of renal colic, for example, may be scared and apprehensive about what is causing the pain, but once they know and understand the diagnosis they can cope reasonably well, knowing that it will soon pass. On the other hand, back pain that might mean the recurrence of cancer is much less bearable. The uncertainty of the pain and its implications can be profound for that person's future.

Suffering, then, is less about pain and more about the meaning or implications of the symptom or illness. It usually involves a feeling of helplessness in the face of a threat to their idea of themselves and/or their world. As Cassell puts it, 'Suffering is experienced by *persons,* not merely by bodies, and has its source in challenges that threaten the intactness of the person as a complex social and psychological entity'(our italics).(2)

In a similar way, parents suffer greatly from the illnesses of their children, especially long-term illnesses such as cancer or congenital disease. It is also hard to sit by and observe the pain and distress of parents or loved ones, especially in terminal illness. Suffering is felt by the whole family, not just the person who is ill. The powerlessness of being unable to relieve the pain or discomfort of others can cause tremendous suffering.

Cassell outlines a comprehensive typology of persons that we will return to in Chapter 2. Disturbance in any aspect of personhood can cause suffering. Doctors need to be curious about patients *as persons,* in order to identify the meaning of their particular suffering.

On the other hand, healing involves the amelioration of suffering. Suffering is resolved if the threat to personal integrity is removed. Following on from Cassell, Egnew helpfully proposes a definition of healing as 'the personal experience of the transcendence of suffering'.(3) Suffering can be transcended through acceptance of the situation or by finding meaning in the experience of suffering. This can happen regardless of whether or not the patient is actually cured or restored to health, and even when the patient knows their illness is terminal.

Suffering is not defined by the diagnosis of a particular disease. Suffering is an experience that is peculiar and specific to each person. Healing must also be specific: whether a doctor can help or not will be specific to that person, the meaning of their illness, and the particulars of the doctor–patient interaction.

Fortunately, most disease does not cause much suffering, as the challenge to the patient's integrity as a person is relatively minor. Patients quickly accommodate a short-term problem such as tonsillitis or a broken bone; they know they will recover their lives fully. As will be noted later, this is known as the 'restitution narrative': it is the common overall storyline in acute illness.

To a variable extent, patients will also resolve the impact of more serious disease on their lives and day-to-day aspirations. An injury causing paraplegia, however, will be a profound challenge to the perceived future of most people. Some patients accommodate such misfortune, reaching a new equilibrium within themselves, while others remain bitter and resentful about their bad luck.

Figure 1.1 illustrates how suffering and healing can be usefully identified as sitting at either end of a continuous scale.(4) For example, a person in major grief is clearly suffering; those around them attempt to facilitate their journey towards some equanimity and inner peace in relation to their loss. Similarly, patients are often quite anguished at the onset of major life-threatening disease such as cancer, stroke or heart attack. Their overall recovery will involve physical treatment but may also entail some revisions of *who they are* as a person.

FIGURE 1.1 WOUNDING AND HEALING

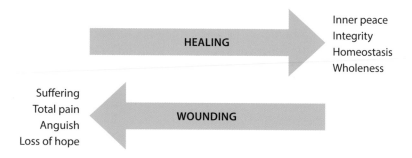

Total pain refers to the combination of physical, emotional and/or spiritual pain.
Adapted from Hutchinson et al.(4)

By placing this continuum over time, it is possible to chart each patient's potential journey towards wholeness and recovery. One of the doctor's tasks is to be conscious of these dimensions and of what is helping or hindering the healing process. Clues to this often lie in aspects of personhood. Being curious and observant of the illness experience and becoming interested in how the patient is doing in relation to their disease is the first step.

VIGNETTE 1.2 GRIEF AND ILLNESS

An elderly woman suffers the loss of her husband of over 40 years. She starts to recover from acute grief but, as is quite common in such situations, develops an intercurrent illness (pneumonia). Her physical recovery from this is quite slow and she requires increased home care. Her daughter comes to stay, encouraging her to resume her previous employment in the local vicarage. This helps her to reconnect back to her original sense of self and identity and she is now able to make the transition to living on her own.

Figure 1.2 illustrates this case as just one example of many healing journeys.

FIGURE 1.2 DIMENSIONS OF HEALING JOURNEY

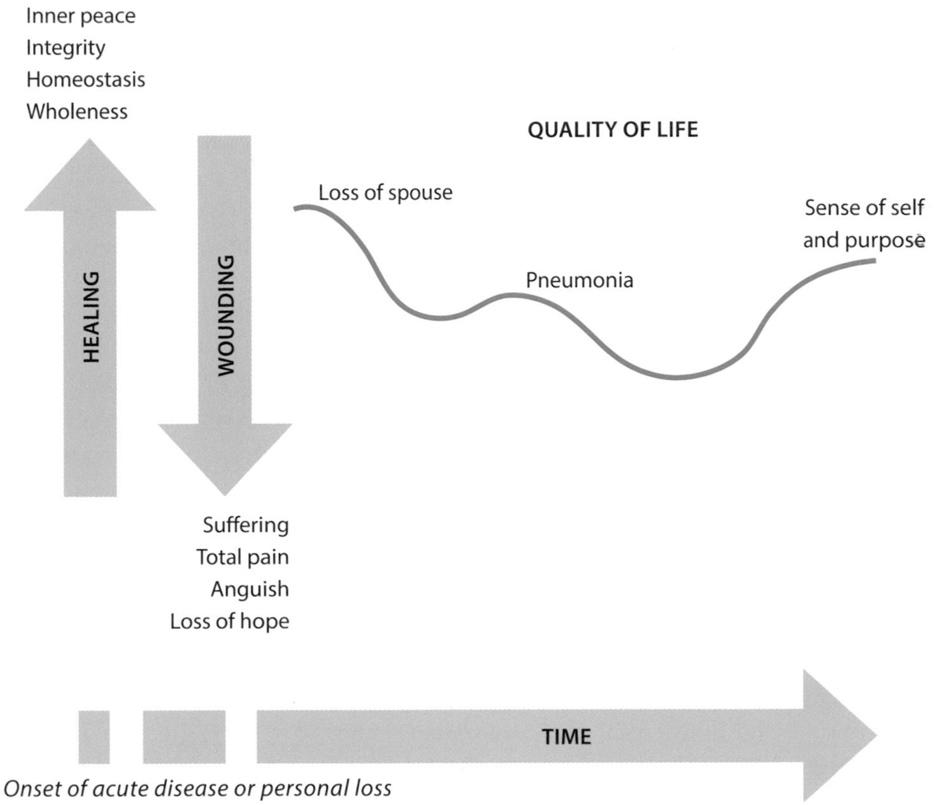

Inner peace
Integrity
Homeostasis
Wholeness

QUALITY OF LIFE

HEALING

WOUNDING

Loss of spouse

Pneumonia

Sense of self
and purpose

Suffering
Total pain
Anguish
Loss of hope

TIME

Onset of acute disease or personal loss

Adapted from Hutchinson et al.(4)

It is fascinating to see how some patients with advanced cancer manage to let go of the idea of cure entirely and embark on a personal journey of discovery about the meaning of their disease. In contrast to restitution, this is known as a 'quest narrative'. (5) Here the action is one of letting go and personal growth. Surprisingly, many such patients comment that having cancer was the 'best thing' to happen to them, as their life was changed for the better.

Mount gives the meaning of healing as 'a relational process involving movement towards an experience of integrity and wholeness, which may be facilitated by the caregiver's interventions but is dependent on an innate potential within the patient'. (6) This useful definition is respectful of each person's capacity for healing, and includes the potential role of the doctor, other health professionals, or family and friends. Before we explore this healing role further, we need to clarify the important distinction between curing and healing.

Curing versus healing

Over the last hundred or so years, the idea that the primary purpose of medicine is to 'cure' has become quite dominant. Historically, the emphasis on a 'cure-based' approach to medical practice is an outcome of the increasing effectiveness of a scientifically based medical practice. While being a powerful curer may be a motivating (if somewhat naïve) idea for early medical students, the reality of clinical practice is quite different. There are many patients who are not curable, many who are dying, and many in whom no disease is actually found. Even though there is much more acknowledgement now of the increasing burden of chronic ('un-curable') disease and the role of community-based health care, the tensions between a 'cure' and a 'care' orientation are still significant and current.

Dr Ellen Fox's insightful and perceptive 1997 article on the 'curative' and the 'palliative' approaches to medical care remains one of the best reviews of this ongoing tension.(7) She asserts that while both models have their place, they are to some extent incompatible. She maintains that the continued, unexamined, and predominant emphasis on cure means that other goals are undervalued, such as 'promoting health, preventing illness and injury, avoiding premature death, restoring functional capacity, relieving suffering, and caring for those who cannot be cured'.

By 'cure', she refers to the eradication of the cause of disease or reversal of the natural history of that disorder. Examples are the removal of an inflamed appendix, successful chemotherapy for leukaemia, or using antibiotics to treat meningitis. Here, the necessary, but exclusive, focus is on the disease of the organ rather than on the person. On the other hand, the palliative care approach, as defined by the World Health Organization, is the 'active total care … of patients whose disease is not responsive to curative treatment'.(7) The attention is on the amelioration of symptoms even if their cause is obscure. The focus is on the whole patient, with their unique social concerns and issues. This approach requires humane qualities and interpersonal skills.

Doctors can be flexible enough to make judicious use of both models in certain circumstances. An acute appendicitis is no doubt cured by appendectomy, as is streptococcal pharyngitis by penicillin. However, ongoing diabetes or arthritis means that a cure is never possible. Symptomatic relief and careful management depend just as much on the patient's personal context as on their underlying disease.

Each model is based on quite different underlying assumptions and values. In brief, the curative way of thinking is analytical and rationalistic. Symptoms are clues to diagnosis; decisions are based on quantitative research; findings can be generalised to other patients, and so on. Subjective, unverifiable, interpersonal or psychological data are thought to be peripheral or even discarded. The palliative model, on the other hand, is more qualitative: subjective, interpersonal, and psychological data are considered equally important.[1]

---

1   We will discuss this more in Chapters 3 and 13. Briefly, the doctor's stance within a 'cure' orientation is located within an objectivist epistemology, and disease is seen to be 'real' as part of a 'modernist' ontology, while research looks for universal laws and applications. A palliative orientation is more subjectivist: illness is viewed as a social construction, with each patient having an individual experience and requiring a unique interpersonal interaction that impacts on illness outcomes.

The next section explores the role of an historical figure who moves between both models – the healer.

Healers in society

Throughout the ages, all societies and cultures have had healers, people with particular abilities and skills who are called upon when someone is sick.(8) They are usually given a special role in their society, sometimes receiving training, sometimes growing into the role through illness of their own. In receiving the patient and offering help, the traditional healer performs an important social role. The story is listened to, the illness is framed with respect to cause, and future events are predicted. The illness is given a context: what before was mysterious or frightening may now be understood.

After this meeting or interaction between sick person and healer, the patient may have to do certain things. He or she might take medicines or herbs, the family may be asked to help, their social supports might be mobilised. The illness is understood within a shared knowledge of causes of illness, while the role of the person who is unwell (the 'sick-role') is discussed and clarified. In brief, the illness is now contained, both personally and socially, within this particular interaction between patient and healer.

The role of healer is not to be taken lightly. Carl Jung, the celebrated psychiatrist and psychoanalyst, identified the healer role as an 'archetype'. Archetypes are inherent and potential forms of human behaviour that are clustered around basic and universal experiences of life: birth, death, separation, and so on.(9) Each has two intrinsic polarities such as father–son, mother–daughter, healer–patient, teacher–learner, individual–collective. Archetypal patterns are 'reinforced by traditional or cultural expectation' and archetypal behaviours are 'most evident in times of crisis'. (10) Illness is a reasonably common form of crisis.

When someone becomes sick, the healer–patient archetype emerges. The patient seeks a healer who can advise and help, while at the same time, the patient's internal capacity for recovery from illness and wound healing will be activated. The doctor–patient relationship is a specific example of the healer–patient archetype.

The doctor thus uses a given and historical set of behaviours designed to facilitate healing in the patient. Furthermore, the 'patient' aspect of the archetype will also be contained within the doctor. The 'wounded healer' is a widespread mythological image referring to the 'patient in the doctor', just as there is always an inner healer within each patient.(11)

What then of modern doctors? Do they fulfil the same social role as traditional healers? We propose that it is helpful to be aware of this symbolic and therapeutic role, even if the tools we now use are quite different from those in more traditional societies. It may be that there are elements of the traditional healer that we can use to augment our modern-day effectiveness.[2]

---

2   We will be discussing some interesting implications of these issues in Chapter 11, which addresses situations where these archetypal roles become problematic.

Traditional healers

In the last 50 years or so, however, the word 'healer' has all but disappeared from medicine, as has the underlying concept of 'doctor as healer'. This is largely due to the increasing emphasis on medicine as science and, more lately, evidence-based medicine. If doctors are capable and effective technicians with powerful interventions at hand, then their interpersonal therapeutic role becomes less important. Yet for several thousand years before modern agents were developed, the doctor was still quite effective. Dixon and others persuasively argue that this was more through their skills in diagnosis and in their use of the therapeutic relationship than through any particular treatment at hand, many of which were inert, or what is now referred to as 'placebo'.(12)

Their review of the 'placebo effect' (a term we will challenge later)[3] illustrates how the doctor can use the 'healing effect' of the doctor–patient relationship. Briefly, this relationship can either augment or hinder the effectiveness of modern treatments, as well as enhance the effect of inert substances.

While Dixon's 1999 article was quite persuasive, the intriguing concept of doctor as healer still remains very much below the medical radar. Doctors tend to reserve the use of the word 'healing' for tissue, organ, or wound healing after trauma, surgery, or other biological intervention. To some extent as well, these words and even the concept of healing have been co-opted by alternative practitioners such as naturopaths and faith/spiritual healers, or are used in relation to recovery from sexual abuse or other traumatic events. Furthermore, the idea of someone 'healing' someone else sounds a little pompous: 'doing something' to your patient while they remain passive, receiving the healing. Perhaps it is this somewhat paternalistic flavour that causes modern doctors to shy away from the term.

Despite these comments, there is a consistent thread within modern medical literature on the doctor as healer. For example, Cassell's *The healer's art* was published in 1976,(13) Brody's *The healer's power* in 1992,(14) Davis-Floyd and St John's *From doctor to healer: the transformative journey* in 1998,(15) and Greaves' *The healing tradition: reviving the soul of Western medicine* in 2004.(16)

Greaves, for example, concurs with Jung in maintaining that all societies need an archetypal healer. He asserts that the modern equivalent is the general practitioner, differentiating this role clearly from that of medical specialists. He draws on Brody's division of the power or authority of the doctor into three components: 'aesculapian' (biomedical), arising from knowledge and skills specific to the profession; 'charismatic', arising from personal qualities and interpersonal effectiveness; and 'social', derived from the status conferred on the doctor by their community.(16)

Traditional or shamanic healers were effective through the social investment and authority conferred on them, despite having limited clinical effectiveness or biomedical power. Given that the focus of general practice is on both the person of the patient *and* their disease, Greaves asserts that the GP's effectiveness, relying as

---

3 Briefly, we believe the term 'placebo effect' has been unhelpful in understanding people's reactions of people to inert substances. We prefer instead the 'meaning response', a term developed by Moerman in his brilliantly insightful book: Moerman D. *Meaning, medicine, and the 'placebo effect'* (Cambridge: Cambridge University Press, 2002).

it does on biomedical and charismatic power located in a community setting, means that GPs are ideally placed to take on the role of modern healer. Their focus can be on the 'healing' of the person, not only through attention to disease details, but also through attention to the person of the patient, with their particular illness experience.

Greaves also maintains that the 'curer' (curing body organ disease) relies on specific and particular use of biomedical skills, whereas the 'healer' relies on the indivisibility of biomedical and charismatic power. The healer can encompass the curer, but the curer cannot necessarily heal.(16)

Greaves's point (echoing Dixon) is that although GPs are the modern equivalent of the archetypal healer, this role has become obscured by the increasing emphasis on doctors as 'technicians of the body'. We argue, however, that a healing role can be utilised by all doctors, regardless of their specialist discipline. It simply depends on an awareness of this potential role, the capacity to take into account the personal issues for the patient, and a combination of both biomedical and charismatic power.

The modern doctor as healer

Discussion about healing in our postgraduate groups usually prompts the following questions: Why choose medicine as a career? What do you value in medicine and what do you hope to achieve? What does being a doctor of medicine really mean to you?

Several writers have considered medicine as a healing profession and the attributes of a healer. The following section summarises ideas from Kleinman, Elwyn, and Colquhoun, doctors who have attempted to answer these questions.

Dr Arthur Kleinman is an American psychiatrist and anthropologist who has researched and written extensively on cultural perspectives in medicine.(17) His seminal book on the experiences of illness includes an insightful chapter about eight different doctors.(18) While almost all were practising hospital-based medicine, they were representative of a variety of philosophies, personal characteristics and approaches to medical work: the self-denying 'devoted servant', the 'burnt-out internist' who had been 'sucked dry' by constant emotional demands, and the 'cynical paediatrician' who practised defensive medicine and doubted any treatment could be effective.

From this ethnographic study, Kleinman draws the following conclusions: a powerful illness in the doctor can lead them into a healer's role and that chronic illness can sensitise the doctor to the experience of suffering; the experiential core of doctoring is a moral domain; doctors can be considered as teachers of moral wisdom; most doctors are somewhere between the healer and the cynic (it may depend on the patient for each doctor); bureaucratic and legal constraints can contaminate the role of the healer, leading to that of technician, filler-of-forms, or even adversary. These are astute and perceptive observations of current doctors at work.

Kleinman also asks how student idealism can change later into corrosive cynicism:

> The professional mask may protect the individual practitioner from feelings of being overwhelmed by patients' demands; but it also may cut him off from the human experience of illness … The very sense of compulsive responsibility essential to the care of acute illness … may, over the long course, create chronic irritability and numbing exhaustion … The practitioner's defences may lead to a self-corrosive negativism or an

iron cage of professional distance from which neither himself nor his family is liberated. (18)

In other words, there are major issues that can act as barriers to becoming a healer. Yet Kleinman also notes that a personal vision and coherence between one's goals and practical work can help doctors escape such depressing outcomes.

Other writers provide personal accounts of medical practice. Dr Glyn Elwyn, a GP and academic from Wales, perceptively discusses 17 consecutive patients, describing each consultation within the context of the patient's life narrative.(19) He describes his attempts to make both biomedical and interpersonal interventions.

Elwyn's article serves to 'normalise' the experience of GP doctoring. He is explicit about the inherent uncertainty within each consultation, noting that he is not sure why some patients are in his surgery, not sure how to encapsulate some problems into biomedical terms, not sure if biomedical knowledge will provide an answer, unclear if interventions are wise in the long term or not, and so on. Elwyn captures the day-to-day dissonance of general practice. He demonstrates the gap or tension between medical training based on a curative model and the reality of daily work.

Dr Glenn Colquhoun, who has written the foreword for this book, is a well-known doctor and poet from Wellington, New Zealand. His 2009 address to the Royal New Zealand College of General Practitioners, 'The therapeutic uses of ache', has become an instant classic.(20) Like Elwyn, he details his own responses to work and patients, making no attempt to distance himself from the task of healing. His story is couched in poetic language, metaphors, and creative images, especially that of ache, 'that point beyond which human beings need faith to function'. He sees his job as listening, hearing people 'love, cry, praise, confess, and ache'.

Colquhoun reveals the personal suffering that allows him to 'sit with' his patients' ache. He describes watching his once-strong father deteriorate and wither from progressive Parkinson's disease, his struggles with his former wife, his doubts over fatherhood. Because he has been sensitised to ache, he allows his patients to reveal their own in his consulting room. His being aware of ache and recognising it, and sometimes sharing that he too has it, means that his patients are not alone: 'People can figure it out from there. This is not doing nothing, ache recognises ache.'

In other words, from being 'wounded' himself, he can act as a facilitator, being respectful of patients' pain and allowing them to figure things out. This stance of professional intimacy is both engaged and at a distance. It maintains respectful boundaries as to who is suffering, the time it will take to recover, and who is doing the work.

Colquhoun touches on issues such as the doctor–patient relationship, the use of therapeutic disclosure, boundaries, and tension between biomedicine and compassion. This is an excellent description of the GP as healer by a modern doctor who is not afraid of this role.

All these writers are exploring the relationship between doctor and patient, where the *person* of the doctor is crucially involved in healing. We return now to the case from Vignette 1.1, this time from the doctor's perspective.

VIGNETTE 1.3 THE NAÏVE ENQUIRER

The management of this patient was handed over to me after the other doctor left. I had heard this patient's dry retching for over an hour, so was curious about what was going on and why there was no response to quite powerful medications.

I entered the consulting room and sat down on a chair opposite the bed. The patient was curled up on her side. Her eyes were wide open and focused. Her friend was sitting near her head at the top of the bed.

After a quick review of her physical status, I was keen to explore her previous episodes of these intractable bouts, looking for clues to better management and perhaps cause. I wondered out loud why she had so many bouts of 'food poisoning'. Alcohol didn't appear to be involved, so I indicated that I wanted to explore family history as possibly being important. The death of her sibling then emerged, which – while clearly significant in her life – was not necessarily linked to these bouts. Her family sounded as if they were still immersed in complex grief. I wondered if these family issues were somehow holding her back from making the normal maturation decisions of a 20-year-old (coming-of-age celebration, career choices, and so on). She revealed she had just fought with her mother a day or so before this current illness.

By this stage she was sitting up. There had been no dry retching whatsoever since I had entered the room. I suggested that she look for any patterns in these bouts of vomiting with respect to personal or family issues, and possibly identify any early warning signs if a further one was brewing.

I felt her rapid improvement was probably due to a combination of the injections and getting some issues into the open, but I also felt we had achieved something quite important. I hoped she would now look at these bouts in a slightly different way, and that there might be some movement in her grief.

From personal experience, I was aware of the nature of grief, how complex it is, and how this can impact on recurrence of illness. While I did not disclose those experiences in this consultation, I found it helpful to have already travelled along that difficult path.

Clearly this patient was distressed by her vomiting, but the additional factor seemed to be the underlying presence of grief. It seemed she was suffering in a number of ways: from the loss of her sister, the effect this was having on her family, and her difficulty in normal individuation. There was also the possibility that these bouts of vomiting were somehow linked to psychosocial triggers.

What was the doctor doing in this vignette? Was he simply encouraging her to work through her grief? If so, would this reduce her suffering? Can he be labelled a 'healer' if his intervention was helpful?

The role of the doctor above seemed to be largely explorative. He was simply being curious about what made this patient quite different from others with vomiting. In doing so, the underlying personal and family issues emerged. The task did not seem to be active in the sense that there was anything the doctor actually needed to do. As it turned out, simply talking was arguably as effective as drug interventions.

In general, we believe that by listening carefully and trying to clarify the meaning of their illness, doctors can help patients define and articulate their suffering. This can occur even when patients have not previously brought such issues to full consciousness. The task is more to encourage and facilitate than to cure. Resolution of suffering depends on what the patient does later, and may take some time to resolve.

The consultation above was effective because the doctor attended to more than her disease, gastrointestinal upset. Potential suffering was identified and explored. This illustrates a broadening of role from that of biomedical curer (of disease) to potential healer (of persons).

While we are not advocating that doctors become psychotherapists, the nature of health professional work means that underlying personal, family and psychological issues are often just below the surface. However, we *are* advocating that the doctor have some degree of psychological awareness. This means being aware both of how personal issues can trigger many physical presentations[4] and of how doctors can themselves be the active therapeutic agent.

An example of this approach can be seen in the work of Drs Michael and Enid Balint, European psychiatrists who explored the doctor–patient relationship within modern clinical practice.(21) Their research was conducted through facilitating and observing GP discussion groups.[5] Balint noticed that the doctor acts as a sort of 'drug', where the doctor carefully prescribes a dose of herself. Adler reinforced this approach more recently.(22) Patients may clarify the nature of their suffering through the doctor's careful acknowledgement and use of empathy and compassion during the consultation. Hidden issues may emerge. Such an approach to history taking can indeed be therapeutic.

As noted at the end of the vignette, the doctor had personal experiences of grief. This leads to discussion of being 'wounded' and its impact on the self of the doctor.

The 'wounded' healer

Looking at the stories from Kleinman and Colquhoun, we might ask: does one have to be 'wounded' in order to be identified as a healer? Certainly some of the doctors described by Kleinman could be called wounded, but what of the majority of doctors who have no obvious scar in their psyche that might have led them towards a helping profession?

There is no doubt that medical students enter medicine for a variety of reasons. Perhaps they want to help others, come from a medical family, or are good at science; perhaps it was expected of them, or – quite often – they apply to medical school for no identifiable reason at all. However, they did not sign up to be a bricklayer, airline pilot or business executive. There must have been something attractive about being in one of the helping professions.

Two common types of wounding are the vicarious experience of illness in a family member, and the personal experience of being unwell or suffering. Both may contribute

---

4 See extended discussion in Chapter 7.
5 Balint encouraged GPs to discuss their patients in considerable detail, including their personal reactions to various patients. This seminal research on the doctor–patient relationship has been enormously influential, being the forerunner of Balint groups, communication skills training, and registrar training in family medicine. See the Appendix for fuller discussion.

to one's choice of career.(23) As noted already, the archetypal role of the wounded healer may contribute to the doctor's capacity for understanding and empathy with patients.(11)

Tying it all together: Reflecting on healing

In our work in postgraduate education for doctors, we often ask GPs to reflect on their work as a doctor, sometimes posing questions about suffering and healing. These GPs mention their difficulties in sitting alongside suffering when medicine has little to offer. Others discuss patients who have symptoms but no identifiable disease. Such reflection usually leads to consistent themes. In particular, GPs often make the following observations about themselves, now that they are in a general practice setting.

First, they stop trying to 'fix things' for their patients. Instead, they realise that in most cases their task, if possible, is simply to modify disease and to stand alongside the patient as their disease progresses. Sometimes patients are cured, but most of their practice is not about making a brilliant new diagnosis or saving lives. They also stop making so many decisions *for* their patients, allowing them more say in treatment options.

Second, they note that their own experience of illness, either personally or in their family, has a large impact on their style of practice. They start to appreciate why they chose medicine in the first place. There are usually links to the ethos of their family of origin and their role in it as peacemaker, resource person, or confidant(e).

Third, they identify what gives them job satisfaction. Often this is related to being of service to others in a wider sense, rather than pride in choosing the correct medications or similar. This is not to say they don't enjoy diagnostic puzzles or their success in treatment!

Fourth, they become more articulate about what they find difficult. This is often related to the illness experience: particular situations where GPs feel powerless to help, where medical theory is ineffective, or where no option is satisfactory.

In other words, these doctors have worked through an initial naïvety about the practice of medicine. Since graduating, and certainly since they entered primary care, they have made substantial shifts in their approach to clinical practice. From being highly theorised, idealistic and goal orientated, they seem to have become more realistic and pragmatic. Their focus is now just as much on persons as on the technical side of medical practice. With this shift, they appear to find more job satisfaction and meaning in their work. They are also less challenged by the absence of disease-based explanations.

These doctors are working through an apparent contradiction within modern medical practice: one of several contradictions that GPs commonly describe, this is the 'contradiction of helping'. Doctors may enter medicine through wanting to help others, but as they realise that their ability to 'cure' disease may be quite limited, they become more realistic and pragmatic. As they lower their sights from wanting a cure for every patient, their effectiveness actually increases: they learn to stand alongside their patients, creating the context for their patient's growth, understanding and mastery of illness.

Conclusion

Societies invest considerable social power in their doctors. This is helpful for individual patients as their illness is both explained and 'held' by the doctor. Furthermore, doctors' treatments are usually augmented by this social investment or covenant. Patients have an internal capacity for healing which doctors can facilitate.

This does imply, however, that doctors know about such healing power and work to use it wisely. While much of clinical practice is routine, it is important to recognise that some patients are suffering, and that their suffering is often hidden. In order to be effective agents of recovery and healing, doctors must be conscious of their role as potential healers, and must work on this with as much enthusiasm and 'scientific rigour' as they do on their biomedical expertise. The end result is wisdom, something not often discussed in medicine, but often apparent in the combined and effective use of the doctor's biomedical skill and social authority.

The role of the modern doctor, especially the GP, is to make judicious use of biomedicine – not as an end in itself, but as a tool *in service* to the patient. The task is to provide small acts of kindness, being aware of what the patient needs. In so doing, the modern doctor can indeed function as a healer. The outcome of thoughtful listening and careful use of the doctor–patient relationship can be the patient's movement towards wholeness and personal integrity – or, in other words, towards healing.

BOX 1.1 USEFUL READING ON SUFFERING AND HEALING

Cassell EJ. *The nature of suffering and the goals of medicine.* New York: Oxford University Press, 1991.

Greaves D. *The healing tradition: reviving the soul of Western medicine.* Oxford: Radcliffe Publishing, 2004.

Dixon DM, Sweeney K, Gray DP. The physician healer: ancient magic or modern science. *Br J Gen Pract* 1999, 49:309–12.

Helman C. *Suburban shaman.* Cape Town: Juta and Co, 2004.

Wellwood J. *Toward a psychology of awakening: Buddhism, psychotherapy and the path of personal and spiritual transformation.* Boston: Shambhala, 2000.

Hutchinson T, ed. *Whole person care: a new paradigm for the 21st century.* New York: Springer, 2011.

Kearney M. *A place of healing: working with suffering in living and dying.* Oxford: Oxford University Press, 2000.

SUMMARY POINTS

- Suffering is experienced by persons, rather than by their diseased organ.
- Healing involves the resolution of suffering in some particular way. It is specific to that person, whereas cure involves just the resolution of disease.
- All societies have designated healers who have a role in attending to the sick. Within modern society, GPs are the closest to this archetypal role.
- The choice of a career in medicine is usually related to underlying altruistic aims of helping others. Personal and family illness can impact on this choice and on ways of being a doctor.
- Modern biomedicine provides the tools to be a doctor, but being able to facilitate healing in patients requires a carefully nurtured doctor–patient relationship.
- Doctors need to learn to juggle both biomedical and interpersonal skills to be effective.
- By working through the apparent contradiction of wanting to help, doctors can become even more effective.
- The 'scientific imperative' of objective observer versus interpersonal engagement with each patient is an ongoing tension. Perhaps the resolution of this tension holds the key to healing.

References

1. Cassell EJ. The nature of suffering and the goals of medicine. *New Engl J Med* 1982, 306(11):639–45.
2. Cassell EJ. *The nature of suffering and the goals of medicine*. New York: Oxford University Press, 1991.
3. Egnew T. The meaning of healing: transcending suffering. *Ann Fam Med* 2005, 3:255–62.
4. Hutchinson TA, Mount BM, Kearney M. The healing journey. In: Hutchinson T, ed. *Whole person care: a new paradigm for the 21st Century*. New York: Springer, 2011. pp.23–30.
5. Frank A. *The wounded storyteller: body, illness, and ethics*. Chicago: University of Chicago Press, 1995.
6. Mount BM. Healing and palliative care: charting our way forward. *Pall Med* 2003, 17(8):657–58.
7. Fox E. Predominance of the curative model of medical care: a residual problem. *JAMA* 1997, 278(9):761–63.
8. Kakar S. *Shamans, mystics and doctors*. Chicago: University of Chicago Press, 1982.
9. Jung CG. *The archetypes and the collective unconscious*. London: Bollingen Series, 1981.
10. Samuels A, Shorter B, Plaut F. *A critical dictionary of Jungian analysis*. London: Routledge & Kegan Paul, 1986.
11. Guggenbühl-Craig A, Gubitz MB. *Power in the helping professions*. New York: Spring Publications, 1971.
12. Dixon DM, Sweeney K, Gray DP. The physician healer: ancient magic or modern science? *Br J Gen Pract* 1999, 49:309–12.
13. Cassell E. *The healer's art: a new perspective on the doctor-patient relationship*. Cambridge: MIT Press, 1976.

14. Brody H. *The healer's power*. New Haven: Yale University Press, 1992.
15. Davis-Floyd R, St John G. *From doctor to healer: the transformative journey*. New Brunswick: Rutgers University Press, 1998.
16. Greaves D. *The healing tradition: reviving the soul of Western medicine*. Oxford: Radcliffe, 2004.
17. Kleinman A. *Patients and healers in the context of culture: an exploration of the borderland between anthropology, medicine and psychiatry*. Berkeley: University of California Press, 1980.
18. Kleinman A. *The illness narratives: suffering, healing, and the human condition*. New York: Basic Books, 1988.
19. Elwyn GJ. So many precious stories: A reflective narrative of patient based medicine in general practice, Christmas 1996. *BMJ* 1997, 315(7123):1659–63.
20. Colquhoun G. The therapeutic uses of ache. Oration. Wellington: Royal New Zealand College of General Practitioners, 2009.
21. Balint M. *The doctor, his patient, and the illness*. London: Pitman, 1957.
22. Adler H. The history of the present illness as treatment: who's listening, and why does it matter? *J Am Board Fam Pract* 1997, 10(1):28–35.
23. Groesbeck C. The archetypal image of the wounded healer. *J Analytical Psychol* 1975, 20(2):122–45

Chapter 2

The World of the Patient

CONTENTS

Introduction

In his oft-quoted and celebrated address to Harvard University medical students in 1927, Dr Francis Peabody lamented that the newer graduates of his generation were not being instructed in how to care for their patients: 'The most common criticism made at present by older practitioners is that young graduates have been taught a great deal about the mechanism of disease, but very little about the practice of medicine – or, to put it more bluntly, they are too "scientific" and do not know how to take care of patients'.(1)

Some 60 years later in 1989, Professor Ian McWhinney started his benchmark chapter on illness, suffering and healing with 'The central tasks of a physician's life are understanding illness and understanding people. Because one cannot fully understand an illness without also understanding the person who is ill, these two tasks are indivisible.'(2)

While separated by many decades, these seminal quotes make a similar point: in order to practise medicine, doctors must approach the patient as a person. In responding to these critiques, undergraduate education has certainly changed. Models of clinical care that include the patient's perspective are now well developed. (3) Medical students are routinely taught basic consulting techniques,[1] which include eliciting the patient's experience of illness.(4)

There is still a problem, however, with the perceived *relevance* of the illness experience in day-to-day clinical work. This is especially the case in secondary care, where patients often have acute or serious organ pathology that requires specific focus and attention. Theoretically, students and physicians might acknowledge the need to see each patient as a person, but there are often many other pressing tasks that take precedence.

This chapter attempts to understand the patient's experience of illness. While not dismissing the need for clinical competence, we propose that acknowledging the 'felt experience' of the patient is helpful – even, at times, imperative. These comments apply in both hospital practice and community settings. Questions that need an answer are:

- What are the generic elements of the illness experience and how can doctors understand, and work with, these elements?
- How can illness be researched?
- What impact does the illness experience have on disease outcomes?
- How important is the 'meaning' of illness, regardless of the context of clinical care?
- How can undergraduate training better prepare doctors to recognise and respond to the illness experience?

Personal stories of illness

How can medical students and doctors learn about illness? One way is to read or to listen to personal stories of what it is like to be unwell. These first-person narratives of illness are called 'pathographies'.(5) They often include discussion of patients' interactions with their health-care professionals (stories that at times are none too flattering), and provide many examples of the distinction between disease (symptoms, pathology, treatment) and illness (ideas, feelings, expectations, personal meaning).

Anatole Broyard(6), for example, was an established writer before he developed prostate cancer. He wished his doctor 'would survey my soul as well as my flesh, to get at my illness, for each man is ill in his own way'. His accounts of his troubles are often hilarious. They are also very revealing, not only of illness, but also of the effect of the doctor on him and his illness:

> You don't really know that you're ill until the doctor tells you so. When he tells you you're ill, this is not the same as giving you permission to be ill. You eke out your illness ... The knowledge that you're ill is one of the momentous experiences in life. You expect that you're going to go on forever, that you're immortal. Freud said that every man is convinced of his own immortality. I certainly was. I had dawdled through life up to that point, and when the doctor told me I was ill it was like an immense electric shock.

---

1   Details of various models of consulting skills are listed in Chapter 6.

… This other, all-too-human doctor took me into an examining room and felt my prostate. It appeared to me that he had not yet overcome his self-consciousness about this procedure.(6)

Norman Cousins, also a writer, was suddenly stricken with severe arthritis.(7) Unable to negotiate his preferred treatment in hospital, he eventually moved out of hospital to set up his own management plan based on high-dose intravenous vitamin C and regular laughter. His perceptive and eloquent story illustrates the idiosyncratic nature of illness and the importance of a doctor who could tailor treatments accordingly.

Another insightful narrative comes from R.F. Murphy, a renowned professor of anthropology whose life was transformed by slow-onset paralysis due to a spinal cord tumour. He provided an extraordinary account of his experiences of 'the body silent'. (8) His book is now a standard text for medical students around the world, and he has made a significant contribution to the understanding of both illness and the social impact of disability.

However, Peabody's comments are probably still relevant: medical students continue to focus on learning about disease to the relative exclusion of learning about persons, while patients continue to grizzle that they are not being listened to, heard, or validated in their experience of illness.

If doctors are not listening, other people certainly are. Patient support groups are now quite common, providing a vehicle for others to hear their individual stories and to provide support. Personal narratives of illness are now being published in books and on the Internet in their thousands.[2] An interesting corollary is that doctors are also starting to share their subjective experiences of doctoring, both in peer groups and through online publishing.[3]

Many doctors have written fascinating stories about being 'on the other end of the stethoscope'. Their experiences help them see medicine in a completely new light, suddenly discovering a new world of illness they had been unaware of. Similarly, they learn that their colleagues – now as their doctors – often struggle to acknowledge or connect with their personal experience.(9) Stetten, for example, was an ophthalmologist facing impending blindness. He lamented how other specialists seemed uninterested in helping him make the most of what little sight he had left.(10)

These pathographies from doctors are particularly interesting. They learn first-hand about the importance of the *subjective* experience of being unwell. Their learning is usually quite belated. It is only after some doctors have had their first heart attack that they realise the importance of listening to their patients and exploring what illness actually means to them.[4]

Disease and illness
It is helpful to distinguish between the twin concepts of disease and illness. This distinction has been readily adopted in general practice(11) and is now one of the building blocks of emerging models of clinical care such as the patient-centred clinical method.(3)

---

2 See for example: http://www.healthtalkonline.org
3 See for example: http://www.pulsemagazine.org/index.cfm
4 See extended discussion on doctors' experience of health and illness in Chapter 8.

Briefly, 'disease' includes all the details about the organ involved, relevant biomedical research, investigations and various current treatments. This is an important and necessary focus for undergraduate training and the acquisition of knowledge. 'Illness', on the other hand, is the lived experience of each person within their particular social context. Illness is a helpful concept, not only because it reminds doctors of the unique person on the other end of the stethoscope, but also because of the emerging evidence of the links between particular aspects of illness and the *outcomes* of disease, whether involving major diseases such as cancer or myocardial infarction, or less immediately life-threatening problems such as arthritis or diabetes.

Research into the illness experience

Why has illness, as a subject in itself, been relatively neglected in clinical practice? Surely how a patient feels about and actually *experiences* his disease would be of great interest to doctors? Or does it make no difference at all? Will each disease continue inexorably onwards, no matter what the patient thinks, feels or does about it? Brohm's archetypal interaction with her breast cancer surgeon illustrates this point: 'I asked the doctor what I could do to help myself. To put myself in the winning half of the statistics. "Nothing," he replied.'(12)

Modern medical practice has been predicated on the scientific model, where the doctor is largely in the role of 'objective researcher' and the patient is the object of study. During the twentieth century, how each patient felt about their illness gradually came to be regarded as largely irrelevant. Similarly, because each person's subjective experience of illness is unavoidably individual and interior, it was much less open to the usual quantitative methods of analysis that have characterised medical science.

Learning about the subjective experience of illness has required the emergence of qualitative methods of enquiry as a valid research method.(13,14) One-to-one personal interviews and focus groups are now legitimate. All aspects of personal experience are being researched more rigorously, using 'phenomenological' methods or 'grounded theory'.(15) Researchers now approach the experience of a particular illness with the same fascination as anthropologists used to explore a new tribe in Africa or South America.(16) Insights from research are gradually being applied to the actual work of doctoring.(17,18)

Links to disease outcomes

Do variations of the illness experience link to the outcomes of disease? Because illness is a subjective experience, this question presents considerable challenges to researchers. Fortunately, Weinman and others have developed a quantitative tool to measure certain aspects of illness, which can now be correlated against a variety of other variables. Their tool is the Illness Perception Questionnaire, first developed in 1996(19) and later revised in 2002.(20) Questions are related to the five major cognitive components listed in Box 2.1.

BOX 2.1 RESEARCHABLE COMPONENTS OF ILLNESS

Identity: comprised of the label of the illness and the symptoms the patient views as being part of the disease

Cause: personal ideas about aetiology which may include simple single causes or more complex and multiple causal models

Timeline: how long the patient believes the illness will last (illnesses can be categorised into acute, chronic or episodic)

Consequences: expected effects and outcome of the illness

Cure/control: how one recovers from, or controls, the illness.

From Moss-Morris et al.(20)

As a result of this research tool, there is now an emerging bank of evidence indicating that how patients think and feel about their illness will indeed have an impact on the outcomes of their disease. Some examples from research abstracts follow.

Recovery after myocardial infarction: 'Patients' initial perceptions of illness are important determinants of different aspects of recovery ... Specific illness perceptions need to be identified at an early stage as a basis for optimising outcomes from rehabilitation programmes.'(21)

Compliance with medication for hypertension: 'Beliefs about specific medications and about hypertension are predictive of compliance. Information about health beliefs is important in achieving concordance and may be a target for intervention to improve compliance.'(22)

Role of carers in schizophrenia: 'Although carers' reactions to schizophrenic illness in a close family member may have important implications for the patient and for themselves, little is known of factors that influence the way carers respond ... Carer cognitive representations of the illness may have important implications for both carer and patient outcomes in schizophrenia.'(23)

Help-seeking behaviour with psoriasis: 'Patients who initially engaged in coping characterized by more expression of emotions, seeking more social support, seeking more distraction, and less passive coping were prescribed a lower number of different therapies, were less anxious, less depressed, and had a better physical health 1 year later. These results have implications for the management of patients with psoriasis, which reinforces current views on integrating psychosocial aspects into clinical care.'(24)

A recent clinical example illustrates these points.

VIGNETTE 2.1 THE CHALLENGE OF DIABETES

I was doing an inner-city GP locum and met a 50-year-old female patient with long-standing diabetes, treated with tablets and insulin. On reviewing the laboratory results, I noticed her diabetic control was poor. So I asked a rather naïve question about her self-

monitoring of blood sugars. She said she wasn't testing at all. This was puzzling to me, as she was at considerable risk of developing complications.

I was wondering about this, but to avoid putting her on the spot, I offered her a couple of options: 'Some people don't test because they don't like the pain of finger pricks, while others don't really want to have diabetes in the first place.' She readily acknowledged it was the latter. Her mother had quite severe diabetes with many complications, dying in her early 70s.

She said that despite her usual doctor 'tut-tutting' every time about her poor control, she just couldn't get around to being more proactive about her disease. I wondered if 'not testing' was a sort of denial of her diagnosis, and that in her rejection of the implications of having diabetes, she was putting herself at risk of complications similar to her mother's.

In this example, the patient's illness experience was dominated by feelings of horror and rejection of her mother's experience. This prevented her being more 'adherent' with usual management and, in turn, her diabetes was out of control. Exploring her illness experience had helped identify the barriers to treatment. When she met the GP again about two years later, she intimated this consultation had been a helpful turning point in her approach to diabetes.

We now consider illness in greater depth by using two slightly different perspectives: the nature of personhood and the concept of narrative. These approaches can help doctors understand how a person might suffer and how patients and doctors together may reconstruct the story or narrative of their experience.

What makes a person

As we noted in Chapter 1, Cassell has made a significant contribution to clinical practice with his focus on suffering and the role of the doctor. He based his ideas on how suffering arises from various aspects of 'personhood'.(25) While any breakdown of personhood into various categories risks being reductionist, these ideas allow the doctor to consider the person of the patient in more detail.

Cassell's 'typology of persons' is paraphrased below. The experience of illness in relation to particular disease will be inextricably linked to the degree of disruption, loss or alteration of one's prior state.

Persons have **personality and character.** Depending on personality, everyone responds differently to symptoms and disease. Some personality characteristics appear to be relatively fixed, while others may change over time.

A person has a **past.** This is all their experiences of life so far. In the medical context, the patient 'brings along' their experience of previous illnesses, doctors and health-care systems to the consultation.

Family. Past experiences of family, including ideas of disease inheritance, will contribute to the sense of meaning that a patient has about their current illness. This may explain why patients respond differently to particular conditions based on their family history.

Culture. There are always cultural determinants to what is perceived to be health or ill health, while responses to symptoms and disease are profoundly influenced by cultural mores. Although ethnicity is a signal for differences in culture, every person has their own culture, shaped by personal life experiences. These factors are best explored on an individual basis, with the doctor enquiring of the patient about the particular significance of symptoms and signs. This is preferable to making an assumption that may be valid for a wider ethnic community, but not apply to that particular patient.

Roles. Every person has a particular set of roles. Those roles may be related to their family function, to their work, or to particular social organisations to which they belong. These roles influence a patient's perception of self and they will be disrupted with illness.

Persons exist in **relationships**. Everyone exists in some form of community and relationship with other people. Not only will an illness impact on a person's ability to function within those relationships, but their relationships will have a significant bearing on how a patient copes and is cared for during an illness. The patient's 'significant other' is the third most important person in the consultation, even if they are not present.

A political being. People have rights, responsibilities and obligations. They participate in society. Their sense of political participation will be impacted on by illness. This is particularly important for sufferers of chronic illness or those with a disability that can reduce their ability to participate fully.

Actions. Related to, but separate from, the sense of political involvement is the idea that a person is defined by their actions. Illness may affect the ability to function in the world. Reciprocally, being unable to do one's usual activities helps define sickness. People identify with their regular and normal activities. Noting this helps doctors think about the impact of being temporarily disabled.

The body. Cassell points out that people have a relationship with their own body, and the presence of disease alters that sense of relationship. They might not be able to trust their own body now, or their body may be altered in a way that changes their sense of who they are.

A secret life. This includes people's fears, desires, loves, hopes and fantasies that can be damaged by the presence of disease.

A perceived future. Just as everybody has a past, being unwell impacts on one's perceptions of the future. This may include concern about work the next day, playing sport in the weekend, or it may be more profound in terms of future goals and aspirations. Loss of a perceived future contributes to patients' anxieties when confronted by life-threatening illness such as cancer.

A transcendent dimension. This is the life of the spirit, religious affiliations, and being in relationship with the wider world. This transcendent or spiritual dimension has potential to both influence and be influenced by the existence of illness. How illness is perceived, and how patients derive meaning or hope for a good outcome, will be directly affected by this dimension.

Cassell's ideas provide a structure for thinking about what might be lost or threatened by being sick, and what other aspects of personhood might provide resilience or aid recovery for a particular patient. These ideas are teachable to students, linking to their sense of a 'common humanity'.

VIGNETTE 2.2 LIFE AND ILLNESS

Graeme, a 45-year-old man, was a fit and well tradesman until about seven years ago when he developed severe multiple sclerosis (MS). He gave up work when he developed painful spasms and became increasingly fatigued. Neurologists had indicated there was essentially no effective medication or long-term cure for his condition.

His wife left him shortly after the onset of this disease. He also became estranged from his two sons who were then of primary-school age. He formed a new relationship with a woman who also had MS, but this was fraught with the difficulty of their combined disabilities. They parted and he shifted towns, now presenting at my practice.

When I first met Graeme, he struggled in from the waiting room using two elbow crutches. He was dishevelled, tall and thin, and had a somewhat agitated air about him, as if desperate to be out of this predicament. He appeared to be resigned and trapped. He told me a little of his story, but basically he just wanted a repeat of his medications (antispasmodic and antidepressant).

Over the next few months I sometimes saw him using crutches; at other times he used a motorised electric wheelchair. He seemed to be physically deteriorating, and looked to be lonely and sad. He told me in great detail of his plans to shift again, this time to a slightly bigger town, in search of company.

Then one day he presented with a caregiver – a pleasant local woman in her 30s. Graeme seemed happier, as though she was his partner. However, I knew that she had her own partner and family, and I was concerned that his approach towards this woman may not be quite appropriate.

At the next consultation the situation was entirely different. The caregiver was forgotten. Graeme had a woman and her teenage daughter now living in his house with him. Also gone were the plans to shift towns. He was happy, out of his wheelchair and back on crutches. However, I held some misgivings. I had met his new partner previously as a patient, finding her rather complicated, seeking medications on behalf of her daughter with headaches. However, Graeme assured me that all was well.

Then there was a crisis. Graeme presented very distressed – the new partner had physically assaulted him, threatened further violence, then left. The police were involved. He was not sleeping, believing she might return. His MS deteriorated. He was in increasing pain and back in the wheelchair. I attended him a couple of times through this period.

Then, at the most recent consultation, he was with a new partner. He seemed happy again, was walking with just one crutch and seemed more buoyant. His new partner also transferred care to my practice but appeared to have significant problems. Physically impaired and needing welfare support, she too seemed to be escaping her social circumstances by shifting towns. Graeme seemed quite oblivious to my concerns.

These encounters between the patient and his doctor reveal many elements of Cassell's typology of person. Before Graeme's multiple sclerosis, he had enjoyed good bodily health, an apparently satisfactory marriage and family life, an occupation that he enjoyed, and, I suspect, a sense of a shared future. Although his story is complex, several components of personhood were disrupted or lost because of illness.

His varying functional capacity seemed now to be linked to his relationships with caregivers and partners.

This story also leads to a further understanding of illness, that of narrative, where the patient's illness experience can be viewed as an ongoing story over time.

Narratives of illness

The concept of the illness *as a story in itself* is now gaining more attention. Examples include the work of Kleinman in his groundbreaking book *The illness narratives*,(26) Brody's *Stories of sickness*,(27) and Hydén, from a sociological perspective.(28)

Particularly in the general practice setting, doctors are constantly listening to and engaging with patients' stories or narratives. Greenhalgh's influential series of articles in the *BMJ* asserts that the clinical method is 'an interpretive act which draws on narrative skills to integrate the overlapping stories told by patients, clinicians, and test results'.(29) Similarly, Donnelly suggests that doctors can do much more than simply 'abstract' all the relevant medical details from the patient's 'history'. Instead they can look for the patient's experience as a story or narrative in and of itself, worthy of focused attention and inclusion in the patient record:

> Narratives of illness in medical records and case presentations in teaching hospitals say surprisingly little about an important matter: what patients understand and feel. Nowadays, medical narratives tend to neglect or objectify subjective experience, including symptoms. Such narratives concentrate, in the manner of chronicles, on events in the exterior, objective world rather than the interior world of the sick. Medical students and physicians will construct more balanced accounts of human illness once they envision these accounts as 'story', a form of narrative that traditionally accesses subjective experience as well as objective events.
>
> ... One can effectively begin the process of transforming medical chronicles into stories simply by asking patients what they know and how they feel about their situation and by documenting the response, using some of the patient's words, in the history of present illness. These actions will identify and preserve important information, facilitate empathy in all care givers who hear or read the history, and signal to everyone the physician's serious interest in patients as persons. Getting the voice of the patient into the history of present illness will not only help to right the medical record, but also help to right the relationship of physician and patient.(30)

Embedded in the term 'narratives of illness' are two important ideas. First, patients continually *construct* ways of communicating their experience to others. They tell their doctor, not by song, poem or dance, but by a spoken story that attempts to convey their illness experience. Second, the doctor can become part of the narrative. Just by being told the story, the doctor engages with that patient's experience and in some way will shape it.

Sometimes a patient tells a particularly distressing story. The doctor listens. Although there is no ready solution, the patient leaves saying that they feel much better and are now able to move forward. The human interaction between doctor and patient has reshaped the patient's experience, perhaps altering the trajectory of illness.

What sorts of stories do doctors encounter? Stories usually have a beginning, a middle and an end, but doctors often listen to a clinical narrative that is as yet incomplete. It can be helpful to stand back from the immediate medical details and see if there is a pattern starting to emerge from the overall storyline. Arthur Frank identifies three particular narratives, eloquently labelled as restitution, chaos, and quest.(31)

The restitution narrative

This is the classical story of illness that follows the natural history of a disease. A patient presents with symptoms; the symptoms and the doctor's findings fit a particular diagnosis (using the biomedical approach); an intervention is used and the patient is restored to their previous state of health. This is the bread and butter of ordinary medical practice. The restitution narrative can be told from either the patient's or the doctor's perspective, but the plot is essentially the same. A subtext is that this is a success story, the triumph of medicine over disease. The restitution narrative is the usual plot of advertisements for popular health remedies.

However, there are potential problems. One is that the patient's symptoms (and possibly their examination findings and investigation results) may not fit with a recognised disease. Without an explanatory model, the patient continues to search for the meaning in their illness, while both doctor and patient become perplexed and frustrated. Patients with chronic fatigue syndrome, for example, may keep looking for reasons *why* they have symptoms. Their endless search becomes the plot of a 'failed restitution' narrative.

Similarly, some patients may not respond 'appropriately' to treatment, even with a known diagnosis. For these patients, the narrative is disrupted, and again, the doctor and patient may become frustrated. This is especially so if the only narrative they know is one of restitution.

The chaos narrative

The chaos narrative is threatening to both patient and doctor. The narrator of the chaos story struggles to put their existence into words. Frank describes the gaping void that is difficult to make sense of or even talk about. Instead of a storyline, there is 'anti-narrative'.(31) The characteristic chaos narrative has no beginning, no end, no resolution, and no restitution. There is simply the painful lived expression of the body going wrong, no rhyme or reason to what is happening. Chronic pain, cultural dislocation, family violence and early stages of cancer can all be examples of the feeling of chaos.

There are potential pitfalls when attending to a chaos narrative, especially if it is not recognised as such. Trying to resolve issues or impose an order on such a story can create further tensions. The patient is sometimes labelled 'a poor historian', who is not telling a 'proper story'. And indeed the patient is not. The story is, if anything, a story of failure to make sense of what is going on. Frank notes that patients are unable to distance themselves from their experience.

The key to helping such a patient, whose illness story and entire life can be chaotic, is first to recognise this particular narrative, then attempt to listen carefully with compassion to the inherent suffering. Correctly identifying the chaos narrative can be freeing for the doctor, as the responsibility to achieve restitution is reduced.

In Graeme's story above, there are short periods of relative stability, followed by major psychosocial upheaval. With elements of both failed restitution and chaos narratives, the doctor is challenged to continue to stand alongside, as Graeme lurches from crisis to crisis.

The quest narrative

In this narrative, rather than simply seeking restitution, the patient seeks to better understand and make more sense of their experience of illness. This search for meaning can be intense and life changing. Being aware of this third type of narrative is crucial if the doctor is to validate and support the patient in their journey.

The quest for meaning is usually more than just searching for information about their condition. It may be a deeply reflective process, including seeking out the experience of other family members, friends or colleagues who have suffered a similar experience.

A slightly different type of quest narrative is sometimes found in patients whose disease or disability can never be restored back to the pre-illness state, and where the patient's view of themselves in the world is profoundly changed. This transformation often takes the form of helping others through their own experience. An example would be a patient's response to a brain tumour or breast cancer. Their whole life is threatened, but in their quest to find meaning for their illness there is a change in personal orientation towards others. In this reorientation, they sometimes express the rather contradictory idea of being 'grateful' to their cancer for having triggered these changes. Perhaps this is the origin of the concept of the wounded healer, a health professional with a shared experience of suffering.

The quest narrative poses quite different issues for the doctor. The quest can be an uplifting narrative that transforms the patient's life through a renewed sense of meaning. The doctor needs to learn how to stand alongside and not interfere.

In summary, it is useful to have a structure for listening to patients' narratives in clinical practice. Asking oneself 'What sort of story is this?' is a start, as the doctor tries to gain an overview of the journey so far. Most patients desire a restitution narrative for their acute illness so they can get back to normal, and fortunately, doctors can often help them achieve this. However, chronic disease is more problematic, as patients usually need to rethink their identity and future. Being prepared to sit with a chaos narrative without feeling compelled to intervene is helpful. And understanding how quest is a valid response to illness allows the doctor to help the patient reach a new understanding of themselves in their world.

Teaching and learning about illness

The most common way of teaching medical students to explore the patient's illness experience is derived from the patient-centred clinical method.(3) Students are instructed to explore the patient's *feelings* and *ideas* about their illness, how it has affected their day-to-day *functioning,* and their *expectations* of the consultation. These questions, remembered through the mnemonic FIFE, are now fully integrated into the Calgary-Cambridge guides to consulting skills.(32)

Requiring students to explore the illness in this formal way has helped the consultation focus more on the patient as person (although there are still issues in translating what emerges into the medical record). The danger in this 'painting by numbers' approach is that students can miss the usual spontaneous cues to these issues and instead ask formal questions such as 'How do you feel about your illness?', even if the patient has been talking about just that already. FIFE is, however, a useful first step for beginners. Many doctors incorporate these concepts less formally, but still cover similar ground.

While students are now being taught about the illness experience in more detail, narrative medicine as a clinical approach is still in its early stages. Some medical schools are starting to explore these concepts in practical ways. Professor Rita Charon at Columbia University, for example, requires her students to write a 'parallel chart' on their patients, noting down any observations about their patients that are not included in the 'normal' clinical record. This includes their own responses to these patients.(33) Subsequent discussion with their tutor helps students to see their patient as a unique person, currently caught in a web of illness that has forced their hospitalisation. These discussions also explore students' own 'journeys through medicine'.

Key points of illness

For graduates, we propose a revised method of exploring the illness experience. This is based on the typology of personhood and the patient's potential for suffering, as well as the concept of narrative. In brief, the task of the doctor is to explore the following four issues:

- Disruption to normal life
- Loss and dependency
- Emotions, including shame
- The meaning of illness.

Disruption to normal life

Every individual has what could be considered a 'normal' existence. Normal patterns of behaviours can be significantly disrupted by illness, depending on the type and severity of the affliction. A minor transitory illness may disrupt bodily function but have little impact on the ability to work or relate to others. Conversely, illness can cause major disruption to normal life. The task of the doctor is to explore its effect on functioning, how important that is to the patient and what it means, and how this problem might be addressed.

Loss and dependency

In both acute and chronic illness, especially where there is more severe disability, patients experience a sense of loss. When a patient is in a chaotic situation, they may not have defined what they have actually lost. In putting words to the void in their existence, the listening doctor can validate that loss. The loss of a perceived future may be particularly painful, even if the patient has not articulated that before meeting with the doctor.

Issues of dependency may severely impact on how a patient views their illness and then copes with it. The idea of being dependent on others for the normal activities of daily living may be particularly distressing to somebody who has always been independent. Particularly when restitution to full health is impossible, it is helpful to acknowledge the struggle the patient is having.

Emotions and shame

Illness will always generate strong feelings, such as fear, anger, even resentment at others for being well. One of these feelings, often buried or hidden, is the shame of certain symptoms or conditions.(34) The disease itself, and the patient's contact with the medical care system, have the potential to increase shame. One such example is HIV/AIDS, where there has been significant social stigma attached to the diagnosis, often not helped by a doctor's reaction to the person with the virus. A more common example is obesity: many patients feel considerable shame about their size despite efforts at weight reduction.(35) Requiring such patients to stand on the scales each time they attend clinic has the potential to induce further shame. Genital symptoms are often associated with shame and may provide a reason for late presentation.(36)

Patients can be overwhelmed by shame about bodily functions, loss of independence, loss of normal mobility, and so on. As shame can be defined as a sense of failure of the entire self,(37) there is a potential for 'failure' in one aspect of personhood to lead to a more general loss of confidence.

Although shame is usually hidden, it may still drive much of the patient's help-seeking or help-avoiding behaviour. While shame may be too delicate an issue to discuss directly, a gentle and accepting manner can facilitate the patient's own acceptance of their condition. Acknowledging and attending to shame can become an important task in some consultations.

Sense of meaning

Every illness will have personal meaning, being the sum of all other aspects of illness. Meaning starts with understanding the disease, its cause, how it might develop over time, and so on. The initial task of the doctor is simply to explain the patient's condition so they can more easily deal with it.

At a deeper level, however, and consistent with the ideas about the quest narrative and the transcendent nature of a person, illness may have changed this person in some particular way. The doctor's task is to help the patient explore the ways in which their condition has altered their view of themself. Meaning is not something that a doctor gives to a patient; rather, the doctor attempts to understand the patient's process of change. In attempting to achieve this, doctor and patient have an iterative conversation: if the patient knows that the doctor knows how it is for them, then there is some degree of empathy. Considerable research in a variety of health professions indicates how helpful this approach can be.(38)

At a practical level, the following exploratory questions can help to elicit these aspects of illness:
- What do you think is happening to you?
- Why do you think this has happened?
- What is it like for you to have this illness?

- What has changed for you because of this?
- Who else is concerned for you, and what are their ideas around this?

Here is a final vignette that illustrates the key points of this chapter, provided by one of our postgraduate students.

VIGNETTE 2.3 LIVING WITH CANCER

I had a patient who was doing rather badly with her cancer. She was really struggling with her side effects from chemotherapy and missing her specialist appointments. I had seen her many times in the last two years and while the prognosis was still quite uncertain, her cancer was very disruptive to her life and to her family. So I eventually asked her: 'What is it like for you having this cancer?'

She immediately burst into tears, saying no one had ever asked her that before. We had a good chat. It turned out she was terrified, not so much of dying, but of her possible mode of death, being dependent on her family, and so on. While she was probably crossing some bridges well before she needed to, we discussed these issues in depth.

The outcome was she became a lot more accepting of her cancer. She returned to outpatients and managed to patch things up a bit with her specialist. She proceeded with the chemotherapy. I now see her more regularly for follow-up, and with a much easier relationship than before.

Once again, this short clinical story illustrates the continuum between suffering and healing. The doctor was able to facilitate this patient's movement towards a degree of inner peace, despite the cancer remaining present.

Conclusion

This chapter has explored the experience of illness from a number of angles. It will help doctors to move into the world of the patient, allowing patients to be heard and validated in the changes to their existence brought on by disease. This approach brings us back to the discussion of the nature of healing in Chapter 1 and reinforces the idea that 'being made whole', or 'healing', may not necessarily equate to the full restitution of a previous state of health.

Alongside the traditional medical task of making the diagnosis and offering treatment options, Peabody in 1927 and McWhinney more recently have both referred to the illness experience as being central to the work of doctoring. In Chapter 6, we outline various models of clinical practice that attempt to both include and address each person's illness as an important task of doctoring.

Having a conversation about what it is like to be unwell usually uncovers many of the issues we have outlined above. If a doctor focuses on the person, medical work need not be boring or tedious. One of the fascinations of clinical practice is the continual surprise in how each patient responds and reacts to their illness.

SUMMARY POINTS

- All doctors can attend to the patient's illness experience, regardless of their context of work.
- Understanding the patient's illness experience is integral to good patient care.
- Personal stories of illness (pathographies) provide insight into the illness experience.
- Considering the different components of *person* is useful in understanding and validating the illness experience.
- Identifying various types of patient narrative (restitution, chaos or quest) helps the doctor identify their own role and tasks more accurately.
- The patient-centred clinical method encourages medical students to explore patients' feelings, ideas, functioning and expectations.
- Considering the illness experience in terms of disruption to normal life, loss and dependency, emotions and shame, and sense of meaning can be helpful for more experienced practitioners.
- The role of the doctor is to help co-construct the narrative of illness.
- Validation of the illness experience can help the patient resolve their personal anguish and suffering.

References

1. Peabody FW. The care of the patient. *JAMA*. 1927, 88(12):877–82.
2. McWhinney I. *Textbook of family medicine*. 3rd edn. Oxford: Oxford University Press, 2009.
3. Stewart M, Belle Brown J, Weston W, McWhinney I, McWilliam C, Freeman T. *Patient-centered medicine: transforming the clinical method*. 2nd edn. Abingdon: Radcliffe, 2003.
4. Silverman J, Kurtz SM, Draper J, van Dalen J, Platt FW. *Skills for communicating with patients*. Abingdon: Radcliffe, 1998.
5. Hawkins AH. Reconstructing illness: Studies in pathography. West Lafayette: Purdue Research Foundation, 1999. *JAMA* 1993, 270(12):1482.
6. Broyard A. *Intoxicated by my illness and other writings on life and death*. New York: Ballantine, 1993.
7. Cousins N. *Anatomy of an illness as perceived by the patient: reflections on healing and regeneration*. New York: Norton, 1979.
8. Murphy RF. *The body silent: the different world of the disabled*. New York: Norton, 2001.
9. Hahn RA. Between two worlds: physicians as patients. *Med Anthr Quart* 1985, 16(4):87–98.
10. Stetten D. Coping with blindness. *N Eng J Med* 1981, 305(8):458–60.
11. Helman CG. Disease versus illness in general practice. *J Roy Coll Gen Pract* 1981, 31(230):548–52.
12. Brohm P. *Gentle giants*. London: Century, 1986.
13. Black N. Why we need qualitative research. *J Epidemiol Community Health* 1994, 48(5):425–26.
14. Denzin N, Lincoln Y. *The handbook of qualitative research*. Thousand Oaks, California: Sage, 2000.
15. Strauss AL, Corbin JM. *Basics of qualitative research: techniques and procedures for developing grounded theory*. Thousand Oaks, California: Sage, 1998.
16. Conrad P. The experience of illness: recent and new directions. *Res Soc Health Care* 1987, (6)1–31
17. Reiser SJ. The era of the patient: using the experience of illness in shaping the missions of health care. *JAMA* 1993, 269(8):1012–17.

18. Rothman SM. *Living in the shadow of death: tuberculosis and the social experience of illness in American history.* New York: Basic Books, 1994.

19. Weinman J, Petrie KJ, Moss-Morris R, Horne R. The illness perception questionnaire: a new method for assessing the cognitive representation of illness. *Psychol Health* 1996, 11(3):431–45.

20. Moss-Morris R, Weinman J, Petrie K, Horne R, Cameron L, Buick D. The revised illness perception questionnaire (IPQ-R). *Psychol Health* 2002, 17(1):1–16.

21. Petrie KJ, Weinman J, Sharpe N, Buckley J. Role of patients' view of their illness in predicting return to work and functioning after myocardial infarction: longitudinal study. *BMJ* 1996, 312(7040):1191.

22. Ross S, Walker A, MacLeod MJ. Patient compliance in hypertension: role of illness perceptions and treatment beliefs. *J Hum Hypertens* 2004, 18(9):607–13.

23. Barrowclough C, Lobban F, Hatton C, Quinn J. An investigation of models of illness in carers of schizophrenia patients using the illness perception questionnaire. *Br J Clin Psychol* 2001, 40(4):371–85.

24. Scharloo M, Kaptein AA, Weinman J, Bergman W, Vermeer BJ, Rooijmans HG. Patients' illness perceptions and coping as predictors of functional status in psoriasis: a 1-year follow-up. *Br J Derm* 2000, 142(5):899–907.

25. Cassell EJ. *The nature of suffering and the goals of medicine.* New York: Oxford University Press, 1991.

26. Kleinman A. *The illness narratives: suffering, healing, and the human condition.* New York: Basic Books, 1988.

27. Brody H. *Stories of sickness.* New Haven: Yale University Press, 1987.

28. Hydén LC. Illness and narrative. *Soc Health Illness* 1997, 19(1):48–69.

29. Greenhalgh T. Narrative based medicine in an evidence based world. *BMJ* 1999, 318(7179):323–25.

30. Donnelly WJ. Righting the medical record: transforming chronicle into story. *JAMA* 1988, 260(6):823–25.

31. Frank A. *The wounded storyteller: body, illness, and ethics.* Chicago: University of Chicago Press, 1995.

32. Kurtz S, Silverman J, Benson J, Draper J. Marrying content and process in clinical method teaching: enhancing the Calgary-Cambridge guides. *Acad Med* 2003, 78(8):802–09.

33. Charon R. *Narrative medicine: honoring the stories of illness.* New York: Oxford University Press, 2006.

34. Lazare A. Shame and humiliation in the medical encounter. *Arch Int Med* 1987, 147(9):1653–58.

35. Silberstein LR, Striegel-Moore RH, Rodin J. Feeling fat: a woman's shame. In: Lewis HB, ed. *The role of shame in symptom formation.* Hillsdale, NJ: Erlbaum; 1987. pp. 89–108.

36. Newton DC, McCabe MP. A theoretical discussion of the impact of stigma on psychological adjustment to having a sexually transmissible infection. *Sex Health* 2005, 2(2):63–69.

37. Jacoby M. *Shame and the origins of self-esteem.* London: Routledge, 1994.

38. Hojat M. *Empathy in patient care: antecedents, development, measurement, and outcomes.* New York: Springer, 2007..

Chapter 3

The Assumptions of Modern Medicine

CONTENTS

Introduction

This chapter will consider the foundational assumptions of modern medical practice. By assumptions, we mean the taken-for-granted rules that underpin the work of the modern doctor. These rules are rarely made explicit, but they guide day-to-day practice. We will explore how these ideas and beliefs in medicine have evolved in the last few hundred years, and how these beliefs are involved in each and every encounter with the patient.

Western medical practice is based on what is known as 'biomedicine', a biological understanding of human anatomy, physiology and physico-chemical processes.(1) Biomedical knowledge helps doctors answer the questions 'What is the matter with this patient?' and, more practically, 'How can I help?' Most of the time the model works very well, and it is one of the reasons that life expectancy has markedly increased in the Western world. But there are clinical situations where the model is less accurate. Having a deeper understanding of the various limitations in these assumptions can then be very useful.

In this chapter, we will look at the way biomedicine evolved as an outcome of expanding scientific knowledge during the sixteenth to eighteenth centuries. We will then discuss how ongoing difficulties with biomedicine led to the development of the 'biopsychosocial' model. We will finish the chapter with a discussion of two major anomalies of medical practice: somatisation and what is known as the 'placebo effect'. Arguably, these anomalies illustrate that biomedicine continues to be the dominant medical paradigm. First, though, a brief history of science.

A brief history of science

In Western Europe at the time of the Reformation, views of the world were undergoing substantial change. The Enlightenment (1600–1800) saw the rise of a scientific approach to understanding nature. Leading thinkers in various fields included Newton (physics), Descartes (philosophy), Galileo (astronomy) and later Darwin (botany and evolution). Superstition was rejected and new knowledge based on rationalism was embraced.

At the same time, religious reformation began to differentiate between the idea of the body and that of the soul. The church retained ownership of the soul, while exploration and understanding of the body became the preserve of the newly emerging domain of science. Over a couple of hundred years, the result was a reduction in the intellectual power of the church. Natural phenomena were no longer attributed to spiritual causes. The scientific revolution also provided more legitimacy to the practice of medicine, affording the profession a virtual monopoly in the management of sickness.

These ideas are encapsulated in what is commonly referred to as Cartesian dualism or the **mind–body split**, a concept attributed largely to French philosopher René Descartes(2) by which the soul came to be equated with the mind. Residing (somewhere) within the body, the mind directed the body to act, but was separate from the body. The mind retained its sacred status as the essence of human existence and the body became a physical object, now subjected to the investigatory processes of science.(3)

Looking back now, it is clear that the revolutionary ideas of Descartes and others were an intellectual tour de force that afforded an unprecedented insight into the workings of nature and why people became unwell. While it is fashionable to be critical of this artificial division between mind and body, the advances in medical science that we all now enjoy are principally due to those radical pioneers who initiated a different way of thinking about nature and the human body.

What is science?

To understand biomedicine in more detail, we first need to outline the assumptions of modern science, as they emerged during the Enlightenment.

Science is *empirical*, meaning that all knowledge is derived from experience: hypotheses and theories must be tested against observations of the natural world, rather than relying on previous assumptions. Empiricism emphasises evidence, especially as discovered through experiments. Science is also based on *realism*, meaning that physical objects in the real world exist independent of the observer or what might be expected to exist. Science is *materialistic*, in that matter and energy are the only things that exist. Finally, science is *positivist*, meaning that positive verification of knowledge is required before it is considered true or authentic; ethical, spiritual and religious speculations are less important as they are difficult to prove or verify.(4)

The corollary of these ideas is that there is an experimental or 'scientific' method. The assumption is that it is possible to understand nature by formulating a specific question and then conducting an experiment. To do so 'scientifically' means the scientist must define and then control various factors involved, introducing only one at a time.

Two further philosophical concepts are **reductionism** and **holism**. Reductionism is the process of seeking ever more basic explanations for phenomena. It helped to differentiate science from quasi-religious explanations, allowing a more empirical and materialistic understanding of the natural world. Holism is the opposite of reductionism. This theory posits that the whole is greater than the sum of its parts. Furthermore, testing a theory (especially about causation) cannot be performed in isolation because other interrelated factors will impact on the outcome. The emerging sciences of the Enlightenment and the early medical understanding of the body were largely based on reductionist principles.

The emergence of biomedicine

The principles of science outlined above afforded a new approach to medicine. This was based on an understanding of the body as the primary basis of disease, quite disconnected from the need for knowledge of the mind or person. As Samson notes: 'Enlightenment medicine reflected a confidence in scientific methods of observation and experimentation to *control* nature and *intervene* to correct ailments that seemed to cut life short.'(3) Biology is the scientific study of living organisms, including humans. Biomedicine, then, is science as applied to normal function and disease within human beings.

Learning about the anatomy of the body was a major feature of early biomedicine. The body became available for dissection and its multiple intricate parts were observed and studied. A dominant and persistent metaphor emerged, that of the body as machine. The body is considered to be a collection of pumps, mechanical levers, physiological processes, and so on.

How do the rules of science relate to the practice of medicine? Similar to the experimental method above, clinical knowledge is based on scientific principles of understanding nature. Biomedicine seeks to understand the biological function (and dysfunction) of the internal organs of the human body. It is reductionist, progressively delving into tissues, cells, sub-cellular components, molecules, and even atoms. It seeks to classify and explain observed clinical phenomena (symptoms, signs, and disease outcomes) by understanding normal and diseased function. As time passed, the focus of biomedicine became the cure of diseases related to organs of the human body.

In biomedicine, explanation is usually linked to an identifiable cause-and-effect relationship. A bacterium called mycobacterium *causes* the disease of tuberculosis, and so on. The model suggests (quite seductively) that it is possible to know how to practise medicine through an understanding of the components of the body and their interaction with a scientifically proven causative agent of disease. Medical education and practice is largely based on this proposition.

This understanding of medical practice has been extraordinarily powerful. Advances in medicine during the twentieth century included: the development of anaesthesia and safe surgical techniques; understanding of microbiology and antibiotics; understanding of immunology, malignancy and the development of effective chemotherapeutic regimes; advances in imaging techniques; and more recently, advances in the understanding of genetics.(5) These are powerful examples of the validity and utility of the scientific method and the place of biomedicine in medical practice.(6)

Biomedicine in practice

The following is a typical biomedical story and its many components will be familiar to practising clinicians.

VIGNETTE 3.1 A HEART ATTACK

Martin is a 62-year-old man, married with two sons in their young adulthood. He has a small block of land and works as a groundsman. Medically, he could be described as an 'arteriopath'. A committed smoker with moderate hypertension and an abnormal lipid profile, he had had a successful angioplasty for arterial ischemia.

One afternoon he presented with an acute myocardial infarction – within an hour he developed all the classical symptoms. He was in considerable distress, but this was managed with oxygen, intravenous morphine and oral aspirin as we arranged ambulance transfer to our base hospital about an hour away. He had an urgent coronary angiogram and three vessels were stented. Despite the timeliness of this treatment, he suffered a full thickness myocardial infarct with some loss of left ventricular contractility on later scanning. He stopped smoking and two weeks later was hankering to get back to work. Although I urged caution, he was back to his full workload in just six weeks.

Dissecting this vignette, it is possible to see biomedicine at work very successfully. The patient had well-defined disease that was understandable with respect to anatomy and physiology. He had presented in a typical way with symptoms and signs that pointed to a particular pathology of internal organs. He was managed in an up-to-date way. The sequence of events is recognisable and teachable. Medical students can learn about the different bodily components contained within this story. Patient management can be considered and critiqued at a professional and institutional level.

As a simple demonstration of utility, the biomedical model has much to offer this patient. Arguably, he is still alive because of biomedical expertise. The model provides a powerful explanation of what happened (although future outcomes are more unpredictable, as we shall see).

The underlying assumptions of biomedicine

In 1984, McWhinney offered a major and influential critique of the biomedical model of clinical practice, identifying several 'rules' or hidden assumptions that underpin it.(7). It is helpful to explore these assumptions with respect to day-to-day clinical practice, identifying both strengths and potential contradictions. The assumptions are outlined in Box 3.1.

BOX 3.1 THE ASSUMPTIONS OF BIOMEDICINE

1. Patients suffer from diseases that can be characterised in the same way as other natural phenomena.
2. A disease can be viewed independently from the person who is suffering from it and from his or her social context.
3. Each disease has a cause and finding it is a major objective of research.
4. Given a certain level of host resistance, the occurrence of disease is explained as a result of exposure to a pathogenic agent.
5. The physician's main task is to diagnose the disease and, wherever possible, to prescribe a specific remedy aimed at removing the cause or ameliorating the symptoms.
6. The physician uses an intellectual tool, the clinical method known as differential diagnosis.
7. Mental and physical diseases can be considered separately, with provision for a group of psychosomatic diseases in which the mind appears to act on the body.
8. Each disease follows a defined clinical course that can be influenced by medical interventions.
9. The doctor's effectiveness is independent of gender or beliefs.
10. The doctor is usually a detached, neutral observer.
11. The patient is usually a passive recipient of the prescribed treatment.

Adapted from McWhinney(7,8)

In our postgraduate courses for GPs, we present these 'rules' to our students for discussion. Usually, there is considerable debate about just how 'true' the assumptions are, or to what extent they still have validity in current clinical practice.

These postgraduate students usually identify the inherent contradiction of the second assumption, that a disease can be considered as 'separate' from the person with it. However, this view or conceptual understanding of disease has been a clever idea or tool within the developing history of medicine. It enabled the early clinicians to 'figure out' all the details of each disease (what causes it, how it affects people, the 'natural progression' without treatment, and so on). The understanding of tuberculosis as a disease, for example, relied on an underlying ontological framework that was able to identify the 'cause' (mycobacterium bacillus) and then to observe and classify its effects on human functioning.

Given the recent shift away from paternalism, our students also quite correctly point out that patients can no longer be considered as 'passive recipients' of care. Likewise, they do not consider themselves to be 'detached' or 'neutral observers' in their interactions with their patients. These GPs in the twenty-first century are often sceptical about such assumptions or 'rules' still having currency in modern clinical practice.

The problem, however, is that if assumptions 1–8 are considered to be relatively true (or at least, useful metaphors), then points 9, 10 and 11 become logical implications or corollaries. For example, if diseases are indeed independent of the person, then the doctor need only focus on or treat the affected organ (using drugs, surgery, and so on). In this depiction of disease, who the doctor is or how they communicate and interact with the patient would become largely irrelevant.

While doctors may no longer take these rules quite so literally, we contend that the successes and triumphs of modern medicine still depend on their continued utility. There are also many medical procedures and routines that demonstrate their continued influence within clinical practice – for example, the structure of the traditional hospital ward round, and research into the natural history of disease.

The biomedical ward round

Ward rounds are a well-structured routine where a group of doctors (and sometimes other health professionals) gather round the bed of each patient in hospital and talk about what to do. Occupying an unchallenged role as the flagship of medical discourse, the ward round remains largely uncontested or problematised. A recent paper, for example, described the 'enduring value of the ward round', noting 'its potential to model professionalism, enhance clinical reasoning and demonstrate the cultural norms of medical practice'.(9)

Ward rounds have been in existence for several centuries, increasing in popularity under the influence of Sir William Osler (1849–1919), known as the 'father of modern medicine'.(10) Medicine in his time was rapidly moving towards a more scientific basis for both practice and training, most of which occurred within hospitals.

Despite recent critiques noting how the patient is largely excluded,(11–13) the modern round still seems quite similar in appearance to that of the early 1900s. Looking carefully at the process, the style of the round remains primarily impersonal: the patient's current biomedical status is conveyed to the head of the team; discussion takes place in front of, but often does not involve, the patient. The doctors' predominant role appears to be that of 'objective observer', while the patient remains the 'grateful and passive recipient of care', being subjected, as Foucault would suggest, to the 'clinical gaze'.(14) These comments are not intended to be critical of the practical utility of the round, nor of the hard-working doctors who conduct it. It is simply that the round still seems to embody the assumptions noted above, without making them explicit.

'Pure' biomedical research

While the profession has now changed considerably, two projects in the middle of the twentieth century also illustrate how the assumptions of science have been a powerful influence on medical research. In the Tuskegee syphilis experiment, conducted between 1932 and 1972 in Alabama by the U.S. Public Health Service, researchers observed the outcomes when syphilis was diagnosed but not treated.(15) Similarly in Auckland, New Zealand, in the 1960s and 1970s, Professors Green and Bonham researched the natural history of cervical cancer.(16) Their protocol first identified patients with carcinoma in situ, then observed their progress over time without medical intervention. As they did not tell their patients about the underlying agenda, their research became a national scandal for the profession in New Zealand and a turning point for the ethics of informed consent.(17)

These two projects illustrate how researchers were applying the rules of science quite literally, even when the subject of experimentation was human beings.(18,19) Since then, other methods of research (cross-sectional and cohort studies) have also been developed to provide information on disease without potentially harming patients.

The limitations of biomedicine

Scientific models gain currency because of their predictive power. From current observations, the scientist attempts to predict what will happen in the future. Turning to the physical sciences by way of illustration, for many centuries Newtonian physics was a superb predictive model about the movement of planets and stars. However, as equipment became more precise, observations gradually began to show discrepancies. A further, more refined, model from Einstein and others was required to explain subtle variations.

Similarly, in medical practice, biomedicine has proved to be an excellent model for understanding the body, especially in acute disease. However, not all clinical observations appear to be explicable, as the next sections demonstrate.

Here is a follow-up encounter with Martin from the earlier vignette, now about three months later. Can biomedicine explain what is happening?

VIGNETTE 3.2 RECOVERY FROM HEART ATTACK

When it was time for re-prescribing his medications, Martin presented with his wife. He appeared a bit dejected: not depressed, just downcast. He seemed like a man for whom awareness of a changed reality was starting to dawn – a reality that he was powerless to change or control. His wife was tense and anxious.

I enquired as to how he was getting on, and his answers to my questions were vague. He didn't have angina; he wasn't overtly short of breath; he just couldn't do what he was used to doing easily, what he expected himself to be able to do. 'After all Doctor, I'm cured, aren't I? – the stents have fixed my arteries, I've stopped smoking, done all the things I'm meant to?'

I asked his wife what her concerns were. 'I don't want him to die', she said. 'Do you think you might die, Martin?' I asked. He wasn't at all shocked by the directness of my question and just said that he wanted to be well again, to be back to how things were previously.

We talked for a while about how his heart had been damaged by the infarction, how it might not ever return to its previous level of functioning. I tried to be positive, pointing out that the stents had been successful and that he was doing well with his non-smoking and getting back to work.

But deep down, I felt that something inside him had changed, perhaps permanently. Martin's loss seemed to be much more than just a few grams of myocardium. His subjective experience was real, but it was very difficult for me, his wife, or indeed Martin himself, to define just what had changed in any 'scientific' sense. These were personal changes that were over and above his myocardial damage.

In this situation, biomedicine now appears to have less explanatory power. We will return to Martin's story in a minute, but first, here are some further observations of clinical practice, each followed by a question (Box 3.2).

BOX 3.2 COMMON OBSERVATIONS IN CLINICAL PRACTICE

1. Mr X was dying of lung cancer, but was able to hang on until after Christmas. *What are the links between the disease, the patient, and the eventual outcome (death)?*
2. The doctor can influence the rate of recovery from the patient's flu-like illness by being confident, clear and definitive about the diagnosis and treatment. *True or false?*
3. Attending a breast cancer support group can help patients survive longer from their breast cancer. *True or false?*
4. The recovery from myocardial infarction depends more on whether the patient feels loved and supported by their spouse than on which particular medication is provided. *True or false?*
5. The Pope has been unwell recently. Millions of people around the world are praying for him. *What underlying assumption is their prayer based on?*
6. The mind (ideas, thoughts, theories) can be considered separate to the body (symptoms, pain, pathology of organs). *True or false?*
7. The oncologist wanted to start chemotherapy on the day the diagnosis was made, but Mr Y wanted to sort out his stress first, to see if the cancer would go away. *What underlying rules is each person following?*

Such questions are quite difficult, asking us to unpick what is tacitly accepted and rarely discussed. In observation 7, perhaps the oncologist believes that treatment will work regardless of what the patient thinks or feels about disease. On the other hand, the patient is convinced there are connections between his personal world and that of his internal organs.

Situations such as these have prompted many clinicians and theorists to look more closely at biomedicine itself, considering whether the model could be expanded or improved in some way.

The biopsychosocial model

In the latter part of the twentieth century, both doctors and patients became more aware of the difficulties described in this follow-up consultation. While the Western world had been swept along by the advances in biomedicine, a sense of dissatisfaction had started to arise, both from the lay public and from within the profession. In Martin's case, the disease was ostensibly cured, but the patient was not. Recognition of various limitations of biomedicine led to the **biopsychosocial model**, first proposed by George Engel, an American physician and psychiatrist.

In his seminal 1977 paper, 'The need for a new medical model: a challenge for biomedicine', (20) Engel proposed a different way of thinking about medical practice. As the name would suggest, this includes considering not only biological issues, but also psychological aspects of human experience in the context of relevant social circumstances.

Engel argued that the disease-centred biomedical model was no longer adequate for the scientific challenge or social responsibility of medicine. He contested physicians' conceptualisation of disease within narrowly defined somatic or bodily parameters, arguing that it was affecting their attitudes and behaviour with patients. Because it was limited to organic elements of disease and neglected the psychosocial determinants of suffering, he felt, medicine was failing patients and society.(20)

Systems theory

Engel based his revised medical model on 'systems theory', which in turn was based on von Bertalanffy's general system theory.(21) Systems theory was a response to the mechanistic and reductive methods of enquiry that characterised eighteenth- and nineteenth-century science (linear cause and effect), proposing instead that a series of self-regulating systems are linked within a well-defined hierarchy. Homeostatic mechanisms maintain the equilibrium of each system in a steady state, although changes in one system will eventually affect the others.

This explanatory model is applicable to complex systems such as the weather, as well as to all living organisms, including humans. The hierarchy of living systems moves from organelle, to cell, to tissue, to organ, to each individual person, to family, and extends out to community and society. Each level is a self-contained system with its own laws and dynamics, while relating directly to the levels both above and below.

Engel applied this concept to the physiological systems of the human body, including the patient's wider context of life and society (Figure 3.1). The biopsychosocial model was the first attempt to acknowledge and include the patient's personal, psychological and cultural factors, linking them to the onset and outcome of disease.

Martin's unwellness in Vignette 3.2 is difficult to define in terms of the biomedical model. However, as we noted in the last chapter, illness may involve disruption or loss of the many different aspects or components of *person*. If one considers the features of his psychological upset and expects to see correlations with other systems, then his disturbed physiological functioning becomes easier to understand. The biopsychosocial model may not instantly lead to a solution, but is a better explanatory framework than the linear cause-and-effect model based more narrowly on organ dysfunction.

Engel's goal was to expand medical expertise so that doctors would become more effective. In this example, Martin cannot be considered in isolation from his wife and family, his tasks in life, his various roles, and perhaps most importantly, his perception of future life. Understanding this patient is incomplete if we restrict ourselves to his disease. While biomedicine has focused on levels *below* that of the person, biopsychosocial medicine leads us to explore the patient's relationships and wider social context. In Figure 3.1, these levels are legitimately connected to the person, their organs and even their cells and molecules.

FIGURE 3.1 SYSTEMS HIERARCHY (LEVELS OF ORGANISATION)

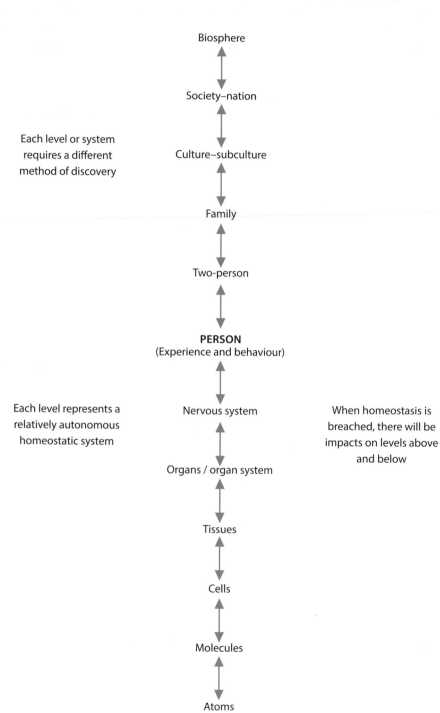

Each level or system requires a different method of discovery

Each level represents a relatively autonomous homeostatic system

When homeostasis is breached, there will be impacts on levels above and below

Biosphere

Society–nation

Culture–subculture

Family

Two-person

PERSON
(Experience and behaviour)

Nervous system

Organs / organ system

Tissues

Cells

Molecules

Atoms

Adapted from Engel(22)

Do these ideas illustrate a change in the fundamental basis of the practice of medicine? Using more philosophical language, has medicine entered a new belief system where the underlying assumptions and epistemology have been altered? Before those questions can be answered, it is helpful to review the concept of paradigms.

Paradigms

A paradigm is a set of received beliefs within a science. This concept was popularised by Thomas Kuhn, the celebrated philosopher of science.(23) An historian, he carefully traced and analysed changes in the scientific frameworks of chemistry, physics, and astronomy over the last thousand or so years. His thesis (now one of the most widely quoted books of the twentieth century) is that all sciences are characterised by particular **paradigms**. These have currency and endure as long as scientists agree on the underlying principles in that discipline, using them to solve the issues at hand. This is identified as the 'normal science' within each paradigm.

However, when sufficiently important observations emerge that challenge those principles, the paradigm comes to a point of crisis. Either the empirical observations of nature are in error, or the underlying principles need to be re-examined, even radically altered. These troublesome observations are called **anomalies**. Given sufficient validity and acknowledgement by scientists, anomalies usually lead to paradigm change. Such change is usually not without its problems, as the older generation of scientists may resist suggested changes quite vigorously. Factions are usually formed, each side armed with evidence about the validity and predictive capacity of their preferred model.(23)

Over time, however, a paradigm change occurs when there is a fundamental alteration in the belief system of that science. The proposed alternative ways of understanding must better explain the anomalies. An oft-quoted example is the shift from Newtonian physics to Einstein's theory of relativity. Put simply, the way in which particles interacted and functioned according to Newton became a less and less viable way of understanding atomic and subatomic physics. The belief system about their interactions was completely transformed. This is an example of a paradigm shift.

While Kuhn did not analyse medical models, many people believe his theory of paradigms is applicable to modern medicine. Certainly McWhinney mounts a strong case for this, but there is debate as to whether the biopsychosocial model is sufficiently different to represent a paradigm shift that is distinctly separate from biomedicine.

Kuhn also observed that paradigm change usually allows the current paradigm to be incorporated into a newer one (Newtonian physics still 'works' in a day-to-day mechanical setting). There is, however, a revised set of assumptions that supersede the older ones. The question here is whether the biopsychosocial paradigm is a true example of paradigm shift: have its assumptions been normalised into the teaching and practice of medicine?

We turn now to common clinical observations that are a poor fit with the disease model (at least as a method of explaining dysfunction and illness). Using the framework above, these are identified as anomalies to the assumptions of biomedicine.(8)

Anomalies to the biomedical paradigm

McWhinney lists several clinical instances that are 'difficult to ignore', especially in primary care medicine. The first is the **specific aetiology** anomaly, where although many people are exposed to the same causal agents of disease such as bacteria, only some people are affected. The implication is that simple cause-and-effect models of disease are inadequate.(8)

Another example is the **mind–body** anomaly, which we refer to as somatisation. This is where patients are unwell, but there is no identified disease. Similarly, the so-called **placebo effect** is where inactive substances appear to have substantial effects on human physiology and functioning. The placebo effect is commonly accepted and accounted for within randomised clinical trials, but this does not necessarily indicate that doctors understand how and why the phenomenon occurs. Neither somatisation nor placebo can be explained using current biomedical theory. We will now outline these two commonly observed phenomena in more detail, before returning to the issue of paradigms in medical practice.

Somatisation: The bane of medical practice

VIGNETTE 3.3   IRRITABLE BOWEL SYNDROME

Mrs Jones has suffered for several years with intermittent diarrhoea and wind. As she is in her mid-50s and has a family history of bowel cancer, I investigated with a barium enema. Her symptoms persisted and although I suspected irritable bowel syndrome, most of my interventions made little difference (antispasmodics, dietary roughage, referrals to specialists, colonoscopy, and so on). She admitted to ongoing stress (her daughter's abusive marriage and her own isolation), but there seemed no effective method of linking her symptoms to her life stresses.

Using McWhinney's assumptions of biomedicine, this patient is 'undiagnosable'. Her bowel is anatomically normal, at least as delineated by various investigatory procedures. There is no 'medical' cause for her symptoms. Further attempts to investigate and treat her condition seem bound to failure. The 'normal' method of diagnosis and treatment is not working.

One of the key rules of biomedicine is that 'mental and physical diseases can be considered separately', perhaps a legacy of the historic split between mind and body during the Enlightenment, when science differentiated itself from the church. As Epstein et al. somewhat wryly note: 'Attempts to force the problem of unexplained somatic symptoms into a 19th-century pathologically based diagnostic system have not been successful.'(24)

Mind–body dualism has been, and continues to be, a significant problem. Patients persistently turn up to their doctor with physical symptoms that appear to have no correlation whatsoever to their internal organs. We noted in the last chapter how Peabody had lamented in 1929 that the newer graduates were not caring adequately for their patients. His address was also an excellent overview of somatisation, as he wanted graduates to notice what was happening in their patients' lives, treating them through an empathic understanding of stress-related symptoms.(25)

Problems with classification and nomenclature

In some reference texts, the definition of 'somatisation disorder' is limited to severe, multi-symptomatic patients who are unresponsive to treatment. We first use the term in a narrow sense to cover single or intermittent presentations of physical or psychological symptoms that are unrelated to single organ disease. In a broader definition, somatisation refers to the contribution of psychosocial factors to both organic and functional illness.(26) For example, patients with known arthritis, asthma or heart disease have flare-ups when under stress.

While the traditional label has been 'psychosomatic' illness, other labels are also in common use: medically unexplained symptoms (MUS), functional disorder, functional somatic syndrome, bodily distress syndrome, somatic symptom disorder, symptom defined illness, and somatoform disorder.

'Medically unexplained symptoms' has become fashionable recently, but as Creed and others point out, '[this] term is in itself a barrier to improved care ... It defines the patient's symptoms by what they are not, rather than by what they are, and it reflects dualistic thinking – regarding symptoms as either "organic" or "non-organic or psychological".'(27)

All these labels are problematic, given the continued 'mind–body split' paradigm that both doctors and patients appear to be using. With this ongoing confusion over aetiology and nomenclature, it is little wonder that these illnesses can be very frustrating.

Practical issues

We use the helpful framework provided by Dr Brett Mann, a GP from Christchurch with a longstanding interest in somatisation.(28) He distinguishes between 'facultative' and 'obligate' somatisers. To explain these terms, he notes that many patients wonder if there are links between their symptoms and their life issues. They present for assessment, simply wanting the doctor to confirm this idea, or else they are quite open to mind–body connections if the doctor suggests it.(29) These people are better known as **facultative** somatisers, as they are flexible in their understanding of aetiology.

On the other hand, Mrs Jones in Vignette 3.3 would be classed as an **obligate** somatiser, unable to consider the idea that her physical symptoms might be linked to ongoing personal distress. She may be largely unaware of her underlying emotions, continuing to present with inexplicable symptoms. The outcome may be more and more investigations and referrals, all of which have costs and potential side effects.(30)

Every specialty has their own set of somatising patients, usually with symptoms that are poorly related to particular organs of the body: irritable bowel syndrome and abdominal pain in gastroenterology; pelvic pain in gynecology; headaches in neurology; chest pains in cardiology; asthma and shortness of breath in respiratory medicine; low back pain in orthopaedics, and so on.(31) However, many patients are not diagnosed with somatisation and often lurch between GP and specialist looking for an explanation and treatment.

We will discuss somatisation in more detail later, but briefly, this phenomenon is not unique to only some patients; *everyone* can somatise. Under acute stress, the human body reacts with sweaty palms, racing heart, even loose bowels. This is because the body is not comprised of discrete 'parts': neural and hormonal connections mean the person and their body are inseparable. Returning to Cassell's typology of the person, all the components of personhood have the potential to cause distress and accompanying somatic symptoms.(32) Under both acute and chronic stress, bodily symptoms can vary from person to person. They can be mild or severe and can be located in any part of the body.

Mann and Wilson have identified four major barriers that prevent doctors being more effective with these patients: lack of appreciation of psychosocial factors within the traditional biomedical model; negative perceptions of such patients arising from the occasional intractable (obligate) somatiser; lack of specific training within undergraduate and postgraduate education; and lack of confidence in psychological skills.(33)

In brief, somatisation is a clinical anomaly as it lies outside the scope of traditional biomedicine. It is a source of significant suffering for both patients and their doctor. We will explore some better approaches to these patients in Chapter 7. In the meantime, we will consider another major anomaly, that of the incorrectly named 'placebo effect'.

The placebo effect = the 'meaning response'

The 'placebo effect' is one of the great misnomers in medicine because, by definition, something that is inert *cannot have an effect*. Academic interest was initiated by Beecher's pioneering 1955 article,(34) where he pondered the age-old observation that people respond to treatments that have no logical basis. Yet by persisting with this particular label, the profession has missed the opportunity to consider this phenomenon more critically. Patients clearly do respond to drugs or other interventions that are 'inert', so better labelling and a deeper understanding are required.

Early explanations were that some patients were 'placebo responders' or that the patient was improving anyway and was thus identified rather unscientifically as a 'spontaneous remission'. Further influential books continued using the same term,(35) but in 2002 Moerman insightfully challenged those prior and naïve explanations, more correctly identifying placebo as a 'meaning response'.(36) Based on extensive analysis of placebo data embedded in decades of clinical trials, he postulated that humans are 'cultural animals' with significant interactions between culture and biology. As in systems theory, organs cannot be considered as separate from the person and their social context.

The meaning response poses considerable challenges for the purist within the biomedical paradigm. Many doctors and patients admit to surprise when they hear, for example, that blue pills are better for anxiety, red pills are better for depression, 'placebo surgery' is effective, or that pain relief also depends on the prescribing doctor's *attitude* to the drug being used.(37) Various placebo observations derived from clinical trials are listed in Box 3.3.

BOX 3.3 RESEARCHING THE PLACEBO EFFECT

Communication studies

- Patients responded better to a new drug for anxiety (meprobamate) if their doctor was instructed to be 'enthusiastic' rather than 'skeptical' about this medication: 'With the enthusiastic doctors, patients taking meprobamate improved more than patients taking placebo, whereas with the skeptical doctors, patients taking placebo tended to improve more than patients taking mepobromate.'(38)

- Many patients in general practice have symptoms but no definitive diagnosis. Thomas randomly assigned 200 such patients to one of four consultations: 'a consultation conducted in a "positive manner," with and without treatment, and a consultation conducted in a "non-positive manner," with and without treatment. Two weeks later he found a significant difference in patient satisfaction between the positive and negative groups but not between the treated and untreated groups. Similarly, 64% of those receiving a positive consultation got better, compared with 39% of those who received a negative consultation (p = 0.001) and 53% of those treated got better compared with 50% of those not treated (p = 0.5).'(39)

Pain relief studies

- Prior to dental surgery, pain and subsequent anxiety from a mandibular injection of local anaesthetic were reduced by giving a placebo tablet prior to the injection. All patients had the same placebo, but information about it varied, either an 'oversell' ('this tablet is very effective') or an 'undersell' message ('this tablet only works for some people'). It made no difference if the injection was given by a technician or a dentist: 'Enthusiastic messages of drug effects produced statistically and clinically significant reductions in postplacebo fear of injection and anxiety state and markedly lower ratings of pain experienced during injection of local anesthetic.'(40)

- Placebo treatment of stable angina was successful in 77 per cent of a group of 35 patients. The average number of attacks of angina before 'treatment' (a placebo pill only, in addition to normal use of nitroglycerin) was 10.6: 'The number of attacks per week decreased by 48% (P<0.0001) during the titration period (8 weeks) and by 77% during the whole 6 months.'(41)

Surgery studies

- In some trials, 'sham' arthroscopy (surgical wound on the knee without exploration of the underlying joint) was found to be just as effective as 'normal' arthroscopy.(42)

- In Sweden, Spangfort did a retrospective review of 2504 operations for sciatic pain resulting from lumbar disc herniation, noting that 346 patients had normal discs at surgery, thus not requiring the usual debridement and excision of degenerative fragments (or in other words, they underwent sham surgery).

Postoperatively, over 70 per cent of these patients had considerable improvement. (43)

- Ligation of the internal mammary arteries was an emerging treatment for angina in the 1950s. In 1959, patients were randomly assigned to a 'treatment' group (ligation) and a 'non-treatment' group (incision of skin only). Eighty-three per cent of the placebo patients had substantial improvement, compared to 67 per cent of patients in the treatment group.(44) In retrospect, it appears that both groups were given a 'placebo' intervention.

- 'Laser revascularisation' is a recent treatment for patients with severe, drug-resistant angina. It involves firing short bursts of laser directly into the myocardium, ostensibly to allow blood to have access to cardiac muscle. It can be performed with open-heart surgery or via a femoral catheter. There is no anatomical explanation for why this new treatment might work, but in the 1990s it was taken up with enthusiasm by cardiologists and patients alike. The first placebo-controlled study divided patients into three groups: high-dose laser, low-dose laser, and a mock or sham procedure. *All* groups showed substantial improvements on subjective and objective measures over six months. The authors concluded: 'Treatment with percutaneous myocardial laser revascularization provides no benefit beyond that of a similar sham procedure in patients blinded to their treatment status.'(45) Notably, the authors did not discuss why this particular treatment has such a strong placebo effect.[1]

Explaining the meaning response

These clinical examples are quite surprising. They challenge commonly held ideas about the human body and how it works. While both patients and doctors expect bodies to behave in a purely anatomical way (blocked arteries will cause angina, unblocking them will relieve it, not unblocking them won't, and so on), these reported observations illustrate the complexity of human functioning.

Many factors impact on a patient's response to a particular medical intervention. In addition to whether a drug (for example) actually works, the meaning response includes the role and social esteem that society gives the doctor, the patient's and doctor's ideas about that particular treatment, various nuances within the doctor–patient relationship, and many other issues such as the patient's cultural beliefs about health and treatments.

Moerman suggests that the 'physician's demeanour' helps to activate the efficacy of surgery and medications, over and above their intrinsic properties. The main aspect of demeanour appears to be the feeling of certainty that the doctor conveys. This includes an assurance that things will turn out well, and includes the doctor's 'deep and abiding commitment to the character and nature of their techniques'.

---

1 Given the data in the box, it would be interesting to do a placebo-controlled trial on Coronary Artery Bypass Grafting (CABG). While this has never been done, it would be surprising if there were not substantial meaning responses from 'sham' CABG.

(36) Believing in the underlying theoretical basis of one's chosen profession may be just as important as the interventions made. This belief is somehow passed on to patients, whose meaning response is enhanced. As an example, Smith and Glass's comprehensive analysis of various modalities within psychotherapy illustrates the similarity of patient outcomes,(46) regardless of the underlying theoretical construct.[2]

A more recent example is a Cochrane review of nonpharmacologic therapies for low back pain: '[S]pinal manipulative therapy is as effective as other commonly used therapies like exercise, standard medical care and physical therapy for the management of chronic low back pain.'(47) The slight advantage of manipulation reported in this trial might arise from the enthusiasm of those who use it, compared to providers who feel quite neutral about various treatments on offer.

Other researchers have also noted how doctors can inadvertently create a 'nocebo' effect (48) or 'negative meaning response'. For example, the patient has a diagnosis of cancer. The news is broken to them poorly without offering hope; they feel they are being avoided by staff; they are told their chemotherapy will make them feel very sick and may not work anyway, and so on. Under the guise of honesty or not instilling 'false hope', the patient's own healing responses and the trajectory of illness are being influenced in a negative way.

The question is no longer *whether* these influences exist. A better question is: can doctors utilise this meaning response more consciously and more effectively in their day-to-day practice? It is interesting that undergraduate training now places greater emphasis on communication skills and the doctor–patient relationship, but most medical schools do not make it explicit that this effort can impact on the patient's recovery from disease through an enhanced meaning response.

'Placebo effect' has often been used to explain how complementary or alternative therapies (CAM) work. Some of these therapies utilise the patients' own internal homeostatic capacities (e.g. meditation, relaxation, massage, etc). Others use active ingredients or agents (e.g. herbal therapy), while still others use an understanding of energetic fields (homeopathy, Chinese acupuncture, Reiki, etc.).

Discussion of the range of CAM modalities is outside the scope of this book, but once a meaning effect is understood by the practitioner as a legitimate goal of any therapeutic intervention, then it is not surprising that many therapies appear to work quite well, over and above any 'active' ingredients. Being listened to and *being understood* by any practitioner will be helpful for patients through this meaning response.

In summary, the meaning response can be elicited by a sincere belief in the modality being used, attending to the doctor–patient relationship, gaining trust and respect and providing a positive spin on the treatment that is being offered. Wise practitioners have always done this instinctively, while doctors who think the patient is somehow separate from their diseased organ may feel less inclined to do so.

---

2 Their conclusion is as follows: 'Few important differences in effectiveness could be established among many quite different types of psychotherapy. More generally, virtually no difference in effectiveness was observed between the class of all behavioral therapies (systematic desensitization and behavior modification) and the nonbehavioral therapies (Rogerian, psychodynamic, rational-emotive, and transactional analysis). On the average, the typical therapy client is better off than 75% of untreated individuals.' One interpretation is that the practitioner's belief in their method is as important as the method itself.

A paradigm change in medical practice?

Now that we have discussed these anomalies, the question remains: is biomedicine still the dominant and prevailing medical paradigm of the twenty-first century?

Using Kuhn's model, paradigms enter a crisis period when anomalies are observed but are not explained by current theory. Given a better explanatory and predictive model, a paradigm change occurs. This may take some time as scientists learn to let go of their previous ideas and adapt to revised concepts. The anomalies have now been accommodated. 'Normal' science will then continue, but using the new assumptions of this particular science.(23)

In medicine, the biopsychosocial model proposed over 30 years ago is potentially helpful, but it has yet to become the working model of clinical practice. Similarly, somatisation and the 'placebo' effect are still outliers to normal clinical practice. Patients with the former are poorly theorised and managed, while the latter is not consciously and deliberately utilised to improve clinical outcomes. In our view, biomedicine is still the predominant paradigm, but there is significant paradigmatic tension and debate.

Conclusion

This chapter is intended to provide a better appreciation of the strengths, contradictions and weaknesses within biomedicine. Biomedicine has been, and still is, extraordinarily effective for acute disease where physical interventions are helpful, but it has less utility in chronic disease or when symptoms are not readily explained. These situations often lead to frustration for both doctor and patient. The prevailing assumptions of biomedicine remain a significant barrier to better medical care for patients with somatisation, and doctors could make greater use of the meaning response.

There is no intention here of being critical of biomedical advances. The rules of biomedicine have been a very useful *metaphor* for researching and treating health issues. The metaphor works extremely well in many situations, also being the basis for medical training in the twentieth century.

Instead, this chapter attempts to help practitioners work through any dissonance or even disillusionment about their clinical work. Such dissonance often occurs when doctors move from hospital to general practice or to family medicine clinics. Here, the anomalies of biomedicine become more apparent, although hospital outpatient and emergency departments often confront similar issues. Common responses to dissonance are to feel inadequate or to blame the patient. A more thoughtful response is to re-examine the model of current practice.

Dissonance can also lead to cynicism. This may arise from a prior and naïve conception of medicine's ability to identify and treat all diseases, or to help every patient. An existential problem might stem from discovering that the received model from medical school does not fit the realities of practice. Many medical students struggle in their transition from pre-clinical theory to clinical training as they attempt to apply the biomedical model to real patients.

Our own resolution to these issues is that the biomedical paradigm is simply a useful tool. The tool is of course not 'real', in the same way that maps of a town or a landscape are not 'real'. Maps – and biomedical conceptions – are useful approximations for what is happening in the real world. The ultimate purpose of medicine, however, is *caring for the patient*. Doctors are fortunate to have a powerful intellectual tool for diagnosing and treating disorders of the body, but their ultimate goal is looking after persons, not just their internal organs.

In terms of the philosophy of modern clinical practice, we have avoided discussion of positivism and post-positivism, terms describing philosophical understandings of the world and our place in it. Many commentators have located biomedicine within a positivist ontology consistent with eighteenth-century science(49) – 'diseases are out there to be discovered', and so on. A postmodern understanding is that the observer influences and shapes the world, including the objects under study. Postmodern medical knowledge can be considered as a 'social construction' and the outcomes of medical care are socially mediated.(50, 51)

In Chapter 1 we mentioned the 'apparent contradiction' in trying to help. Discussion with many GPs about paradigms, biomedicine and anomalies has led to another contradiction, this time about medical science. Doctors learn a great deal about the body, much of it under the banner of science and scientific knowledge. However, the practice of medicine includes a considerable degree of 'unscientific' uncertainty and unpredictability. Yet as doctors learn to let go of their 'scientism' (an unrealistic belief in the utility or application of science to individual patients), they become more accurate and observant – and more scientific – in their interactions with patients. Their clinical effectiveness increases as they learn to use biomedicine more judiciously.

It is helpful to appreciate that biomedicine is conceptually innovative, but has its limitations. Being more objective about the method we use gives us a more thoughtful perspective about patients and their problems, our involvement with them, and the realities of illness. We would like doctors to be wise as well as knowledgeable.

SUMMARY POINTS

- Much of clinical work is based on biomedicine, which in turn is embedded within the scientific paradigm.
- Biomedicine is focused on the classification and management of disease.
- Classically, biomedicine views disease as being separate from the person of the patient, while the doctor is a detached observer or scientist.
- The biopsychosocial approach recognises the role of psychological and social determinants of illness.
- Somatisation is an anomaly of biomedicine that is more readily approached and understood within a biopsychosocial approach.
- The 'placebo effect' is a misnomer and is better thought of as a 'meaning response'.
- Biomedicine has been in a state of paradigmatic tension for nearly 50 years: this is yet to be resolved.
- Many doctors have a sense of dissonance as they realise how clinical practice differs from theory.
- Learning about the underlying assumptions of biomedicine helps to create a more realistic perspective.
- Realising that biomedicine is just a useful tool helps doctors become even more effective.

References

1. Lock M, Gordon D, eds. *Biomedicine examined*. Dordrecht: Kluwer Academic, 1988.
2. Descartes R, Moriarty M. *Meditations on first philosophy: with selections from the objections and replies*. New York: Oxford University Press, 2008.
3. Samson C. Biomedicine and the body. In: Samson C, ed. *Health studies: a critical and cross-cultural reader*. Malden: Wiley-Blackwell, 1999. pp. 3–21.
4. Little JM. *Humane medicine*. Cambridge: Cambridge University Press, 1995.
5. Collins FS, Patrinos A, Jordan E, Chakravarti A, Gesteland R, Walters LR. New goals for the US human genome project: 1998–2003. *Science* 1998, 282(5389):682.
6. Angell M, Kassirer JP, Relman AS. Looking back on the millennium in medicine. *N Engl J Med* 2000, 342(1):42–49.
7. McWhinney I. Changing models: the impact of Kuhn's theory on medicine. *Fam Pract* 1984, 1(1):3–9.
8. McWhinney I. *Textbook of family medicine*. 3rd edn. Oxford: Oxford University Press, 2009.
9. Ker J, Cantillon P, Ambrose L. Teaching rounds: teaching on a ward round. *BMJ* 2008, 337:a1930.
10. Osler SW. *The principles and practice of medicine*. New York: Appleton, 1892.
11. Fletcher KE, Rankey DS, Stern DT. Bedside interactions from the other side of the bedrail. *J Gen Int Med* 2005, 20(1):58–61.
12. Launer J. Doing the rounds. *Q J Med* 2003, 96(4):321–22.
13. Sweet GS, Wilson HJ. A patient's experience of ward rounds. *Pat Educ Couns* 2010, 84:150–51.
14. Foucault M, Martin LH, Gutman H. *Technologies of the self*. Amherst, MA: University of Massachusetts, 1988.

15. Thomas SB, Quinn SC. The Tuskegee syphilis study, 1932 to 1972: implications for HIV education and AIDS risk education programs in the black community. *Am J Pub Health* 1991, 81(11):1498.

16. Green G. Is cervical carcinoma in situ a significant lesion? Int Surg 1967, 47(51):1–7.

17. Cartwright SR, Mackay EV. *The report of the committee of inquiry into allegations concerning the treatment of cervical cancer at National Women's Hospital and other related matters.* Wellington, NZ: Government Printing Office, 1988.

18. Paul C. The New Zealand cervical cancer study: could it happen again? *BMJ* 1988, 297(6647):533.

19. Corbie-Smith G. The continuing legacy of the Tuskegee syphilis study: Considerations for clinical investigation. *Am J Med Sci* 1999, 317(1):5–10.

20. Engel GL. The need for a new medical model: a challenge for biomedicine. *Science* 1977, 196(4286):129–36.

21. Von Bertalanffy L. *General system theory: foundations, development, applications.* New York: George Braziller, 1968.

22. Engel GL. The clinical application of the biopsychosocial model. *Am J Psych* 1980, 137(5):535–44.

23. Kuhn TS. *The structure of scientific revolutions.* Chicago: University of Chicago Press, 1962.

24. Epstein RM, Quill TE, McWhinney IR. Somatization reconsidered: incorporating the patient's experience of illness. *Arch Int Med* 1999, 159(3):215–22.

25. Peabody FW. Landmark article March 19, 1927: the care of the patient. *JAMA* 1984, 252(6):813.

26. Broom B. *Somatic illness and the patient's other story.* London: Free Association Books, 1997.

27. Creed F, Guthrie E, Fink P, Henningsen P, Rief W, Sharpe M, et al. Is there a better term than 'medically unexplained symptoms'? *J Psychosomatic Res* 2010, 68(1):5–8.

28. Mann B. Generalism: the challenge of functional and somatising illnesses. *NZ Fam Phys* 2007, 34(6):398–403.

29. Peters S, Rogers A, Salmon P, Gask L, Dowrick C, Towey M, et al. What do patients choose to tell their doctors? Qualitative analysis of potential barriers to reattributing medically unexplained symptoms. *J Gen Int Med* 2009, 24(4):443–49.

30. Barsky AJ, Orav EJ, Bates DW. Somatization increases medical utilization and costs independent of psychiatric and medical comorbidity. *Arch Gen Psychiat* 2005, 62(8):903–10.

31. Fink P, Rosendal M, Olesen F. Classification of somatization and functional somatic symptoms in primary care. *Aust NZ J Psychiat* 2005, 39(9):772–81.

32. Cassell EJ. The nature of suffering and the goals of medicine. *N Engl J Med* 1982, 306(11):639–45.

33. Mann B, Wilson HJ. A new approach to somatisation in general practice. Forthcoming, 2013.

34. Beecher HK. The powerful placebo. *JAMA* 1955, 159(17):1602–06.

35. Shapiro AK, Shapiro E. *The powerful placebo: from ancient priest to modern physician.* Baltimore: Johns Hopkins University Press, 1997.

36. Moerman DE. *Meaning, medicine, and the 'placebo effect'.* Cambridge: Cambridge University Press, 2002.

37. Moerman DE, Jonas WB. Deconstructing the placebo effect and finding the meaning response. *Ann Int Med* 2002, 136(6):471.

38. Uhlenhuth E, Rickels K, Fisher S, Park LC, Lipman RS, Mock J. Drug, doctor's verbal attitude and clinic setting in the symptomatic response to pharmacotherapy. *Psychopharm* 1966, 9(5):392–418.

39. Thomas K. General practice consultations: is there any point in being positive? *BMJ* 1987, 294(6581):1200–02.

40. Gryll SL, Katahn M. Situational factors contributing to the placebo effect. *Psychopharm* 1978, 57(3):253–61.

41. Boissel J, Philippon A, Gauthier E, Schbath J, Destors J. Time course of long-term placebo therapy effects in angina pectoris. *Europ Heart J* 1986, 7(12):1030–36.

42. Moseley JB, Wray NP, Kuykendall D, Willis K, Landon G. Arthroscopic treatment of osteoarthritis of the knee: a prospective, randomized, placebo-controlled trial. *Am J Sports Med* 1996, 24(1):28–34.

43. Spangfort EV. The lumbar disc herniation: a computer-aided analysis of 2,504 operations. *Acta Orthop Scand Suppl* 1972, 142:1–95.

44. Cobb LA, Thomas GI, Dillard DH, Merendino KA, Bruce RA. An evaluation of internal-mammary-artery ligation by a double-blind technic. *N Engl J Med* 1959, 260(22):1115–18.

45. Leon MB, Kornowski R, Downey WE, Weisz G, Baim DS, Bonow RO, et al. A blinded, randomized, placebo-controlled trial of percutaneous laser myocardial revascularization to improve angina symptoms in patients with severe coronary disease. *J Am Coll Card* 2005, 46(10):1812–19.

46. Smith ML, Glass GV. Meta-analysis of psychotherapy outcome studies. *Am Psychol* 1977, 32(9):752–60.

47. Bronfert G. High quality evidence that spinal manipulative therapy for chronic low back pain has a small short-term greater effect on pain and functional status compared with other interventions. *Evid Based Med* 2012, 17(3):81–82.

48. Helman CG. Placebos and nocebos: the cultural construction of belief. In: Peters D, ed. *Understanding the placebo effect in complementary medicine*. Edinburgh: Churchill Livingston, 2001. pp. 3–16.

49. Lyng S. *Holistic health and biomedical medicine: a countersystem analysis*. New York: University of New York Press, 1990.

50. Mattingly C, Garro LC. *Narrative and the cultural construction of illness and healing*. Berkeley: University of California Press, 2000.

51. Wilson HJ. The myth of objectivity: is medicine moving towards a social constructivist medical paradigm? *Fam Pract* 2000, 17(2):203–09.

Chapter 4

The Doctor–Patient Relationship

CONTENTS

Introduction

So far in this book we have discussed the illness experience of the patient and the underlying assumptions of the modern doctor. This chapter introduces the concept of the doctor–patient relationship, the meeting point between the world of the patient and the world of the doctor. Key aspects of this relationship are the capacity to listen attentively and respectfully and the capacity to engage and respond.

We also explore why 'relationship' has not been a central aspect of modern clinical practice, proposing instead that it is necessary in all clinical settings: general practice, specialist practice, and secondary and tertiary care. Relationships matter: they make the difference between good and not-so-good consultations, they impact on disease management, and they contribute to the doctor's sense of self and job satisfaction. Chapter 5 then develops these ideas further, examining the doctor's 'heartsink' experience when the relationship becomes problematic.

It is only recently that medical students have been taught about consulting or relationship skills. We start this chapter with some observations and insights from a student training session, then discuss the links between relationship and patient outcomes. This is followed by the importance of listening(1) and of emotional intelligence. The second part of this chapter introduces various frameworks for conceptualising relationships, including discussion of the use of power. We end with the benefits of relationship-centred care for both patient and doctor.

VIGNETTE 4.1 A TRAINER'S PERSPECTIVE

I am watching senior medical students interview a simulated patient.[1] Their task today is to take a medical history. Various sub-tasks known as micro-communication skills are related to both medical content and interpersonal process: a good introduction, eliciting the patient's agenda, using open questions, doing a review of systems, exploring the symptoms and past medical history, being empathic, and so on. The actor scores each student at the end of the consultation based on whether she would return to see them again. I also score the interview on various medical points as well as observations about interviewing skills.

Without it being planned, my chair had somehow been placed so that I was more directly opposite the actor than the student, and I was able to watch her face and body language quite closely. As I observed a series of consultations (18 students in total), she became more and more immersed in her role. It became easier and easier to see how she was responding to different students. While her presenting complaint was upper abdominal discomfort, the major background issue seemed to be the problem of her partner being away at sea quite regularly: she felt quite 'fragile' at present, which may or may not have been connected to her physical symptoms. With some students she opened up and talked openly about her fragility; with others the subject was never broached at all.

I found this to be quite fascinating: what were those students doing who were able to reach and discuss this delicate personal point? The actor was quite consistent: she made a series of 'offers' about her current use of antidepressants and her history of depression. Some students picked up on these offers and asked another question or explored some more, but others didn't. As I watched, I realised the actor and the better students were sort of 'dancing' together: she would offer, the student would respond; she would give a bit more; he would acknowledge and listen some more; closer and closer they got to her point of pain.

As they danced in this way, she became more open, her face and voice softer. Although she was talking about a potentially painful area, she became more engaged and energised: she seemed more authentic.

For the students she danced with, she indicated she would return again: with others she was more guarded. This capacity for a deeper engagement by students seemed independent of how thorough or not they were with their other medical tasks (history of present illness, review of systems, etc.). This deeper engagement was probably achieved through identifiable micro-skills such as reflection, use of silence, acknowledging feelings,

---

1 A simulated patient is an actor who is provided with a detailed patient scenario. Students' consulting skills are thus examined in a standardised way.

*and so on, but these students seemed to be doing more than just 'painting by numbers'
– something perhaps to do with being genuine. I felt these students genuinely wished to
engage and understand, to be intrigued by this person, to be curious about what makes
her tick and why she had come along today.*

*In short, these consultations (even with an actor with a script) were the start of a
significant relationship where the patient has trust in the doctor and, having trust, is able
to reveal and discuss current and important issues. The actor was following a well-written
scenario, but at times I think she surprised herself at the depth of her disclosure. While
none of the students offered any solutions, I wondered if their engagement and listening
was in some way therapeutic. Nothing of course had changed for the patient except that
she was putting into words something which previously had only been felt. Someone else
had listened, and so her experience of her illness (and perhaps even its meaning) had been
acknowledged and validated. She had been 'heard'.*

The marginalisation of relationship training

After World War II, there was growing discontent with some aspects of medical
practice. Here is a typical comment from 1968, where 'art' refers loosely to relationship
skills:

> The 'art' of medicine has been the topic of much discussion, but has never been
> subjected to scientific scrutiny. Whereas other aspects of medical practice are included
> in the physician's training, the approach to the patient is expected to be on the basis
> of intuition, and it is traditionally only learned by precept and by experience … In
> addition there is daily testimony to the discontent of the community with the medical
> care offered. Most especially, there is criticism aimed at the lack of warmth and
> humanity in the available medical care … Care of the doctor–patient relation has for too
> long been left to chance; because of its importance to general practice it must now be
> examined, defined, and taught, for only then can it be practiced efficiently.(2)

The final remarks quoted above are insightful. Apart from rather vague references
to attributes such as 'bedside manner', relationship skills have, at least until recently,
been taken for granted. It was not until near the end of the twentieth century that
medical students were trained in consulting skills, and even now, most current
practitioners do not use a specific method or technique for analysing and improving
their interpersonal interactions with patients.

As we stated in Chapter 3, the underlying assumptions of biomedicine have tended
to exclude 'relationship' as an important or worthy focus within modern clinical
practice. The dominant metaphors of biomedicine have been 'body as machine',
'doctor as scientist', and 'patient as passive recipient'. The classical stance of the doctor
has largely been that of 'objective observer': the patient 'exhibits' particular features
that require academic and scientific observation. In this framework, examination and
tests are considered against a known body of diseases, and eventually the patient is
informed of the likely diagnosis and the best current treatment.

In other words, the epistemology of *science* (the relationship between the scientist
and his or her object of study) that underpins biomedicine had been transposed onto

the *interaction* between the doctor and the patient. The corollary was an expectation that the doctor would keep the patient at a distance, perhaps out of concern for 'becoming over-involved' and/or 'losing scientific objectivity'. From the patient's perspective, however, such a doctor could be perceived as remote or distant, regardless of their technical competence. So while the doctor was endeavouring to be professionally objective or 'not-in-relationship', the patient's not uncommon perception was that 'he doesn't listen to me' or at worst, 'he doesn't care': indeed, the opposite of 'no relationship'.[2]

Medical students have always been faced with this particular dilemma: they are required to learn the essential 'facts' of medicine using the traditional scientific approach, but they are also required to develop some expertise in how to interact and 'be with' their patients. As Dobie notes, this task requires a different style of learning: 'Medical students enter medical school hoping to have good relationships with their patients. Along with residents, however, they are exposed to a hidden curriculum that places the acquisition of biomedical knowledge above and at times at odds with development of the awareness and relationship skills important to the patient-physician relationship.'

Dobie makes a good case for educational change that will 'encourage development of the communication and relationship-building skills throughout the medical education process. This will require a paradigm shift to a culture where teachers and learners are willing to consciously attend to their relationships and to work on self-awareness and mindfulness while they also master the biomedical knowledge required of the profession.'(3)

Nevertheless, not everyone agrees that the interaction between doctor and patient is so important. Many doctors consider that the biggest influence on patient outcomes will stem from disease processes set against the competence and technical expertise of the doctor: making the correct diagnosis, choosing the best available treatment, and so on. Such discussions are often conducted somewhat dualistically: 'I would rather have a brilliant but remote or even rude surgeon, than a kindly but incompetent one,' and so on. To resolve this impasse, we need to look for evidence.

Listening and medical outcomes

There is clearly a problem in trying to 'prove' that relationships actually matter. One of the most important components of relationship is high-quality communication. Fortunately, there is now a considerable amount of data on the ways in which quality of communication is linked to outcomes of care. Stewart analysed 21 studies published between 1983 and 1993 that looked at various aspects of communication. She concluded: 'The quality of communication [in both history and management] was found to influence patient health outcomes. The outcomes affected were, in descending order of frequency, emotional health, symptom resolution, function, physiologic measures (i.e., blood pressure and blood sugar level) and pain control.'(4)

---

2   There is a sense, however, in which 'detachment' is a subtle but appropriate component of the doctor's engagement: this will be discussed at the end of this chapter.

Further studies in the 1990s also illustrated the links between medical communication and various health outcomes such as empathy,(5) adherence,(6) and reducing the incidence of complaints.(7) In 2001, Di Blasi et al. did a further systematic review, identifying and revising 25 (single-blind) randomised controlled trials. They noted that 'One relatively consistent finding is that physicians who adopt a warm, friendly, and reassuring manner are more effective than those who keep consultations formal and do not offer reassurance.'(8)

Listening appears to have three main functions: enabling the doctor to make an accurate diagnosis; developing and maintaining a good doctor–patient relationship; and acting as a healing and therapeutic agent.(1,9) As we noted in Chapter 2, human beings have a fundamental need to express themselves and to be heard and acknowledged. In itself, listening is part of the treatment, not simply a method of eliciting sufficient information for the diagnosis (Figure 4.1).

FIGURE 4.1 THREE MAIN FUNCTIONS OF LISTENING

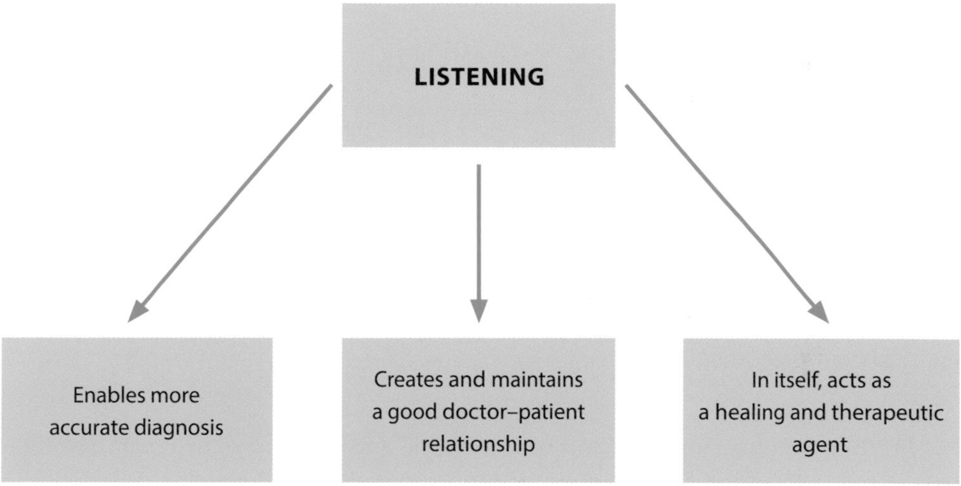

Adapted from Jagosh(1)

How does listening have an impact on health outcomes? Both direct and indirect pathways are outlined in more detail in Figure 4.2.

FIGURE 4.2 PATHWAYS TO HEALTH OUTCOMES

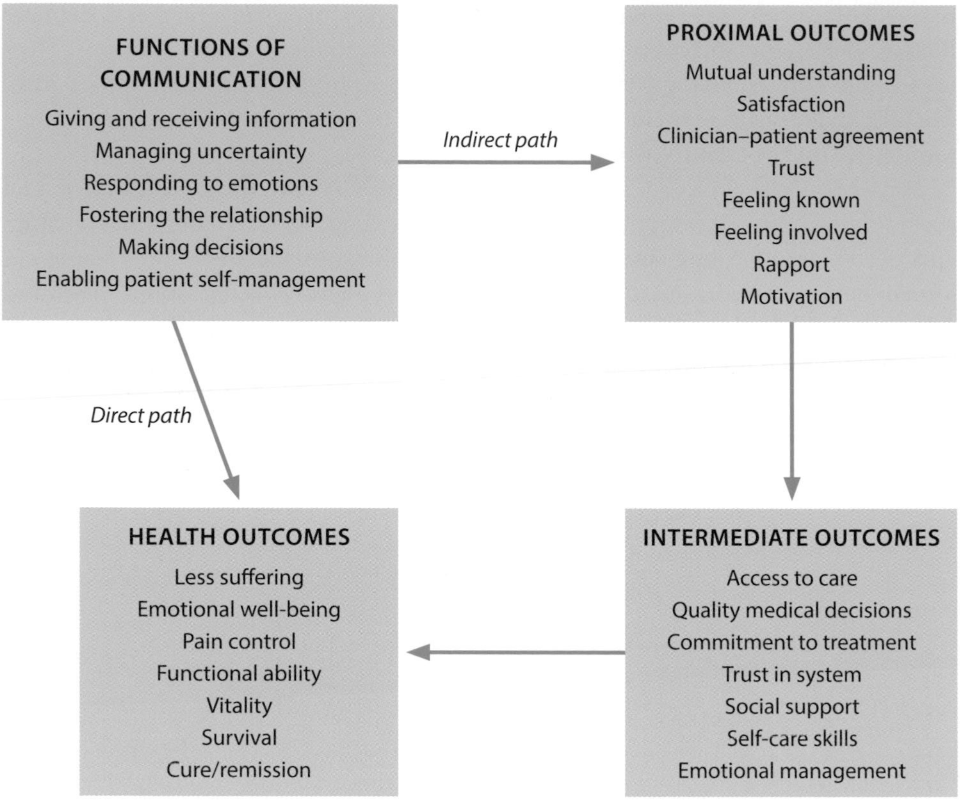

FUNCTIONS OF COMMUNICATION Giving and receiving information Managing uncertainty Responding to emotions Fostering the relationship Making decisions Enabling patient self-management	**PROXIMAL OUTCOMES** Mutual understanding Satisfaction Clinician–patient agreement Trust Feeling known Feeling involved Rapport Motivation

Indirect path

Direct path

HEALTH OUTCOMES Less suffering Emotional well-being Pain control Functional ability Vitality Survival Cure/remission	**INTERMEDIATE OUTCOMES** Access to care Quality medical decisions Commitment to treatment Trust in system Social support Self-care skills Emotional management

Adapted from Street et al.(10)

Starting with the top left-hand box, the style and pattern of the communication between doctor and patient may provide immediate benefit through a direct path to health outcomes: a patient with new and worrisome symptoms can be reassured and relieved by a simple explanation of their symptoms. This may lead to fewer negative emotions (fear and anxiety) and an increase in positive ones (hope and optimism). Communication also produces **proximal outcomes** (upper right box) such as better understanding of the problem or feeling heard and being understood. In turn, these proximal outcomes can lead to **intermediate outcomes** such as having trust, returning for follow-up, adherence to treatment, and better emotional management. These in turn can eventually lead to better **health outcomes** in terms of physical, mental, social and spiritual health.

Returning to the dualistic dilemma (the rude versus the kindly surgeon), the available evidence suggests that technical and interpersonal competencies are synergistic in their capacity to facilitate recovery from illness or interventions such as surgery. Yet, while doctors have highly developed knowledge and technical expertise, their practical skills in relationships are usually developed through trial and error and role modelling from others, without the benefit of more rigorous or focused training. This is in contrast to other health professional training such as psychotherapy or counselling, where the focus – and indeed therapeutic modality – is the *relationship itself* between therapist and client.

The links between psychological therapy and medicine

The current understanding of the role of listening within the doctor–patient relationship owes much to psychological theories developed during the twentieth century. The American psychologist Carl Rogers, for example, was influential in identifying the attributes of relationship that were critical for interpersonal therapy. The three main tenets of person-centred therapy are congruence (genuineness and honesty with the patient), unconditional positive regard (respect for and acceptance of the client) and empathy (the capacity and intention to try to understand what the patient feels and experiences, or 'Does the doctor know what this has been like for me?').(11)

As we will also see in Chapter 6, these tenets have been widely incorporated into various models of consulting such as patient-centred medicine(12) and the Calgary-Cambridge guides to communication skills.(13) These models encourage students to use various micro-communication skills in order to develop respect and gain trust, as well as to 'reflect back' to the patient their understanding of the various aspects of the illness experience.

Rogers's underlying assumption was that everyone has an 'actualising tendency': the inbuilt motivation to develop one's full potential. Expressing ideas and experiences honestly and authentically (whether in writing or with another person) and being listened to attentively and deeply helps to access one's capacity for living. This may explain why patients can find the doctor's respectful listening so profoundly helpful.

Listening as therapeutic

The capacity for listening is one of the key ingredients of relationship. Talking, both as listener and as 'listened to', affects both parties. Physiologically, a finely tuned therapeutic relationship appears to work through reciprocal responses between doctor and patient. Adler has identified this as the 'sociophysiology of caring': empathic attunement appears to be accompanied by physiological reductions in blood pressure, cortisol levels and so on.(14) He concludes that the act of taking the history can be therapeutic in itself, especially if the doctor listens attentively without judgement, acknowledging the tensions and issues within the illness experience.(9) Perhaps these physiological responses explain the observed changes in the actor's demeanour and affect that were described at the start of this chapter. Along the same lines, Haidet and Paterniti write of 'building' rather than 'taking' a history(15) where the presenting complaint is acknowledged and validated as the patient's story emerges.

There is extraordinary power in being listened to attentively and respectfully, more so if the listener is someone with considerable social authority such as the modern doctor. An older phrase was 'bearing witness'.[3] This experience has long been

---

3 We distinguish between attentive listening as a form of 'bearing witness', and the use of this phrase in religious circles where one is present physically to 'bear witness' to a rite of passage or ceremonial ritual.

known to be healing in itself: Wellwood(16) and later Adamsick(17) have both written extensively about the 'power of unconditional presence' and its capacity to validate and support. An example is the following account from Dr Lucy O'Hagan from New Zealand after attending a workshop on listening:

> As GPs we spend our day listening to stories. Every patient arrives in the room with a story. Sometimes we re-interpret these stories in terms of diagnosis and we make plans that will alter the course of these stories. Sometimes there is no diagnosis but there is always a story. Even with diagnosis and treatment there is a story. It is through listening to and telling stories that humans make sense of their lives and each other.
>
> What I learned in this workshop was the power of the 'silent witness'. When I told my own stories it was fantastic to have the listener not respond, but to just listen. But, as health professionals, when we listened, we found it very uncomfortable not to respond. I learned that when we sit in the unknown, the mystery of someone else's story, something curious happens. Something below the radar, outside the scope of words which is incredibly valuable to the story-teller.(18)

Further to listening skills, doctors also need the capacity to engage and respond empathically to the patient. This is because illness is usually accompanied by a range of feelings and powerful emotions. Patients are often in pain or their disease comes with significant implications for their health and their future. Their doctor's response to their feelings becomes highly significant. Doctors need to manage relationships that may be laden with emotional content, which requires them to develop what is known as emotional intelligence or 'EQ'.

Emotional intelligence or 'EQ'

Emotional intelligence is so named to distinguish it from intellectual intelligence (IQ). EQ is defined as 'the ability to monitor one's own and others' feelings and emotions, to discriminate among them, and to use this information to guide one's thinking and actions'.(19) For doctors, these would seem to be important skills or capabilities when interacting with patients, their families, or other health providers. Most of us, however, have not had specific training for this skill. As one US research article notes:

> Most students are selected in to medical school based on history of academic and cognitive successes, yet each possesses a unique emotional make-up that reflects personal life experience, coping skills, and core values and beliefs. To be able to practice medicine, the student must have the ability to understand the views and needs of a wide variety of people, remain sensitive and empathic to patient concerns, and be able to keep his or her personal emotional reactions in perspective, handle stress, and promote social responsibility – all concepts that the EQi attempts to measure. We believe the first step is for students to examine and understand their own emotional intelligence, which will, if developed, assist them in the ability to identify and accept the views of their patients.(20)

Other writers and researchers have criticised the conceptual basis of EQ, suggesting it is too narrowly focused on individuals.(21) Lewis et al. reframe EQ as the 'sensitive and intelligent problem-solving activities emerging from deliberate, structured group learning' (whether that is working in a clinical team, meeting with families, or tutorial groups). In other words, EQ is the group climate, atmosphere, shared affect, or 'culture' of the group, that allows or does not allow respect for others, expression and facilitation of connection and/or feelings. It is the 'intelligent' part of behaviour in group settings.(22)

Domains of EQ

Salovey and Mayer identified five domains within EQ:

- **Knowing one's own emotions** (self-identifying a feeling as it happens, e.g., 'I am feeling upset, angry, sad, hungry, nervous, embarrassed, disappointed, etc.')
- **Managing emotions** (the ability to handle feelings so they are appropriate to the situation, e.g., not lashing out verbally in response to anger, which may be in response to fear)
- **Motivating oneself** (marshalling emotions in the service of a goal, e.g., delayed gratification to achieve long-term goal, being disciplined, knowing when to be meticulous or obsessive, knowing when to be pragmatic or let things go)
- **Recognising emotions in others** (empathy, social awareness, noticing what others are feeling, noticing different feelings in a group, who is being dominant, submissive, embarrassed, etc.)
- **Handling relationships** (skill in managing emotions in others, being respectful, sitting with difficult emotions in others without stopping or 'fixing' them, being aware of the time-course of emotions such as grief).(19)

When things go badly in a consultation, a common sequence of events will be that a patient triggers a range of feelings within the doctor, who may or may not be aware of them. In response to these feelings, a doctor can behave in particular ways towards that patient: this is the 'managing emotions' domain listed above. For example, in response to a 'somatising' patient, clinical actions might include referring the patient to other doctors, doing more tests, or prescribing more medications (see further discussion in Chapter 7). There might well be a 'good rationale' for each of these decisions, but the point here is to be more thoughtful about the background emotional drivers of clinical behaviour.

An important observation of EQ is that it involves learned competencies: one is not necessarily born with these skills.[4] Traditionally, medical students have not been taught how emotions arise as part of normal doctoring, nor how to use them effectively within their work. Instead, the prevailing ethos has been to deny and suppress feelings.

A short anatomy lesson

Given the structural anatomy of the human brain, suppression of feelings is near

---

4   In terms of 'knowing one's own emotions', a simple guide is to use the acronym 'HALTS'. That is, when things are not going well, 'stop' or 'halt' and try to identify what the main feeling actually is. The predominant issue might be feeling Hungry, Angry, Lonely, Tired, or Scared. It is amazing how even very intelligent people may not be aware of these basic emotions on a minute-to-minute basis, nor of how to respond to them.

impossible. This is because there are three *types* of brain within humans: the first is the **brain stem**, which is remarkably similar in structure and function to that in reptiles. This brain is responsible for the unconscious control of physiological processes: heart beating, lungs working, stomach and bowels functioning, hormones being secreted, growth occurring, and so on. These processes continue without conscious awareness.

Second, the **limbic brain** includes the hippocampus, amygdala, septum, and fornix. These structures only started to develop when mammals began to evolve away from reptiles. Because mammals have to look after their young (in contrast to reptiles, which usually lay their eggs and then just wander off), this second brain evolved in order to develop longer-term relationships between adults, protect offspring, enable child rearing, and so on.(23) The limbic brain has the capacity for feeling and emotions, which are used for bonding and social control via a complex set of behavioural and other communication signals within the same species.

The third brain is the **neocortex**, found only in the more advanced mammals such as primates. It adds extra skills like language, writing, planning and reasoning or, in other words, the capacity for abstract thought or conscious thinking.

While these three types of brain in the human are housed in the same skull and work together, they continue to have separate functions. The brain stem organises all the normal bodily processes, the limbic area provides emotional responses, and the neocortex helps the person to reason and think about what is happening. All brains work all the time: every action and event will trigger activity in all three. In response to danger, for example, there will be increased pulse rate and breathing, the subjective feeling of fear, and an understanding of why there is danger.

Because humans know they think, they tend to believe that thinking is the only way to know or apprehend the world, avoiding the expression of emotions. However, the biological structure of the brain is such that low-intensity feelings (and sometimes more powerful emotions) are happening all the time. A good analogy for the relationship of the emotions and the intellect is the elephant and the rider: most of the time, the rider is in control and directs the elephant where to go, but sometimes the elephant wanders off on his own accord and the rider simply has to hang on.

The implications of EQ for medical practice

Doctors are not immune to feelings and sometimes experience strong emotions as part of their work. They are in an interpersonal situation or relationship with every patient and so their limbic brains will be activated. When things go well, there may be a range of feelings such as curiosity, engagement, genuine regard, even quiet satisfaction at having helped. When diagnosis is difficult, or the patient is rude or offensive in some way, there can be feelings of disappointment, sadness, anger, regret, or many other feelings that can be hard either to own or to process.

Feelings can also be used as a diagnostic tool. Sometimes, feelings within the doctor are simply mirroring what the patient is feeling about their illness or situation, including feelings that the patient may be unaware of. At other times, feelings arise from doctors' own ambitions and desires (to be helpful, to take away pain, to relieve suffering, and so on).

There are many situations when our efforts to help are thwarted in some way (patients who die after surgery, complain about their standard of care, shift to a 'better' doctor, or continue to have chronic pain, and so on). In these situations the feelings and responses of the doctor can become overwhelming: learning how to handle these powerful emotions can help prevent frustration and eventual burnout. Awareness of *what* is being felt allows us to consider *why* it is happening.

The overall aim of developing EQ is to provide doctors with both analytical and emotional skills so that they can care more effectively for patients. Of course there are times when the doctor has to put aside or 'bracket' their feelings and emotions and, for a short time at least, concentrate entirely on technique (e.g. surgery) or intellectual analysis (e.g. diagnostic puzzle, or review of research findings to decide on management). During the rest of clinical practice, however, doctors are acutely involved with patients, families, students, and other health professionals. These are human-to-human activities requiring the skills of emotional intelligence. The trick is to know how to use our feelings and emotions, rather than to avoid them.

VIGNETTE 4.2 THE REQUEST FOR A TERMINATION

In 1978, the celebrated psychiatrist and psychoanalyst Dr Tom Main gave a seminal lecture to the Balint Society of the UK. He described a consultation between a rather pushy young patient wanting a termination and her female doctor who was quite reluctant to approve of her request.(24)

As initially described to the Balint group, this doctor found the consultation difficult.[5] Although she had 'no objections in principle' to abortion, she found herself trying to talk this particular patient out of the idea, perhaps because both doctor and patient were of similar age and because of her love of children. She was, however, met with intransigent insistence by this patient with a 'rock-solid hard-luck story'. However 'nicely' they tried, the two of them argued quite insistently. The doctor then did an unnecessary vaginal examination; the patient persisted in wanting a referral; the doctor gave in.

Main provided three levels of analysis of the doctor's *subjective* experiences within this consultation and how she was making use of them. On an initial level of understanding, the doctor responded instinctively to this patient, behaving in ways that were a bit out of character, but not really knowing why. Main then offered a different interpretation, where the doctor's subjectivity could have been valued as a *source of information*: on this level of awareness, the doctor would have been more conscious of her own affective responses to this patient, noting them as being rather curious at the time ('I tried to frighten her, I wanted her to get married, I asserted my doctorhood', and so on).

A third level of understanding would be what Main referred to as a *disciplined subjectivity*. A doctor with this capacity for self-awareness would provide a more nuanced interpretation of those same feelings and subjective experiences, wondering further about the hard-luck story and how it was being used by her patient. She would note how this woman had perhaps triggered her own sense of sibling rivalry, given

---

5   In Balint groups, doctors typically discuss their more problematic patients: often, the issue is less of disease and more about interpersonal issues. The origin, process, and outcomes of Balint group work are discussed in more detail in the Appendix.

that she (the doctor) loved babies and couldn't bear the idea of someone like herself wanting a termination. She might also have noticed how she *tried* to like the patient, but found herself not quite managing to do so. Similarly, she would have wondered why she needed to appease the patient near the end.

Main pointed out that these interactions with patients are complex and difficult and require considerable conscious work if the nuances and subtle interactions going on between doctor and patient are to be used effectively. He also proposed that the doctor has 'defences' against involvement or engagement with the patient; inevitably, at times such engagement can be challenging and even painful. We will come back to the idea of defences against engagement and disciplined subjectivity in the next chapter, on the 'heartsink' experience; but first, the next sections discuss various models of the doctor–patient relationship and the issue of power.

Models of the doctor–patient relationship

In 1956, Szasz and Hollender proposed three main models of the doctor–patient relationship: **activity-passivity**, guidance-cooperation, and mutual participation. (25) Their analysis remains pertinent. In the first model, the physician is active and the patient is passive: treatment or therapy takes place irrespective of the patient's contribution. This model remains quite appropriate in emergency situations, in surgery and in intensive care where patients are entirely dependent on their doctors for survival, at least in the short term; it is perhaps less appropriate when various treatment options are available. The older style of paternalistic medical care was largely based on this model.

The second model, **guidance-cooperation**, is where the patient seeks help and cooperates with the guidance offered by the physician. The degree of doctor guidance depends on the balance of power within the relationship, and we will discuss this further below.

The third model is one of **mutual participation**. The doctor and patient seem to have approximately equal power and are mutually interdependent: they both need each other and engage in activities that are satisfying and of value to both parties. The physician helps the patient to help themselves. This is the model that one might see in the management of chronic disease.

Power in the relationship

Szasz and Hollender's characterisation of the doctor–patient relationship indicates that there may be times where the patient has very little power or control in the interaction. The field of bioethics has contributed to discussion about these issues through ethical analysis of autonomy, paternalism, beneficence and non-maleficence ('first do no harm'). Rather than simply looking at power in terms of its negative connotation of having control or even seeking dominance over patients, Brody introduces the idea of 'power over disease'. He emphasises the positive value of a doctor being powerful in this way, highlighting the fine line between using power against a disease and using power against a patient.(26) He notes that the patient *wants* the doctor to have agency or power to fight the disease.

Beneficence may be defined as trying to do good for someone else or at least to avoid doing harm. One criticism of beneficence is that it may still include an element of paternalism, where the doctor's perspective of what constitutes good or harm may dominate the relationship. Pellegrino and Thomasma(27) introduced the idea of beneficence-in-trust, in which the physician remains obligated to provide benefit to the patient, but where the physician must take into account the patient's own values and desires in order to determine what that benefit is.

Brody points out that power can be owned, aimed and shared. By 'owned', he means that power has to be recognised and accepted and that the person exercising it must be accountable for its use.(26) 'Aimed' means that the goal for which power is being used should be openly and easily stated. Finally, 'shared' power means that it is used responsibly because neither party has a monopoly on it. Considering the doctor–patient relationship as one of shared power allows this abstract notion to be conceptualised more easily into the medical context.

Stewart et al. note that shared power in decision-making allows doctor and patient to find common ground, and that shared power includes a readiness of the doctor and patient to become partners in care, where both doctor and patient are experts: the doctor is expert in the practice of medicine and the patient is expert in the particulars of their illness and their own context.(12) The idea of shared power could also be thought of as a 'therapeutic alliance'. Put simply, doctor and patient are allied in their quest to engage in effective therapy for the benefit of the patient.

Rapport, respect and trust

The capacity to listen effectively and to respond to patients' emotional cues also contributes to other key attributes of a doctor using EQ skills, such as rapport, respect, and trust.(28) These are different from scientific objectivity or distancing oneself from the patient, as they help the doctor acknowledge the patient's suffering. To care is to be engaged with the patient, which includes the idea of an emotional connection. This connection is important: the illness may have caused an 'emotional disconnect' for the patient that a therapeutic doctor–patient relationship has the potential to restore. Although engaging at an emotional level with a patient's suffering can be difficult and challenging, remaining *uninvolved* requires doctors to 'build up protective shells to suppress their feelings'. Suppression denies the doctors' humanity and natural emotional responses.(12)

Trust is reciprocal. Patients need to feel respected by the doctor in order to trust, and doctors need to trust that the patient is representing their experience accurately and honestly. Mutual honesty and trust contribute to building a caring relationship. As consultations build up over time, the doctor–patient relationship will also evolve. Maintaining a therapeutic relationship with trust and ongoing caring allows deeper and sometimes important issues to become evident. The next story illustrates these attributes during day-to-day clinical work.

VIGNETTE 4.3 LAURA AND PETER

Laura, aged 34, was a new patient to the practice. She had presented a couple of times previously with her son James, the youngest of her three children, then aged about 20 months. These were straightforward consultations, and Laura appeared to be coping well.

Then one day she presented with a constellation of symptoms that included tiredness, lack of enjoyment of life, tearfulness and feelings that she was not a good wife and mother. She admitted to these feelings being present for several months, and steadily worsening. Her initial smiles dissolved into tears as she told her story. She couldn't relate her feelings to anything in particular, admitting only to being busy with the children and saying that she had been grumpy with her husband. We talked around these issues as well as about my tentative diagnosis of depression. Laura agreed to think about it and decided to return with her husband for a follow-up consultation.

My analysis of our doctor–patient relationship was that the fundamentals of rapport, respect and trust were present: these had allowed disclosure of Laura's current suffering, and opened the door to diagnosis and further developments.

About 10 days later, Laura re-presented with her husband Peter. I had not met Peter before, and he was quite guarded in his interaction with me. He was not hostile, just seeming a little defensive. However, the atmosphere between Laura and Peter was tense, and I had a sense that there were unresolved problems between them that I had previously been unaware of.

As we talked, several issues emerged. Laura and Peter were virtually living apart – Peter's work kept him out of town during the week and they came together only at weekends, with Laura having responsibility for all of the childcare during the week.

Then Laura became more upset, and blurted out that much of the stress between them was due to some large debts that she had incurred and had kept hidden from Peter. He said he felt this was dishonest and felt angry and betrayed. Both were clearly uncomfortable with Laura's disclosure.

At this point, there were two separate doctor–patient relationships to consider (and the couple's own relationship as well). Her disclosure suggested that Laura trusted me, but it was made before Peter and I had established an effective relationship. He was not prepared for this, and felt put on the spot. I wondered if he felt shamed by his wife's actions, so I now focused the consultation on Peter, offering that this situation must be difficult for him, and giving him the opportunity to be respectfully heard. We talked for a while about how depression might have influenced Laura's behaviours, how Peter felt being in this (now altered) marriage, and the struggle he felt meeting their financial obligations.

Two weeks later I met with Laura again, this time by herself. She told me that they had gone home and 'talked and talked for the first time in ages'. She felt that Peter had started to understand a little of how she was feeling, and that he had affirmed his commitment to her and the children. She felt supported, and that she was starting to 'feel like her old self again'.

These consultations indicate minute-by-minute attention to what is happening in the room. While powerful feelings are being discussed, the doctor is able to monitor his own reactions and attend to both patients carefully and gently. If the doctor had not listened respectfully, Laura may not have felt 'known' or been able to trust the doctor sufficiently to bring along her husband. Achieving these proximal outcomes led to better communication between husband and wife and better emotional well-being. It is likely that both Laura and Peter now feel comfortable in approaching the GP again for future problems.

Benefits for the doctor in attending to relationship

There are substantial benefits to the doctor from attending more consciously to relationship. Generally speaking, students often choose medicine as a career because they want to help others. With the emphasis on medicine as a science, they learn how to objectively appraise their learning and the facts of the discipline. However, they also learn to distance themselves from patients, largely for fear of becoming 'over-involved' or 'losing objectivity'. Instead of medical schools nurturing students' capacity for engagement with patients, there is evidence that emotional blunting actually increases as they progress through training.(29)

Doctors gain their job satisfaction from two main sources: technical competence and proficiency (i.e., astute diagnosis, well-planned and executed treatment), and their patients' respect and gratitude. The latter requires engagement with patients in a thoughtful and nuanced way, identifying any blocks and barriers. Barriers (or defences) to these connections are often due to the doctor's own underlying feelings that have not been identified and examined. Trying to increase emotional distance can be counterproductive, as this can evoke further demanding patient behaviours.(30) There is also considerable research on cynicism and burnout in doctors, relating it to emotional overload, lack of communication skills and subsequent lack of connection to patients and to colleagues.(31)

Increasing one's capacity for engaging with others is a central feature of emotional intelligence or EQ.(19) However, this particular framework has not been routinely used in undergraduate training.(22) While many doctors are quite perceptive interpersonally, this has usually been learned by trial and error rather than by design.

Doctors can be coached into a greater capacity for listening, exploring illness and developing therapeutic relationships through a wide range of methods. The subsequent outcomes of deeper engagement with patients can be considerable. Making significant empathic and caring connections with patients contributes to meaning – not only for them, but also for the doctor. This capacity for engagement also helps doctors to reconnect back to their original purpose for doing medicine.(32,33)

Conclusion

Attending to relationship issues is not an optional activity in medical practice. Awareness of feelings and of the need for emotional intelligence is just as important as the biomedical imperative for accurate diagnosis and management of disease. The doctor–patient relationship affects not only the care that the patient receives, but also the satisfaction and sense of meaning that doctors derive from their work. We will return to these ideas at the end of the next chapter, on the 'heartsink' experience, which is when the relationship becomes more difficult.

SUMMARY POINTS

- Biomedical competence and interpersonal skills are not either/or options. Both are required and are synergistic in facilitating patient care.
- Listening can be therapeutic in itself.
- Emotional intelligence can be taught and learned; EQ skills increase doctors' capacity for effective listening and empathy.
- Models of the doctor–patient relationship include activity–passivity, guidance–cooperation and mutual participation. Relationships can also be examined through ethical principles such as autonomy, paternalism and beneficence.
- 'Power' in the doctor–patient relationship includes the doctor being powerful over disease. Shared power allows doctor and patient to find common ground and become partners in care.
- Key components of the doctor–patient relationship are empathy, respect, trust and continuity of care.
- Enhancing the doctor–patient relationship improves patient outcomes of care and contributes to the doctor's sense of meaning.

References

1. Jagosh J, Boudreau J, Steinert Y, MacDonald M, Ingram L. The importance of physician listening from the patients' perspective: enhancing diagnosis, healing and the doctor-patient relationship. *Pat Educ Couns* 2011, 85(3):369–74.
2. 1. Korsch BM, Gozzi EK, Francis V. Gaps in doctor-patient communication: 1. Doctor-patient interaction and patient satisfaction. *Pediatrics* 1968, 42(5):855–71.
3. Dobie S. Viewpoint: Reflections on a well-traveled path: self-awareness, mindful practice, and relationship-centered care as foundations for medical education. *Acad Med* 2007, 82(4):422–27.
4. Stewart MA. Effective physician-patient communication and health outcomes: a review. *Can Med Assoc J* 1995, 152(9):1423–33.
5. Roter DL, Stewart M, Putnam SM, Lipkin M, Stiles W, Inui TS. Communication patterns of primary care physicians. *JAMA* 1997, 277(4):350–56.
6. Cecil D, Killeen I. Control, compliance and satisfaction in the family practice encounter. *Fam Med* 1997, 9:653–57.
7. Lichtstein DM, Materson BJ, Spicer DW. Reducing the risk of malpractice claims. *Hosp Pract* 1999, 34(7):69–72, 75–76, 79.
8. Di Blasi Z, Harkness E, Ernst E, Georgiou A, Kleijnen J. Influence of context effects on health outcomes: a systematic review. *Lancet* 2001, 357(9258):757–62.
9. Adler H. The history of the present illness as treatment: who's listening, and why does it matter? *J Am B Fam Pract* 1997, 10(1):28–35.
10. Street Jr RL, Makoul G, Arora NK, Epstein RM. How does communication heal? Pathways linking clinician–patient communication to health outcomes. *Pat Educ Couns* 2009, 74(3):295–301.
11. Rogers C. *Client-centered therapy: its current practice, implications and theory*. London: Constable, 1951.
12. Stewart M, Belle Brown J, Weston W, McWhinney I, McWilliam C, Freeman T. *Patient-centered medicine: transforming the clinical method*. 2nd edn. Abingdon: Radcliffe Medical Press, 2003.

13. Silverman J, Kurtz SM, Draper J, van Dalen J, Platt FW. *Skills for communicating with patients.* Abingdon: Radcliffe, 1998.
14. Adler HM. The sociophysiology of caring in the doctor patient relationship. *J Gen Int Med* 2002, 17(11):883–90.
15. Haidet P, Paterniti DA. 'Building' a history rather than 'taking' one. *Arch Inter Med* 2003, 163(10):1134–40.
16. Wellwood J. *Toward a psychology of awakening: Buddhism, psychotherapy and the path of personal and spiritual transformation.* Boston: Shambhala, 2000.
17. Adamsick C. More questions than answers: spirituality, psychotherapy, and awakening. *Thresh Educ* 2003, 29(1):23–26.
18. O'Hagan L. A world of ideas: http://owl.rnzcgp.org.nz/file.php/1/A_World_of_ideas_-_lucy.pdf
19. Salovey P, Mayer JD. Emotional intelligence. *Imagination Cognit Personality* 1990, 9:185–211.
20. Wagner PJ, Jester DM, Moseley GC. Use of the Emotional Quotient Inventory in medical education. *Acad. Med* 2001, 76(5):506–07.
21. Locke EA. Why emotional intelligence is an invalid concept. *J Organiz Behav* 2005, 26(4):425–31.
22. Lewis NJ, Rees CE, Hudson JN, Bleakley A. Emotional intelligence in medical education: measuring the unmeasurable? *Adv Health Sci Educ Theory Pract* 2005, 10(4):339–55.
23. Lewis T, Amini F, Lannon R. *A general theory of love.* New York: Random House, 2000.
24. Main T. Some medical defences against involvement with patients. *J Balint Soc* 1978, 7:3–11.
25. Szasz TS, Hollender MH. A contribution to the philosophy of medicine: the basic models of the doctor-patient relationship. *Arch Intern Med* 1956, 97(5):585–92.
26. Brody H. *The healer's power.* New Haven: Yale University Press, 1992.
27. Pellegrino E, Thomasma D. *For the patient's own good: the restoration of beneficence in health care.* Oxford: Oxford University Press, 1988.
28. Usherwood T. *Understanding the consultation: evidence, theory and practice.* Buckingham: Open University Press, 1999.
29. Williams C, Cantillon P, Cochrane M. The doctor–patient relationship: from undergraduate assumptions to pre-registration reality. *Med Educ* 2001, 35(8):743–47.
30. Bakker AB, Schaufeli WB, Sixma HJ, Bosveld W, Van Dierendonck D. Patient demands, lack of reciprocity, and burnout: a five-year longitudinal study among general practitioners. *J Organiz Behav* 2000, 21(4):425–41.
31. Ramirez A, Graham J, Richards M, Cull A, Gregory W, Leaning M, et al. Burnout and psychiatric disorder among cancer clinicians. *Br J Cancer* 1995, 71(6):1263–69.
32. Remen R. Educating for mission, meaning and compassion. In: Glazer S, ed. *The heart of learning: Spirituality in education.* New York: Penguin Putnam, 1999. pp. 33–49.
33. Remen RN. Practicing a medicine of the whole person: an opportunity for healing. *Hem Oncol Clin N Am* 2008, 22(4):767–73.

Chapter 5

The 'Heartsink' Experience

CONTENTS

Introduction

In Chapter 4 we outlined the importance of the doctor–patient relationship in clinical practice. Attending to this relationship improves outcomes of care, achieved through patients being heard, feeling respected, and developing trust. Sometimes a patient may not be able to express their concerns adequately or is unaware of their own feelings; if their doctor listens adequately and has sufficient emotional intelligence (EQ), the patient's experience, or even the trajectory of their illness, can be altered. Both students and practising doctors can learn how to improve their listening skills and emotional intelligence.

However, relationships do not always go well. Sometimes the doctor and the patient just can't seem to figure out how to 'be with' each other: there might be a clash of personalities, or strong feelings are not identified or expressed. This chapter explores why this happens and introduces the concept of the 'heartsink' experience. This is when the doctor's heart 'sinks to the floor' in relation to a particular patient. Whether within the consultation, during the ward round, or even on seeing a particular name in the appointment book, the doctor might feel inadequate and overwhelmed as she contemplates yet another session with this patient who has persistently refused to get better, take their medication, or who exhibits any number of behaviours that the doctor finds difficult.(1) One of us (HW) outlines his own journey towards a better understanding of these issues in Box 5.1.

   Rather than labelling such a patient as 'heartsink', it is more accurate to identify this process as arising *within* the doctor. This is because not all doctors will respond in the same way to that particular patient. Furthermore, there is usually a complex interchange of feelings under way between the two parties, doctor and patient. While it is helpful to realise that one is in a 'heartsink' experience, labelling it as the patient's problem can be counterproductive.

BOX 5.1 BECOMING AWARE OF RELATIONSHIPS IN MEDICAL PRACTICE

When I first graduated in the late 1970s, I really had no idea that this concept of doctor–patient relationship even existed. Sure, I got on well with some patients and not so well with others, but apart from grizzling about some of them, I was oblivious to any academic literature on this subject. I certainly had no idea that the patient's health outcomes might be influenced by factors over and above my diagnostic competence and prescribing skills.

As I shifted into general practice, however, I found that ambulatory patients were quite different from the bedbound, horizontal ones I had encountered in hospital. Many of them seemed to be their own boss entirely and I had to choose my words carefully if I was to have an influence. At worst, some of them simply up and left, either during consultations that went badly, or when they found another doctor. I remained quite puzzled as to what was happening, having no framework with which to analyse these events.

In the late 1980s, I enrolled in a communication skills course for GPs which was quite helpful, then joined a small supervision group with Dr Brian Broom, the well-known specialist and doyen of mind–body medicine. We focused largely on our most 'difficult' or 'heartsink' patients, and it was enlightening to realise that others had struggles similar to mine. After a year, however, I stopped group supervision in favour of one-to-one meetings with a psychotherapist, Mr George Sweet. This was fascinating: because he was not a doctor, there was no point in talking medical details. Instead, we talked about my own responses to various patients. I suddenly discovered that there was such a thing as the doctor–patient relationship. Excited, I went to the medical library to look it all up, finding, of course, that at that time, texts on this were few and far between.

Over the next two years, I basically 'took' all the patients I had struggled with into this form of supervision: the alcoholics who had frustrated me, the young patients in abusive relationships that I was troubled about, the dying patient whom I was anxious about visiting, and so on. The more I did this, the less they seemed to worry me. Instead, these 'difficult' patients became more and more interesting.(2)

The 'heartsink' concept opened many doors for my own development, as I tried to identify my naïve expectations of practice and how these patients were not fitting the mould.

Before considering this idea of 'heartsink' further, it is useful to explore two important processes: transference and countertransference. These contribute to the emotional and behavioural disconnect often seen in the 'heartsink' experience.

Transference and countertransference

Transference is when someone transfers, transposes or redirects their problems from a previous relationship onto another person. A common example, especially given the potential power imbalance, is for the doctor to be seen as an authority figure. The patient might react to the doctor as if she was a parent, teacher or policeman, who in the past had been authoritative or controlling towards them. For example, an adolescent might switch off from discussing his health issues with an older doctor (seen by him as a powerful parent or similar). Other adolescents who had not experienced such parental control would be less likely to react in that way. The transference reveals information about the patient.

It is worth noting that transference is present *all the time*: on meeting someone new, our behaviour will be based, initially at least, on previous knowledge of others and our interactions with them. Strong transference becomes problematic when it becomes a dominant or fixed way of interacting. Doctors need to be aware that at times they will be on the receiving end of the patient's transference, which can be either positive or negative. At times, it can be helpful to take a conceptual pause in the consultation, to consider what is actually going on.

> **VIGNETTE 5.1** IDENTIFYING AND RESPONDING TO TRANSFERENCE
>
> *A female teenager is consulting with her doctor about contraception. The doctor suggests she start the oral contraceptive pill when she has her next period. However, she is adamant that she wants to start the pill today. When he asks why, she becomes angry and accuses him of prying into her life.*
>
> *This interaction between doctor and patient might be based on her transference of previous authority figures who were intrusive and controlling. If the doctor is open to this idea, then he can disrupt the transference by saying (figuratively) that he is not those other persons. For example, 'It seems like we are having trouble in talking through all the issues related to contraception. Perhaps you are thinking I might become a bit critical or judgmental of you, but that is not the case. At present, I am your doctor and you are asking me (even employing me temporarily) for my technical advice and expertise.' This adult-to-adult interaction might break the flow of transference. It might also help prevent the doctor becoming defensive towards or critical of his patient.*

Just as patients may have transference towards the doctor, the doctor may also make a similar sort of projection and see the patient as though he was someone significant in her own life. For example, she might suddenly become quite diffident about advising treatment for an older patient, as if he were her own parent. This response is the doctor's transference, and in this case it tells us more about the doctor than about the patient. In most medical texts, this is called **countertransference** to distinguish it from those projections arising from the patient.

Transferences either way are generally unconscious. A clue to picking up transference is often the intensity of the feeling, which can be quite powerful or elemental: adulation, fear, hate, or even lust.(3) It is important to notice such feelings, so as to avoid acting on them in the moment. Analysis can come later, as part of reviewing one's day or reflective practice.

In addition to the above examples, the psychotherapy literature includes a more nuanced use of the term countertransference. This is the more subtle feeling created inside the doctor as a result of just *being with* the patient. This is more than simply becoming aware of the patient's emotional state (recognising for example, that the patient is sad or depressed). With countertransference, it can be as though a feeling has been injected into the doctor, something that at the time seems quite odd or unexpected.

VIGNETTE 5.2 COUNTERTRANSFERENCE

A patient consults his doctor with ongoing headaches. They have met before about this, and each time the patient seems to resist the doctor's ideas for treatment. He seems quite combative towards the doctor, even criticising her approach to practice. He is disappointed in her for not helping, for not seeing his headaches as they really are. In contrast to her usual demeanour, the doctor starts to feel inadequate and ineffective.

Here, the doctor is starting to feel what it is like for the patient, a life of conflict and warfare ending in perpetual defeat. These feelings are generated within her, but arise from the patient's general orientation to the world. Other doctors might have similar feelings when seeing this patient, too. These feelings might be clues about what his life is like, perhaps revealing his relationships to other significant figures.

If the doctor can simply observe and stay with her initial response, she may wonder if this is how he is with everyone else as well, accusing and blaming them for how he is feeling.

VIGNETTE 5.2 CONTINUED

However, the doctor starts to get irritated and annoyed with him for being so combative. She starts to outline in detail how she has tried mightily over several years to provide some help but that he has rejected all her suggestions. She starts to lose her temper; he feels hurt and storms out of the room …

The doctor is now reacting to the patient with frustration, annoyance and rejection. Note that her behaviour is *in response* to her earlier feelings of inadequacy and uncertainty (whether identified or not). If the doctor is open to thinking about the links from transference of feelings to behavioural responses, then her actions might be a further clue to this patient's world: this is how he usually experiences others around him.

Psychotherapists are trained to use such emerging feelings in the consultation as a diagnostic tool: 'What do these emerging stirrings or feelings tell me about this patient?' These professionals are trained not to react or respond to those feelings, but instead to observe and stay curious about them. On the other hand, the untrained or junior doctor might respond with irritation, frustration or even anger towards such a patient who 'takes so much of my time, doesn't get anywhere, and who probably doesn't have a proper disease, anyway!' Or, in other words, she blames the patient for her own feelings of inadequacy.

In psychotherapy, working with transference is part of the treatment. By identifying and working with the patient's feelings, the therapist tries to reorientate the patient towards others in the world, a sort of re-parenting of primary relationships. In medicine, there is no such orientation. For example, patients are generally observed to be adherent to treatment or not, and any wondering about the background to such behaviour falls outside the medical model. Education for 'better' adherence is primarily aimed at the patient's behavioural change, rather than being therapy in itself.

Transferences and countertransferences are simply ways of trying to construct a conceptual framework for very complex back-and-forth interactions between two people, especially when both may bring their past relationships with them into the room. Just as the meaning of a disturbing dream is initially quite obscure, so it is that odd or powerful feelings in the consultation indicate unconscious ideas and feelings that require further work to elucidate. The trick to such consultations is to discuss them with others, gradually developing more intuition and acceptance about the ups and downs and nuances of the doctor–patient relationship. Most of us have one or two of these more striking interactions per week; as we shall see later in this chapter, working on them can become a journey of discovery.

The 'heartsink' experience

Summarising so far, 'heartsink' or 'difficult' patients are those who seem to induce reactions 'felt in the pit of your stomach when their names are seen on the morning's appointment list'.(4) These patients may generate feelings of frustration, irritation, dislike, sadness, hopelessness or inadequacy. There can even be a sense of shame about such responses, or concerns about being 'unprofessional'. Such a mixture of complex feelings can be difficult to sort out and work through.

However, the 'heartsink' experience is very common: most doctors have between 5 and 10 such patients at any point in time. Various characteristics of the doctor's practice have been shown to increase the numbers of 'heartsink' patients per doctor, including their perception of their workload, not being satisfied in their job, and lack of training in counselling or communication skills.(5) Many types of patients and behaviours can induce these feelings, so it is difficult to produce a one-size-fits-all analysis.

Some 'heartsink' patients will be transposing old relationships onto the doctor. In other cases, the patient may remind the doctor of a problematic relationship from her past. Yet again, the doctor may feel – and be reacting to – countertransference in relation to particular psychodynamic processes in the patient. Strongly negative feelings towards the patient are thus quite complex and can be difficult to sort out.

Clark and Croft(6) list groups or types of patients where the 'heartsink' phenomenon' is quite common. Note that the descriptors originate from the *doctor's* perception of these particular patients. Mostly, the doctor's responses reveal unexamined countertransference arising from various interpersonal features of these patients:

Challengers These are patients who are highly controlling and who challenge the doctor's authority or expertise. They tend to be regarded negatively by doctors, who may become defensive or feel threatened.

Clingers In contradistinction to challenging patients, these people can make continual demands on the physician, often leaving the doctor feeling as though they have been 'sucked dry'. The physician's countertransference responses include distancing themself from the patient, avoiding contact and potentially leaving these patients in their worst possible predicament, feeling even more abandoned.

Self-destructives These patients may have a history filled with failure, disappointment and suffering. They can induce in their doctor a feeling of needing to protect and care, although such patients can then respond with resistance. Countertransference here can be twofold, starting with taking too much responsibility for the patient, and then shifting towards rejection of the patient or even hostility towards them.

Incommunicatives Difficulty in communicating with a patient for whatever reason (language or cultural barriers, impaired intellect, inability to understand explanations or instructions) may induce countertransference responses of impatience and frustration, and behaviours including avoidance and rejection of these patients.

Somatisers Somatisation is an anomaly to biomedicine. Not surprisingly, these patients often induce in their doctor various feelings such as defeat, helplessness, anger or frustration (see also Chapter 7).

Challenging biomedical conditions Severe and difficult diseases in the patient can elicit negative responses in doctors, such as being frustrated or feeling helpless and incompetent. In turn these feelings may negatively impact on how doctors behave towards these patients and their families, at times delaying seeing them or avoiding them completely.

The list above provides a summary of the types of patients who quite often generate countertransference in their doctors. Linking back to Chapter 3 and the assumptions of modern medicine, these patients could be viewed as 'breaking the rules'. For example, they might not have a clearly identifiable disease that the doctor can attribute to a well-known aetiology; they are not 'grateful and passive recipients' of medical care'; mind and body do not seem to be separate; or the doctor is unable to feel powerful or in control.(2) If doctors are unaware of these subconscious rules that guide their clinical work, then it is not surprising that they react to certain patients with impatience, irritation, or even rejection. This is where emotional intelligence can be applied to clinical work.

A typical 'heartsink' experience is listed in Vignette 5.3. The doctor's thinking and feeling responses are listed in brackets.

VIGNETTE 5.3 A 'DIFFICULT' PATIENT OR 'HEARTSINK' EXPERIENCE

A 25-year-old patient consults her doctor, complaining of fatigue [Am feeling a bit curious, could be anaemia, depression, or thyroid problems]. *She has been unemployed for several months, having lost her job as a checkout operator because 'her boss kept picking on her'* [Hmm, wonder what the background to all that was?]. *She admits to feeling sad and hopeless after her boyfriend 'dumped her' for one of her close girlfriends* [Feeling a bit sorry for her, she looks quite lost and alone]. *The doctor listens carefully, suggesting she look for further work* [Good to keep her mind off that boyfriend]. *At the end of the consultation she also raises the pain of her chronic back problem, asking for some pain relief* [Why didn't she raise this at the beginning if it is such a big issue?]. *The doctor is running late by now so suggests she returns for a further consultation.*

The doctor notes that she misses the next appointment [Am not surprised really, but feel bit irritated as we could have used that appointment for another patient], *but she then turns up a week later without an appointment. He agrees to consult with her* [This is against my better judgment, but let's see what is going on] *and they discuss her back pain, which started with falling off her bike two years ago. Examination reveals a rather stiff lumbar spine but no focal neurological signs. She asks for some stronger pain relief now, indicating that she borrowed a morphine tablet from a friend and that this was helpful* [Feel quite thrown by this and confused; not sure now about the whole story].

Once again the consultation takes some time, the doctor struggling to get to grips with each problem as it arises. The doctor asks how she is going in looking for further work. She then asks for a sickness benefit to cover her time off work, backdated to when she lost her job. [Getting very annoyed now with this patient, who always seems a step ahead of me. I can't backdate a certificate that far, still not sure if she is actually taking drugs or not, this is all too confusing …] *The doctor abruptly ends the consultation by saying she'd better come back for a proper consultation.* [Hope she never returns …]

This doctor started quite well, but became caught up in the patient's transference of dependency. His helpful suggestions prove ineffective and he becomes overwhelmed with her requests, feeling unable to sort them as they arise. Instead of directly clarifying whether she is seeking drugs or not, he ends the consultation with a sort of half-dismissal as he lets her decide if she will return. This is a 'heartsink' sort of consultation: vague feelings are transferred from one person to another; the medical tasks become confused and unclear; the outcome remains uncertain; the doctor blames the patient for his feeling of being so ineffective.

The use and misuse of labels

Labelling the patient appears to help the doctor gain some distance from the uncomfortable or painful feelings that a patient might evoke. 'Gallows humour' provides some relief from these situations, best portrayed in the darkly satirical novel *The House of God*, where epithets such as GOMER[1] are used and the object of clinical work is to avoid any interaction with patients at all.(7)

In 1978, Groves went so far as to identify a range of patients as 'hateful'. His list includes 'dependent clingers, entitled demanders, manipulative help rejecters, and self-destructive deniers'.(8) Yet rather than helping doctors work through these labels in a more nuanced way, Groves's paper appeared to legitimise such stereotyping. Linehan(9) and Clarke and Croft(6) have both noted the inherent fallibility of such logic, attributing a motive to someone because of how they make you feel: the fact that

---

1   'GOMER': 'Get Out of My Emergency Room'

the professional *feels* manipulated does not mean that the patient *intended* to influence others artfully, shrewdly, or fraudulently.(9)

Labels may identify and characterise the sort of problem that a doctor may be facing, but they do not provide a helpful way forward. Stereotyping usually leads to disengagement and rejection, denying that patient the opportunity for more helpful care. Labels are simply another defence against potential therapeutic engagement.

Making better use of 'heartsink' reactions

Noticing our own negative reactions to patients in a more conscious way can be very helpful. O'Dowd recognised the importance of acknowledging the existence of negative feelings about a patient – at least to oneself, but ideally to others as well. His suggestions for ameliorating such strong reactions included engaging more with the patient and their family to find out just who they are and what is going on; formulating a management plan and being explicit about who is involved in management and care; and setting limits on the way in which the patient presents and engages with the practice.(10)

Mathers and Gask also came up with some useful questions for GPs to ask of themselves: 'What is the real problem? What am I hoping to achieve? What sources of support do I have access to? How realistic are my expectations of myself? How realistic are my expectations for my patient? Am I guilty of undervaluing what I have achieved so far? What is my plan of action now?'(1) Being clear about the problem and being realistic about the outlook may be very useful in starting to look at the doctor–patient relationship and eventually improving the quality of care.

The 'heartsink' experience is usually where the doctor struggles to perform in their usual competent way. It is important to realise that these problems are always the doctor's issue, not the patient's. Some doctors find the more difficult biomedical conditions to be just that, rather than a challenge to their personal competence. Others are comfortable with incurable disease such as cancer and find managing such patients to be no different from any other. Some doctors feel quite relaxed when consulting a severe somatising patient who has 'terrorised' other colleagues for years. In other words, 'heartsink' reactions are not compulsory with these patients.

In the final section of this chapter, we explore links between doctors' professional relationships with patients and their sense of purpose or meaning.

Disciplined subjectivity and the search for meaning

The patient comes to the doctor with their problems and issues, usually presenting with physical symptoms, although there are often other personal, family or work-related issues in the background. The task of the doctor is to help the patient, using both biomedical and interpersonal skills. As we noted in Chapter 2, one of the central challenges of the illness experience is to find meaning: it is helpful if the doctor can explore the patient's experience of illness, helping them to articulate in words what might not yet have been spoken out loud.

Does the doctor have to do this each time, no matter how trivial the presenting problem? It is hard to conceive of a biomedical problem that does not have some element of illness experience: the 'sprained ankle in cubicle two' does not sound like a particularly biopsychosocial problem, yet it would be difficult to extract this ankle from the person who has it. The interaction with the patient must always be with the person. Quite often there are only minor issues of meaning that need to be attended to; but, at the very least, doctors need to have the capacity for deeper engagement with each patient. While this may not be required in every consultation, the doctor must be ready for the moment if and when it arrives.

Sitting with the patient's illness experience and the inevitable transfer of complex feelings and emotions can be trying and difficult; it is easier to avoid or even shut down such encounters with the patient. Trying to reach an elusive moment of professional intimacy requires courage and a willingness to travel where the journey is unknown and where dangers certainly lurk. Doctors use many defences against such intimacy, including labelling patients as 'neurotic', 'heartsink', 'borderline', and so on. These manoeuvres help to create a distance between doctor and patient so that the doctor is not overwhelmed; however, such patients do not gain the benefit of a respectful, listening ear. Perhaps the 'thick-file' patient has never really been listened to, so keeps presenting in the vain hope that one day a breakthrough might just happen.

The doctor's capacity for deeper engagement requires focused training, as the defences are there for good reasons. Instead of reacting instinctively and unknowingly to provocative challenges, the doctor can retain her sense of self and poise. She can use a disciplined subjectivity, where feelings in the doctor are observed and examined as useful sources of information about the patient. Rather than engagement being avoided for fear of being overwhelmed by emotions, the therapeutic relationship will benefit from a more nuanced understanding of the concept of detachment. The more one critiques and examines one's own reactions and responses to patients, the more it is possible to sit with greater degrees of suffering. Doctors are thus better able to provide a 'contagious equanimity' in the face of serious disease that is immensely fortifying for the patient.(11) While this is clearly a deep degree of engagement, it also contains a considerable level of detachment.

Adler also noted that 'compassionate equanimity ... can be good not only for the health of the patient but also for the health of the doctor.'(11) As we will see in Chapter 8, job satisfaction is linked to the doctor's capacity for rewarding engagement with patients, as well as to the prevention of burnout.(12) In short, the skilful doctor–patient relationship is meaningful for both patient and doctor: attending to this aspect of clinical work is beneficial for all.

Conclusion

The 'heartsink' experience is a useful door into the world of feelings, self-awareness, and the unidentified goals and assumptions of clinical practice. How can we enhance the doctor–patient relationship for the benefit of both doctors and patients alike? One method involves the concept of reflective practice. We discuss this further in Chapter 10, where we outline what reflective practice is, then describe various techniques that can be used to enhance the doctor–patient relationship. These techniques include working with others in peer and Balint groups, one-to-one supervision, retrospective consultation analysis from script or video, peer observation, making written notes, reflective writing, specific coaching from tutors, and so on. Balint groups are particularly suited to exploring 'heartsink' experiences; this method is discussed in more depth in the Appendix.

SUMMARY POINTS

- Both patients and doctors can transfer feelings onto each other. This can make for quite complex interactions. Labelling the patient is often a clue to countertransference.

- The 'heartsink' experience arises within the doctor. This may emerge when patients 'break the rules' of biomedicine.

- Emotional intelligence (EQ) allows doctors to monitor their own feelings and emotions, and to use the information to guide their thinking and actions.

- To derive meaning from their work, doctors gain job satisfaction from being technically competent and through engagement with patients.

- 'Disciplined subjectivity' allows doctors to engage with patients' experiences of illness without being overwhelmed. It also enhances the personal and professional meaning of clinical work.

- The 'heartsink' experience can be a useful trigger for reflecting on one's approach to and expectations of clinical work.

References

1.   Mathers NJ, Gask L. Surviving the 'heartsink' experience. *Fam Prac* 1995, 12(2):176–83.
2.   Wilson HJ. Reflecting on the 'difficult' patient. *NZ Med J* 2005, 118(1212).
3.   Usherwood T. *Understanding the consultation: evidence, theory and practice*. Buckingham: Open University Press, 1999.
4.   Ellis CG. Making dysphoria a happy experience. *BMJ* 1986, 293(6542):317–18.
5.   Mathers N, Jones N, Hannay D. Heartsink patients: a study of their general practitioners. *Br J Gen Pract* 1995, 45(395):293–96.
6.   Clarke R, Croft P. *Critical reading for the reflective practitioner*. London: Butterworth-Heinemann Medical, 1998.
7.   Shem S. *The house of God*. New York: Richard Marek, 1978.
8.   Groves JE. Taking care of the hateful patient. *N Engl J Med* 1978, 298(16):883–87.
9.   Linehan M. *Cognitive-behavioural treatment of borderline personality disorder*. New York: Guilford Press, 1993.
10. O'Dowd TC. Five years of heartsink patients in general practice. *BMJ* 1988 Aug 20–27, 297(6647):528–30.
11. Adler HM. The sociophysiology of caring in the doctor–patient relationship. *J Gen Int Med* 2002, 17(11):883–90.
12. Linzer M, Visser MR, Oort FJ, Smets E, McMurray JE, de Haes HC. Predicting and preventing physician burnout: results from the United States and the Netherlands. *Am J Med* 2001, 111(2):170–75.

Chapter 6

Models of the Consultation

CONTENTS

Introduction

Over a hundred years ago, Sir James Spence, the eminent British paediatrician and author, defined the consultation as follows: 'The essential unit of medical practice is the occasion when, in the intimacy of the consulting room or sick room, a person who is ill, or believes himself to be ill, seeks the advice of a doctor whom he trusts. This is a consultation, and all else in the practice of medicine derives from it. The purpose of the consultation is that the doctor, having gathered his evidence, shall give explanation and advice.'(1)

In primary care and in some specialist outpatient fields, such as internal medicine, oncology or psychiatry, the consultation forms the basis of clinical practice. Although hospital-based doctors consult with patients during ward rounds, the style of consulting in that context is quite different from general practice. Furthermore, medical specialists may think of other tasks that define their work: operative technique, interpretation of X-rays, latest knowledge in a particular field, and so on.

For general practitioners, however, the unit of work is the consultation. This is where they listen to and address patients' concerns, using their particular knowledge and skills in the service of the patient. The purpose of this chapter is to describe and analyse the consultation in detail. While this will be especially helpful for doctors making the transition to general practice, enhanced consulting skills are useful in all medical contexts.

We will explore five medical frameworks, starting with the traditional medical model and concluding with what is known as 'whole person care'. These emerging models help to conceptualise the tasks of clinical practice, allowing in-depth analysis of the consultation itself. This analysis helps doctors answer the question 'What is happening here?' in each moment of consulting, a form of reflection that we will explore more in Chapter 10.

Although these revised clinical models are a substantial improvement on the traditional one, all of them struggle with the problem of 'illness without disease' or 'somatisation', a common situation that requires particular consulting techniques. Chapter 7 explores this important issue, proposing a revised model of consulting so that both patient and doctor can more fruitfully proceed with history, investigation and management.

The traditional or linear model

Spence's description above embodies what one might call the 'traditional' or 'linear' approach to performing a consultation, one that is familiar to all doctors trained in Western medicine. In basic terms, it involves taking a history from a patient, enquiring about other aspects of the patient's functioning, performing an examination, arranging and reviewing investigations, and using appropriate treatment. The content is the medical facts and observations that link to disease-based problems.

This linear approach – or 'gathering evidence', as Spence put it – is found around the world in the hospital record. The standard format covers the presenting complaint, past medical history, family history and so on, proceeding to 'interrogation' of organ systems, systematic examination and investigations (Figure 6.1). By working through these steps methodically and accurately, the doctor will arrive at the diagnosis and, ideally at least, resolve the problem.

FIGURE 6.1 THE MEDICAL INTERVIEW – TRADITIONAL MODEL

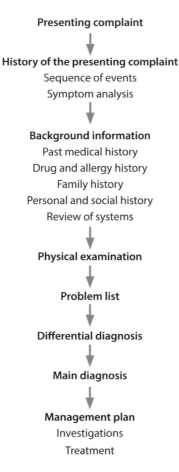

Presenting complaint

↓

History of the presenting complaint
Sequence of events
Symptom analysis

↓

Background information
Past medical history
Drug and allergy history
Family history
Personal and social history
Review of systems

↓

Physical examination

↓

Problem list

↓

Differential diagnosis

↓

Main diagnosis

↓

Management plan
Investigations
Treatment

This model has become the standard medical approach to disease in the Western world, but it only emerged as a coherent and standard method in the late nineteenth century. It took many decades of trial and error to find a system that could differentiate between all the diseases that were being discovered and classified in that era.

Vignette 6.1 illustrates the ongoing utility of this model.

VIGNETTE 6.1 THE BROKEN ANKLE

Belinda was a 40-year-old woman who attended my practice about 12 hours after slipping down an icy doorstep at home and hurting her ankle. Weight-bearing was now painful and she had swelling. Paracetamol had been marginally effective for pain relief. Her usual medications included an antidepressant and gabapentin for chronic pain syndrome. She had previously been dependent on narcotics. At home she had two teenage children and was separated from her partner. Physical findings were consistent with an inversion injury of the ankle with difficulty weight-bearing, lateral joint swelling and localised lateral malleolar tenderness. Differential diagnosis included ankle sprain or fracture. X-rays were obtained and no fracture was seen. She was managed with pain relief (avoiding narcotics), ankle strapping and a referral to physiotherapy.

This is biomedicine in clinical practice, illustrating the various steps of the traditional model. In this example, this model can be used as a guide for teaching the principles of ankle injury management to trainee doctors. Through close observation, it is possible to assess the competence of the attending doctor and to assess the outcome of medical care over time.

However, the traditional patient record above did not include any instructions to the doctor or trainee as to *how* they should interview the patient to elicit that information, or how to develop a therapeutic doctor–patient relationship. The formal medical record was a list of facts, observations and deductions (or diagnosis). It was not explicit about interpersonal processes or precisely *how* the consultation might be properly conducted. Because there were no such inherent instructions, each generation of doctors learned such skills from their seniors by observation or role modelling: a sort of tacit transmission of behaviours and competencies without their being made explicit.

A sense of deeper engagement with the person of the patient – with Belinda herself – is also missing. The traditional model has acknowledged some components of person that might relate to Belinda's presentation or treatment, but it struggles to operationalise the idea of how to care for her *as a person*.

Changing patterns of disease

The current medical emphasis on diagnosis and treatment is quite understandable, given the extraordinary development of biomedicine as an effective therapeutic modality. For millennia, the biological causes of major diseases were largely unknown and their natural history contributed heavily to morbidity and mortality. Childhood illnesses, for example, were often fatal. Biomedical advances helped to identify the cause and outcome of diseases such as stroke and cancer or infections like tuberculosis. Biomedicine therefore became useful as an explanatory model of acute disease. Where a biological remedy became particularly effective, such as streptomycin for tuberculosis, the interaction between doctor and patient became less important.

In the last hundred years, however, the patterns and prevalence of disease have changed significantly. The success of biomedicine has meant that childhood deaths are largely preventable, most infections are no longer fatal, and initial treatment for cancer or heart disease is quite effective. The outcome of the advances in biomedical science is that chronic disease now accounts for much of the current burden of health care. There are now many complex, multi-organ, degenerative or incurable conditions for which there is no simple biological cure.

Patients with these conditions now consult their doctors with long-term illness, often with intermittent exacerbations. Treatments need to be monitored for both helpful and adverse effects, and adjusted accordingly. In these situations, there is more interplay between the person of the patient and their disease. As Norton and Smith maintain, the more the patient's problems deviate from a very narrowly defined acute disease (with clear cause and treatment), 'the more the doctor's style will influence the process and outcome of treatment'.(2) In other words, these more complex consultations require closer attention to the interaction between doctor and patient. In particular, they require careful listening.

As we noted in Chapter 4, there is now considerable evidence from both random-ised trials and cross-sectional studies establishing links between communication skills within each consultation and the health outcomes of patients. This is especially so with chronic disease, where the influence of psychosocial factors is considerable and where long-term management is required.(3, 4)

Street et al. suggest there are both direct and indirect routes to health outcomes.[1] They identify both 'proximal' and 'intermediate' patient outcomes, which in turn impact on long-term health and well-being. Proximal outcomes include the patient's understanding of their condition, as well as the degree of trust and agreement between doctor and patient. Intermediate outcomes include better adherence to treatment and improved skills in self-care. The implication for clinical practice, they argue, is as follows: 'Clinicians and patients should maximize the therapeutic effects of communication by explicitly orienting communication to achieve intermediate outcomes (e.g. trust, mutual understanding, adherence, social support, self-efficacy) associated with improved health.'(5)

The links between communication skills and health outcomes have been demonstrated only recently, although intuitively it is clear that listening and responding respectfully to each patient is likely to be more effective. If we take these links seriously, consultations need to have a dual focus: not only on good biomedical skills, but also on precisely *how* we elicit information from the patient, *how* we convey the diagnosis, and *how* we negotiate treatment ideas with the patient, taking into account their ongoing responses. The importance of listening and its impact on health outcomes is the rationale for focusing on how each consultation might be conducted.

In the rest of this chapter, we review four recent models of the consultation that explicitly incorporate listening and communication skills, each model building on the previous one.

Biopsychosocial medicine

As we noted in Chapter 3, the biopsychosocial model was the first coherent attempt to broaden the concept of disease beyond that of biomedicine. This model was proposed by psychiatrist and physician George Engel in 1977.(6) His influential critique of the 'excessively narrow' focus of biomedicine was based on three problems: dualism (mind–body separation or body-as-machine), where the person of the patient was excluded; reductionism, where anything that could not be objectively verified at the level of molecular or cellular processes was ignored or devalued; and the illusion of objectivity, where doctors denied their influence on the doctor–patient interaction.

While influential, Engel's model remains quite theoretical.(7) It exhorts the doctor to take more account of who the patient actually is, noting the links between their life narrative, their ideas and feelings, and their current medical problems. However, it is not readily operationalised into practical tasks that the doctor can undertake within each consultation.

---

1 See Figure 4.2, page 74.

Patient-centred clinical method

In terms of putting biopsychosocial theory into practice, McWhinney and his colleagues at the University of Western Ontario propose a transformed clinical method.(8) The 'patient-centred clinical method' (PCCM) is so named to differentiate it from the traditional doctor-centred model that interprets the patient's illness only from the doctor's perspective of disease and pathology. PCCM attempts to provide a more practical vehicle by which doctors can synthesise the world of the patient with the tasks of the doctor; it has become the how-to of biopsychosocial theory.

This approach is also called 'patient-centred clinical interviewing', as the doctor has the responsibility to elicit two sets of content from the patient's story – the traditional biomedical history and the patient's experience of their illness.(9) The model is based on the integration of two frameworks: that of disease, and that of illness (Figure 6.2).

FIGURE 6.2 INTEGRATION OF TWO FRAMEWORKS: DISEASE AND ILLNESS

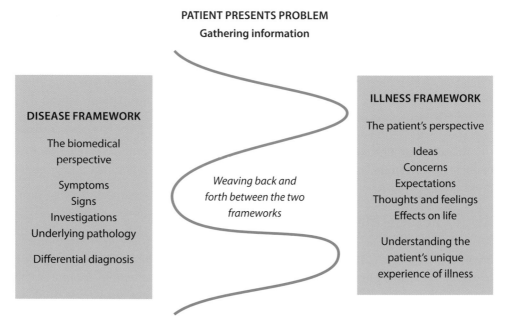

Adapted from Stewart M et al.(8) and Silverman et al.(10)

In this model of consulting, the patient presents to her doctor with problems or cues to both disease (symptoms and signs of organ-based disease, laboratory results etc.) and illness (the patient's ideas about what is happening, what she wants from the doctor, her expectations of the illness, her fears and feelings around it, and how the illness has impacted so far on her life). The doctor's task is to explore both disease and illness, and as noted above in Figure 6.2, he weaves back and forth between these two aspects of the problem. The authors also identify six 'interactive components' within the consultation (Box 6.1).

BOX 6.1 SIX INTERACTIVE COMPONENTS OF PCCM

1. Exploring the disease and illness experience
   A. Differential diagnosis
   B. Dimensions of illness (ideas, feelings, expectations, and effects on function)

2. Understanding the whole person
   A. The person (life history and personal and developmental issues)
   B. The context (the family and anyone else involved in or affected by the patient's illness, the physical environment)

3. Finding common ground regarding management
   A. Problems and priorities
   B. Goals of treatment
   C. Roles of the doctor and patient in management

4. Incorporating prevention and health promotion
   A. Health enhancement
   B. Risk reduction
   C. Early detection of disease
   D. Ameliorating effects of disease

5. Enhancing the doctor–patient relationship
   A. Characteristics of the therapeutic relationship
   B. Sharing power
   C. Caring and the healing relationship
   D. Self-awareness
   E. Transference and countertransference

6. Being realistic
   A. Time
   B. Resources
   C. Team building

Adapted from Stewart et al.(8)

This overall model is illustrated in Figure 6.3, with the six interactive components listed at the top and bottom of the flow diagram.

FIGURE 6.3 THE MEDICAL INTERVIEW – PATIENT-CENTRED CLINICAL METHOD (PCCM)

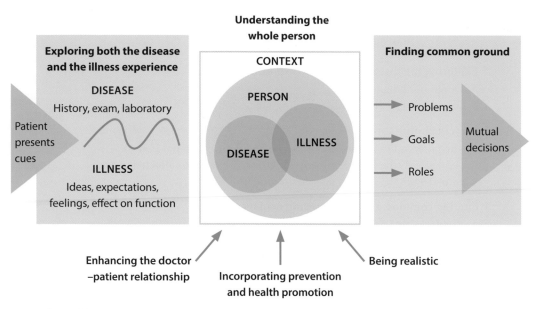

Adapted from Stewart et al.(8)

In this model, the patient presents cues to both disease and illness, which are represented by overlapping circles that are contained within the person (their life, their past medical history, their social supports, their dreams for the future, and so on). The person is further contained (and constrained) within the overall context (the setting of the interview, available resources, society, and so on).

Through mutual discussion and negotiation, the doctor and patient agree on the nature of the problem, the goals of treatment, and which roles and tasks each will take from now on. The outcome of the consultation is that mutual decisions have been predicated on the nature of the problem, set against the background of the patient's illness and the overall context.

During the course of the consultation, the doctor needs to attend to how their relationship is progressing. This requires personal self-awareness, using the basic tools of effective relationships – unconditional positive regard, empathy and genuineness – as essential requirements for the task of consulting.(8) Incorporating prevention and health promotion again builds on this sense of collaboration between doctor and patient, and places preventive health-care measures into the context of the patient's life. The doctor also needs to be realistic about what he can achieve, and who else might need to be involved.

As noted above, the patient-centred method has helped to operationalise the principles of biopsychosocial theory. As a conceptual framework for considering how social, psychological and behavioural dimensions of illness might be considered, the patient-centred method has had a major influence on medical practice, particularly in the general practice setting. While not medicalising human suffering or placing the responsibility on physicians for solving patients' existential issues, this method allows the physician to accurately identify the source of the patient's distress, noting that factors other than organic disease might be implicated.

The model also clarifies good doctoring technique, recognising the complexity of the task of consulting. While many exemplary doctors have not been taught this model explicitly, their practice often illustrates a patient-centred approach. It can be observed in a wide range of medical settings, not just in general practice.

Our own experience of this model dates back to the mid-1990s, when we first started teaching undergraduate students in their general practice rotations at the University of Otago. From clinical experience, we knew that incorporating knowledge of the patient as a person was essential to good medical care. We wanted to pass on these insights about the realities of practice, but we struggled to come up with conceptual models or diagrams that would include the doctor's agenda (making a diagnosis) and the patient's agenda (why they were consulting, who they were as a person).

Fortunately, Professor Judith Belle Brown was visiting our university, and also contributing to the Canadian book on patient-centred care at that time.(8) When she presented us with the diagrams we have used in this chapter, we realised that they illustrated an excellent conceptual model that could address the multiple tasks of consulting. We have since incorporated this model into undergraduate and postgraduate teaching.

However, younger students are often not so enthusiastic. Their immediate challenge is to gain sufficient biomedical knowledge to pass their examinations; discussion about conceptual models of consulting seems rather abstract and peripheral. For them, the term 'patient-centred' is not intuitively obvious: it does not explicitly describe what the doctor is required to do and it is commonly and naïvely confused with just giving patients what they want. Finally, while the patient's perspective is very helpful (ideas, concerns, expectations, feelings, effect on function), students often struggle to incorporate these points into the consultation, other than tacking them on if they remember.

Partly in response to these generic issues, a further influential model was jointly developed by educationalists in Canada and the UK in the late 1990s. Known as the Calgary-Cambridge guides, this model provides students (and doctors) with step-by-step consulting tasks, so that communication skills are more seamlessly incorporated into the necessary biomedical enquiry and discussion.(10,11)

Calgary-Cambridge guides

This method is more explicit about how to combine traditional medical content with the *process* of consulting. Because it is relatively comprehensive, it can be used in all medical interviews, regardless of context. The model is based on emerging quantitative evidence that supports effective communication and listening skills. The distinction between disease and illness remains at the centre of gathering information, while the usual biomedical content (functional enquiry, past medical history, social and family history, and so on) is included in a logical way.(10)

The guides outline a precise communication process with the following six stages:
1. Initiating the session
2. Gathering information
3. Providing structure
4. Building relationship
5. Explanation and planning
6. Closing the session

 For each of these steps, there are various skills or activities that the doctor may choose to use. The authors are quite clear that the guides 'present a repertoire of skills to be used as required, not a list to be slavishly followed in every encounter'.(12) They directly address the various elements of listening, including giving and receiving information, managing uncertainty, responding to emotions, fostering the relationship, making decisions and enabling patient self-management.(5) Box 6.2 lists examples of particular 'process skills' which may be used to achieve these listening objectives. The reader is referred to the entire guide for more detail.

BOX 6.2 CALGARY-CAMBRIDGE GUIDES: COMMUNICATION OR PROCESS SKILLS

Process skill numbers below relate to those in the guides

Initiating the session
1. Greets patient and obtains patient's name
2. Introduces self, role, and nature of interview; obtains consent if necessary
3. Demonstrates respect and interest, attends to patient's physical comfort

Gathering information
8. Encourages patient to tell the story of the problem(s) from when first started to the present in own words (clarifying reason for presenting now)
9. Uses open and closed questioning technique, appropriately moving from open to closed
14. Periodically summarises to verify own understanding of what the patient has said; invites patient to correct interpretation or provide further information
17. Actively determines and appropriately explores:
    patient's ideas (beliefs re cause);
    patient's concerns (worries) regarding each problem;
    patient's expectations (goals, what help the patient had expected for each problem);
    effects (how each problem affects the patient's life).
    [These points are often referred to as 'FIFE']
18. Encourages patient to express feelings

Providing structure

19. Summarises at the end of a specific line of enquiry to confirm understanding before moving on to the next section

20. Progresses from one section to another using signposting, transitional statements; includes rationale for next section

21. Structures interview in a logical sequence

Building relationship

23. Demonstrates appropriate non-verbal behaviour

27. Uses empathy to communicate understanding and appreciation of the patient's feelings or predicament: overtly acknowledges patient's views and feelings

28. Provides support: expresses concern, understanding and willingness to help; acknowledges coping efforts and appropriate self-care; offers partnership

Explanation and planning

33. Checks and chunks: gives information in manageable chunks, checks for understanding, uses patient's response as a guide to how to proceed

34. Assesses patient's starting point; asks for patient's prior knowledge early on when giving information, discovers extent of patient's wish for information

43. Relates explanations to patient's illness framework: to previously elicited ideas, concerns and expectations

44. Provides opportunities and encourages patient to contribute; to ask questions, seek clarification and express doubts; responds appropriately

59. Encourages questions about and discussion of potential anxieties or negative outcomes

66. Obtains patient's view of need for action, perceived benefits, barriers, motivation

70. Encourages patient to be involved in implementing plans, to take responsibility and be self-reliant

71. Asks about patient support systems, discusses other supports available

From Silverman et al.(10)

The guides are also availailable at http://www.skillscascade.com/handouts/ CalgaryCambridgeGuide.pdf/

These guides also offer a revision of the 'content' of the medical interview. Building on the PCCM model, the patient's perspective is again included, while the 'negotiation' of discussion about treatment is now more explicit. The presenting complaint is re-labelled as the 'patient's problems', which may or may not be limited to physical symptoms. Changes to the traditional model of medical content (Figure 6.1) are now underlined in Figure 6.4.

FIGURE 6.4 THE MEDICAL INTERVIEW – CALGARY-CAMBRIDGE REVISED MODEL

PATIENT'S PROBLEM LIST

EXPLORATION OF PATIENT'S PROBLEMS

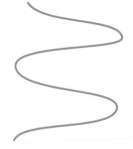

Disease – medical perspective	**Illness – patient's perspective**
Sequence of events	Ideas and beliefs
Symptom analysis	Concerns
Relevant systems review	Expectations
(to symptom)	Effects on life
	Feelings

BACKGROUND INFORMATION – CONTEXT
Past medical history
Drug and allergy history
Family history
Personal and social history
Review of systems

PHYSICAL EXAMINATION

DIFFERENTIAL DIAGNOSIS – HYPOTHESES
Including both disease and illness issues

PHYSICIAN'S PLAN OF MANAGEMENT
Investigations
Treatment alternatives

EXPLANATION AND PLANNING WITH PATIENT
What the patient has been told
Plan of action negotiated

Adapted from Silverman et al.(10)

The guides and the revised medical content are summarised in an 'expanded framework', where medical details are now incorporated within the steps of the communication process (Figure 6.5). We have included here some examples of identified skills under 'Gathering information' and 'Explanation and planning'.

FIGURE 6.5 CALGARY-CAMBRIDGE EXPANDED FRAMEWORK:
OBJECTIVES AND TASKS

PROVIDING STRUCTURE

Making organisation overt

Attending to flow

INITIATING THE SESSION

- Preparation
- Establishing initial rapport
- Identifying the reasons for the consultation

GATHERING INFORMATION

Exploration of the patient's problems to discover the:
- Biomedical perspective
- Patient's perspective
- Background information – context

PHYSICAL EXAMINATION

EXPLANATION AND PLANNING

- Providing the correct amount and type of information
- Aiding accurate recall and understanding
- Achieving a shared understanding: incorporating the patient's illness framework
- Planning: shared decision-making

CLOSING THE SESSION

- Ensuring appropriate point of closure
- Forward planning

BUILDING THE RELATIONSHIP

Using appropriate non-verbal behaviour

Developing rapport

Involving the patient

From Silverman et al.(10)

In brief, this conceptual model of the interview between doctors and their patients is now quite different from the older paternalistic framework, where the doctor decided what the problem was and told the patient what to do. Ideally, there is now input from both parties and the outcome is the end result of a process of negotiation.

Like a sport such as tennis, medical communication is a learned skill: good tennis players, for example, understand what they are trying to achieve and, through practice, master the necessary hand–eye coordination. Players usually spend hours on micro-skills (serve, backhand, volleys, etc.) before putting it all together in a game against an opponent. Similarly, good communication requires practising a range of micro-communication skills, such as learning to use certain phrases at particular points in time. While at first this may feel and look like painting by numbers, it is through skills-based practice that students become proficient at consulting.

The Calgary-Cambridge guides illustrate a substantial shift in the approach to learning how to conduct a consultation. Over 60 per cent of medical schools in the UK use these guides as the basis of consultation training,[13] as they are a useful vehicle by which consulting skills may be both taught and analysed. Both students and faculty can now explicitly identify what the student or doctor is actually doing, moment by moment within each consultation. Rather than students gradually picking up consulting skills over time, students can now be coached into using phrases or terms that they may not instinctively use.

Whole person care

To summarise the chapter so far, various influential leaders over the last 50 years have proposed quite substantial changes to the traditional medical model. In the 1970s, Engel proposed the biopsychosocial theory to acknowledge the impact of psychological and social factors on both disease and treatment,[6] while McWhinney developed the patient-centred clinical method.[14] More recently, the Calgary-Cambridge guides have provided a framework for learning consulting skills, incorporating both biopsychosocial theory and a patient-centred approach. [10,11] These models have also incorporated the significant work of Helman[9] (who clarified the difference between disease and illness), Cassell[15] (who urged doctors to identify and respond to patient suffering), and Balint (who explored the influence of the doctor–patient relationship).[16]

These newer models have had a considerable impact around the world on both clinical practice and undergraduate training. Whole person care[17] is the latest to emerge, building on gains from those listed above. It is particularly suited to palliative care or when the patient is suffering in some way. Doctors are encouraged to integrate the physical aspects of personhood along with psychosocial or existential issues, and to better understand how to respond to suffering experienced by the whole person. [17]

Whole person care: general concepts

Speaking generally, a patient visits a doctor with a problem: chest pain, fatigue, a sore back, unhappiness and so on. Using biomedical science, with its understanding of the anatomy and physiology of the human body, the modern doctor takes a history, does an examination, orders tests, then comes to a diagnosis, usually based on a particular internal organ. The disease is identified and effectively differentiated from the patient. This diagnostic process is outlined in Figure 6.6.

FIGURE 6.6 THE CONSULTATION PROCESS: BIOMEDICINE

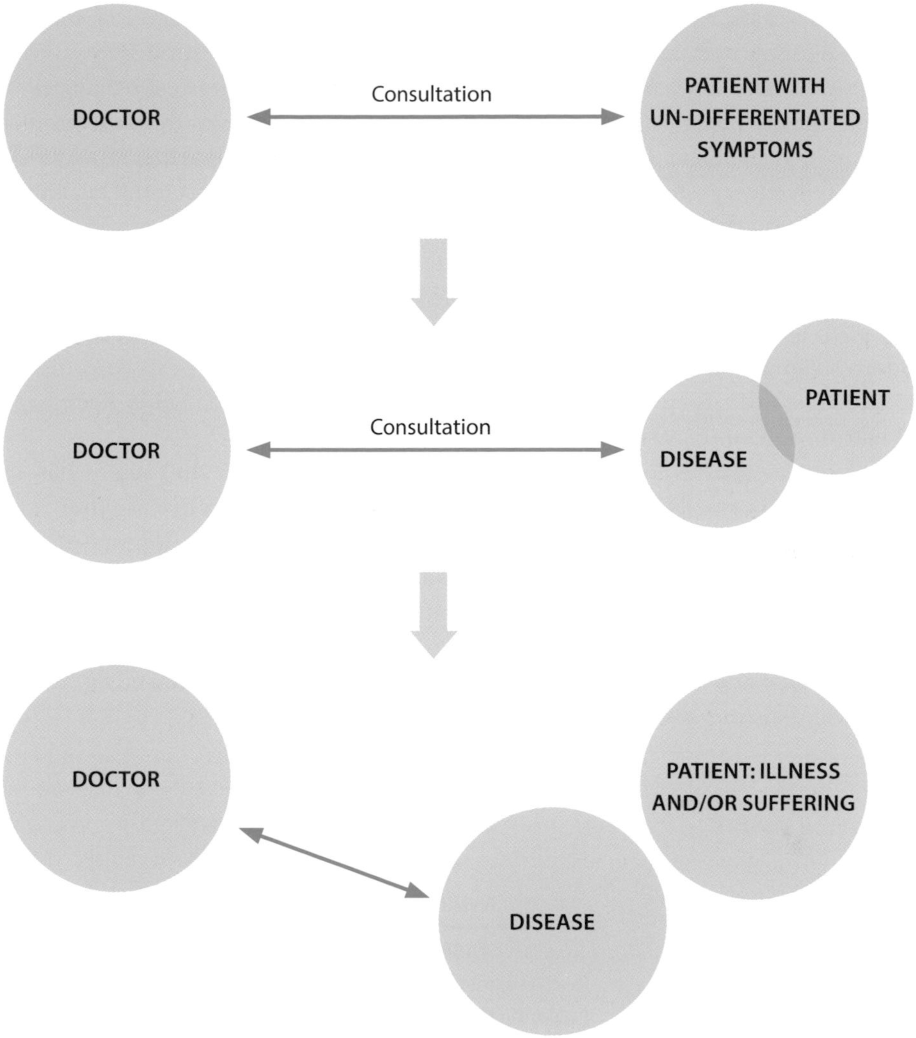

Adapted from Hutchinson and Brawer(18)

While of course the patient's heart or back or problematic organ is never really separate from that person, this conceptual trick is very useful. Separating the disease from the patient clarifies the nature of the problem, validates the patient's concerns, and provides some objectivity for both patient and doctor. The cause of the problem is identified: blocked arteries, abnormal cells, a damaged intervertebral disc, and so on. Furthermore, students can study each disease as if it is an independently real and separate entity from the person who has it. Conversely, where there is 'no disease' (for example, chronic fatigue syndrome or somatisation disorder), patients have great difficulty in justifying and coping with their illness. Doctors may also have difficulty in understanding why the patient remains unwell.

The utility of this conceptual differentiation between disease and person is illustrated by the problem of alcoholism. Long regarded as a moral failing by the medical profession, many people are now substantially helped by attending meetings of Alcoholics Anonymous (AA). In a narrowly defined biomedical model, it is difficult to find a particular diseased organ that might be causing this pattern of behaviour. Yet by labelling it as a disease, patients are able to separate themselves from the problem. The identified problem now leads to treatment: joining and participating in AA. Patients 'in recovery' shift from a life of personal suffering and substantial health risks to a much greater degree of inner peace and wellness. The healing journey of such patients is well documented.(19)

The modern doctor, however, has tended to focus more on the disease than on the person who carries it. This is not surprising, given the increasing effectiveness of modern diagnosis and treatment. Just as patients want their doctor to be competent and effective, so do doctors want to become experts in their chosen fields. Focusing on and learning about diseases takes considerable time and energy.

A problem thus emerges for the modern doctor. He (or she) really has two relationships to consider: his knowledge and skills in relation to disease (the details or content of medical work), and the doctor–patient relationship (Figure 6.7). The goal with the former is cure, or at least modification of the disease process. The goal with the latter is modification of the illness experience through relief of suffering, professional guidance, support and long-term care. As we noted in Chapters 1 and 2, the overall goal of this interpersonal relationship is greater tolerance and equanimity in the face of disease and suffering.

FIGURE 6.7 THE TWO RELATIONSHIPS AND TASKS WITHIN MEDICAL PRACTICE

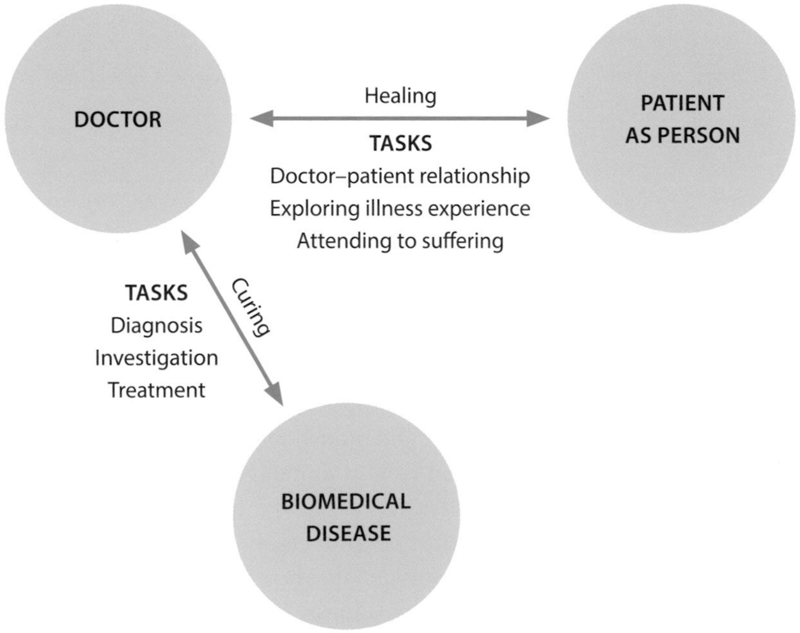

DOCTOR

Healing

PATIENT AS PERSON

TASKS
Doctor–patient relationship
Exploring illness experience
Attending to suffering

TASKS
Diagnosis
Investigation
Treatment

Curing

BIOMEDICAL DISEASE

Adapted from Hutchinson and Brawer(18)

The problem is that the doctors' two tasks (one in relation to the disease and the other in relation to the person with illness) have quite different characteristics. Again using the conceptual trick that the disease is separate from the person, the doctor's focus on disease uses data derived from empirical research within a positivist tradition. When both doctor and patient are focused on the possibility of being cured from disease, the patient's goal is to regain full function and to return to their previous state of health.

The relationship with the person of the patient and modification of the illness experience require a completely different set of characteristics. The doctor is more akin to a qualitative researcher who is doing phenomenological research. Respect, genuineness and positive regard are basic characteristics of such relationships. The contrast in these different relationships is illustrated in Table 6.1. Although the newer models of clinical practice that we have already discussed make a similar distinction between disease and illness, this particular model is more explicit about the different ways of thinking that are required (also referred to as 'epistemology').

TABLE 6.1 THE CLASSIC MEDICAL DICHOTOMY

		GOAL RE CURE OR DISEASE MODIFICATION	GOAL RE ILLNESS AND/OR RELIEF OF SUFFERING
PATIENT	Possibility	Being cured of disease	Relief of suffering
	Action	Holding on to normal	Letting go
	Goal	Survival	Growth
	Narrative	'Restitution'	'Quest'
DOCTOR	Task	Diagnosis, investigation, treatment	Listening, acknowledgement facilitation, support
	Communication	Medical content (disease)	Relationship
	Epistemology	Scientific, rational (objectivist)	Complexity, narrative (subjectivist)
	Validity	'Real'	Meaning response (placebo)

Adapted from Hutchinson and Brawer(18)

The whole person care model usefully reminds the doctor of two main tasks: identification and management of disease on the one hand, and attending to the person of the patient on the other. Returning to the continuum that we outlined in Chapter 1 (see Figure 1.1, page 18), the central goal of clinical practice (attending to patient suffering) is once again restored. Biomedicine is now better viewed as a very useful tool in service of this goal.

Whole person care thus requires a 'whole person doctor' who is open to interpersonal engagement with the patient within the context of their family and culture. This judicious professional engagement requires accurate monitoring of his or her interpersonal interactions: personal awareness, reflective practice, and professional development are required.

Implications for medical education

Undergraduate medical students need focused tuition in both disease and illness, as outlined in these more recent models of clinical practice. Quite correctly, the modern doctor has been trained to remain rather detached from the patient's disease, but acknowledgement of the illness (and facilitation of healing) requires a more nuanced engagement between the doctor and his or her patient.

Students need to study both patients as persons and the various types of illness experience. Crucially, such goals of practice need to be formally legitimised within faculty documents, as otherwise they become marginalised as optional add-ons to the default setting of disease training. As future clinicians, they need to provide sufficient time within each consultation to attend to illness and suffering.

Jagosh et al. contend that 'physician listening is an under-researched, under-evaluated yet crucial skill in medical training.'(20) Consultation models help students become more conscious about their process of consulting. This self-conscious awareness applies in all medical contexts where patients are being cared for, whether in the emergency department, a hospital bed, or in general practice.

For the last hundred or so years, the predominant emphasis in training has been on medicine as an objective science. The ethos of training has only recently started to change, with the impact of consultation training, professional development, reflective practice and so on. However, both faculty and students are at times rather uncomfortable with the idea that medical practice is a series of therapeutic relationships, and it is uncommon for faculty to explicitly discuss the additional goal of healing, as usefully outlined in the whole person care model.

Conclusion

By widening the tasks of the consultation to include listening and the person of the patient, these new consulting models are changing the face of clinical practice. There is a caveat, however: while these models are helpful, even necessary, they are not sufficient to guarantee a high quality of care. This is because listening without genuine caring or authenticity is likely to be felt and noticed by the patient, even if subliminally. The doctor needs to be emotionally present and ready to fully engage with the patient in their problems and long-term care. While the Calgary-Cambridge guides and other models have created a considerable advance in how medical care is delivered, they cannot guarantee that the student or practising doctor will be authentic in their listening and engagement.

The question 'What is happening now in this consultation?' is a useful reflective tool. It helps the doctor to identify both content and process within a consultation. The doctor needs to use biomedicine consciously to make diagnoses and suggest a range of treatments. The doctor also needs to explore the patient's illness experience and attend to suffering. Awareness of models of clinical practice helps the doctor to identify what they are doing moment by moment. This reflective question also leads the doctor to review the nature of the doctor–patient relationship, both at any instant in time, and in terms of how it evolves over a succession of consultations.

As mentioned earlier, there is a further issue that these models of consulting do not completely address: this is the major problem of somatisation. In Chapter 7, we will explore this issue in more detail, offering a modified framework for clinical reasoning.

SUMMARY POINTS

- The consultation between doctor and patient is the basis of all medical practice, but there is more emphasis on consulting skills within primary care and family medicine.
- The traditional or linear model is based on biomedicine and fails to incorporate the person of the patient (and the doctor) into medical care.
- The patient-centred clinical method is a way of operationalising the biopsychosocial theory.
- The Calgary-Cambridge guides explicitly incorporate listening and relationship skills into consulting skills, based on a patient-centred model of clinical practice.
- Whole person care is conceptually easy to understand. It usefully identifies two main tasks of clinical practice, acknowledging the continuum from suffering to healing.
- Models of consulting help to analyse effective and not-so-effective consulting.
- 'What is happening now in this consultation?' is a useful reflective question.

BOX 6.3 USEFUL READING ABOUT CONSULTING MODELS

McWhinney IR. *Textbook of family medicine*. 3rd edn. Oxford: Oxford University Press, 1997. (The foundational textbook on modern general practice.)

Stewart M, Belle-Brown J, Weston W, McWhinney I, McWilliam C, Freeman T. *Patient-centered medicine: transforming the clinical method*. 2nd edn. Abingdon: Radcliffe, 2003. (This textbook outlines the patient-centred clinical method, with helpful chapters on many related topics.)

Silverman J, Kurtz S, Draper J. *Skills for communicating with patients*. 2nd edn. Oxford: Radcliffe, 2003.

Kurtz SM, Silverman J, Draper J. *Teaching and learning communication skills in medicine*. Oxford: Radcliffe, 1998. (The definitive textbook on communication and consulting skills.)

Kurtz S, Silverman J, Benson J, Draper J. Marrying content and process in clinical method teaching: enhancing the Calgary-Cambridge guides. *Acad Med* 2003, 78(8):802.

Neighbour R. *The inner consultation: how to develop an effective and intuitive consulting style*. Oxford: Radcliffe, 2005. (Chatty and accessible books designed to increase awareness of one's consulting style.)

Neighbour R. *The inner apprentice: an awareness-centred approach to vocational training for general practice*. Oxford: Radcliffe, 2005.

Usherwood T. *Understanding the consultation: evidence, theory and practice*. Buckingham: Open University Press, 1999. (A succinct and helpful book on many aspects of the consultation.)

Hutchinson T, ed. *Whole person care: a new paradigm for the 21st century*. New York: Springer, 2011. (This is the most coherent book on this emerging model.)

References

1. Spence JC. *The purpose and practice of medicine: selections from the writings of Sir James Spence*. Oxford: Oxford University Press, 1960.
2. Norton K, Smith S. *Problems with patients: managing complicated transactions*. Cambridge: Cambridge University Press, 1994.
3. Rao JK, Anderson LA, Inui TS, Frankel RM. Communication interventions make a difference in conversations between physicians and patients: a systematic review of the evidence. *Med Care* 2007, 45(4):340–49.
4. Griffin SJ, Kinmonth AL, Veltman MWM, Gillard S, Grant J, Stewart M. Effect on health-related outcomes of interventions to alter the interaction between patients and practitioners: a systematic review of trials. *Ann Fam Med* 2004, 2(6):595–608.
5. Street RL Jr, Makoul G, Arora NK, Epstein RM. How does communication heal? Pathways linking clinician–patient communication to health outcomes. *Pat Educ Couns* 2009, 74(3):295–301.

6. Engel GL. The need for a new medical model: a challenge for biomedicine. *Science* 1977, 196(4286):129–36.
7. Borrell-Carrió F, Suchman AL, Epstein RM. The biopsychosocial model 25 years later: principles, practice, and scientific inquiry. *Ann Fam Med* 2004, 2(6):576–82.
8. Stewart M, Belle Brown J, Weston W, McWhinney I, McWilliam C, Freeman T. *Patient-centered medicine: transforming the clinical method*. 2nd edn. Abingdon: Radcliffe, 2003.
9. Helman CG. Disease versus illness in general practice. *J Roy Coll Gen Pract* 1981, 31(230):548.
10. Silverman J, Kurtz S, Draper J. *Skills for communicating with patients*. 2nd edn. Oxford: Radcliffe, 2003.
11. Kurtz SM, Silverman J, Draper J. *Teaching and learning communication skills in medicine*. Oxford: Radcliffe, 1998.
12. Kurtz S, Silverman J, Benson J, Draper J. Marrying content and process in clinical method teaching: Enhancing the Calgary-Cambridge guides. *Acad Med* 2003, 78(8):802–09.
13. Silverman J. The Calgary Cambridge guides: The 'teenage years'. *Clin Teach* 2007, 4(2):87–93.
14. McWhinney I. Changing models: the impact of Kuhn's theory on medicine. *Fam Pract* 1984, 1(1):3–9.
15. Cassell EJ. The nature of suffering and the goals of medicine. *N Engl J Med* 1982, 306(11):639–45.
16. Balint M. *The doctor, his patient, and the illness*. London: Pitman, 1957.
17. Hutchinson T, ed. *Whole person care: a new paradigm for the 21st century*. New York: Springer, 2011.
18. Hutchinson T, Brawer J. The challenge of medical dichotomies and the congruent physician–patient relationship in medicine. In: Hutchinson T, ed. *Whole person care: a new paradigm for the 21st century*. New York: Springer, 2011. pp. 31–44.
19. Davis D. Women healing from alcoholism: A qualitative study. *Contemp Drug Prob* 1997, 24:147–54.
20. Jagosh J, Boudreau J, Steinert Y, MacDonald M, Ingram L. The importance of physician listening from the patients' perspective: enhancing diagnosis, healing and the doctor-patient relationship. *Pat Educ Couns* 2011, 85(3):369–74.

Chapter 7

Illness Without Disease

CONTENTS

Introduction

'Somatisation' is a common explanation for why patients can present with physical symptoms that do not correlate well with their internal organs. It is an excellent example of an anomaly to the paradigm of biomedicine, where data or observations do not seem to fit the predominant (biomedical) conceptual model. Somatisation is just one of several categories of 'illness without disease', which we will clarify shortly.

Somatisation highlights how frustrating it can be for the doctor when a patient presents with symptoms or illness that do not easily fit into medical theory. The doctor may have no idea how to proceed with the patient, especially when all possibilities of disease seem to have been excluded. In this chapter we will grapple with this anomaly and suggest how 'illness without disease' can be better integrated within the diagnostic process.

To use a building analogy, the house of medical practice has a stable foundation based on the concept of the disease model, a model that has been extraordinarily powerful and successful in identifying and combating the problems of ill health in the last two to three centuries. The more recent models of consulting that we discussed in Chapter 6 are helpful improvements, offering a better understanding of the doctor–patient relationship, the role of listening, and the tasks of clinical practice.

However, somatisation continues to be an important issue that has yet to be adequately addressed. Apart from whole person care, the 'default' end point of consulting is still to identify 'disease'. This is then followed by 'disease treatment'. In other words, the underlying biomedical assumptions have not been challenged. While we are certainly not advocating any radical change in the utility of the disease model for most patients, the problem is that many unwell patients *simply don't have disease*, at least as currently defined. What then for both patient and doctor? What do they do when they reach the end of their nicely communicated interview, but find there is no foundation to stand on, no way forward?

For example, doctors may be thinking about possible psychosocial origins of the problems, but are often quite diffident in raising those possibilities, perhaps for fear of offending the patient. Two common responses (even if not stated overtly) are that 'you are making it all up' or that 'it is all in your head'. While the doctor may not actually say these things, the patient may think he is thinking it, and sometimes these ideas may even be held by the patient themselves. Neither of these attitudes, which usually arise from the doctor's frustration and sense of powerlessness, are of any use whatsoever in the delivery of care. The somatising patient is often a 'heartsink' experience for the doctor, as explained in Chapter 5.

In a *broad* sense, somatisation refers to the contribution that psychosocial factors can make to both 'organic' (diseases of organs) and 'functional' illness, the latter situation being where no structural abnormalities can be found.(1) Using a more *narrow* definition, the term also covers single or recurrent presentations of physical symptoms that are unrelated to diseases of internal organs. We will focus largely on the narrow definition in this chapter where symptoms arise from known psychosocial origins. While many doctors imply there is 'nothing serious going on', these illnesses are very common and range from mild to quite severe and debilitating.

Other terms for somatisation in current use are 'medically unexplained symptoms' (MUS), 'functional disorder' and 'functional somatic syndrome'. In our view, MUS is better reserved as an *initial* summary of a presenting problem if organ-based disease is not immediately apparent.

The whole person care diagrams presented in Chapter 6 provide a starting point for thinking about somatisation. As already noted, the biomedical model uses the conceptual trick of 'separating' the disease from the patient. This separation provides some objectivity about the nature of the problem. However, it is precisely the opposite of what is required for the somatising patient. Here, both patient and doctor must look for possible connections between the person's life and their symptoms. We suggest that resolving the artificial gap between the person and their 'disease' is the key to effective management (Figure 7.1).

FIGURE 7.1 THE APPROACH TO THE SOMATISING PATIENT

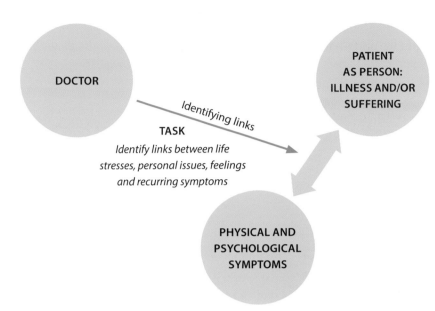

After Hutchinson and Brawer(2)

While most people are aware of their inner feelings in response to the ups and downs and stresses of daily life, others are less aware, developing bodily symptoms instead. These symptoms can mimic disease of internal organs (low abdominal pain for cystitis or appendicitis, dizziness for middle ear disease, and so on). Generally, the doctor's task is to help the patient make links between their symptoms and their intercurrent issues, as well as to coach them towards better recognition of day-to-day feelings.(3)

Prevalence

As far back as the 1970s, Howie(4) and Thomas(5) pointed out that the spectrum of disease in primary care is quite different from that of hospital-based practice. Many patients in primary care never receive a diagnostic label: the incidence of 'medically unexplained symptoms' is between 25 and 50 per cent of consultations. To illustrate its extent, the cost to the national health system in the UK from somatising illness is estimated to be over £3 billion per year.(6)

Somatisation can account for bodily symptoms in all parts of the body (Box 7.1), hence the large numbers of somatising patients in hospital outpatient clinics: up to 30 per cent in neurology, 20 per cent in cardiology and 50 per cent in gastroenterology.(7)

BOX 7.1 COMMON EXAMPLES OF SYNDROMES WHERE SOMATISATION SHOULD BE CONSIDERED

Irritable bowel syndrome (IBS)	Chronic fatigue syndrome (CFS)
Non-specific chest pain	Premenstrual syndrome
Non-ulcer dyspepsia	Tension headache
Temporomandibular joint dysfunction	Insomnia
Atypical facial pain	Hyperventilation syndrome
Globus syndrome	Chronic pelvic pain
Chronic low back pain	Dizziness
Interstitial cystitis	Tinnitus
Pseudo-seizures	

Adapted from Henningsen et al.(8)

Fortunately, the problem of somatisation is now attracting increasing interest: Box 7.2 contains abstracts from representative review articles.

BOX 7.2 SOMATISATION OR 'MEDICALLY UNEXPLAINED SYMPTOMS': REVIEW ARTICLES

'Several definitions of somatization exist and try to deal with the fundamental problem that a large group of patients present with physical symptoms for which a conventional pathology cannot be identified. However, the concept remains somewhat confusing. The prevalence of somatization is high in general practice. Nevertheless, patients do not receive proper treatment and risk iatrogenic somatic fixation and harm, the doctor–patient relationship is often negatively affected, and the overall healthcare system suffers from high expenditure on unnecessary physical investigations and treatments.' *Rosendal et al.(9)*

'Many people present with medically unexplained symptoms. For example, more than a quarter of primary care patients in England have unexplained chronic pain, irritable bowel syndrome, or chronic fatigue, and in secondary and tertiary care, around a third of new neurological outpatients have symptoms thought by neurologists to be "not at all" or only "somewhat" explained by disease. This is not a problem just in developed countries – in Bangladesh, only a third of women with abnormal vaginal discharge had evidence of infection. These disorders are important because they are common and they cause similar levels of disability as symptoms caused by disease. If not treated properly they can result in large amounts of resources being wasted and iatrogenic harm.' *Hatcher and Arroll(10)*

'Medically unexplained symptoms (MUS) are the presenting features in up to a quarter of primary care consultations … They are common throughout the world in all ages and can cause disability as severe as those which originate from organic pathology. The diversity of the presenting symptoms and the associated diagnostic uncertainty make them difficult to manage. Doctors can feel incompetent in their diagnostic and communication techniques and the patient can feel that he/she is not being taken seriously.' *Rolfe(6)*

While these articles adequately describe the extent of the problem and the nature of the distress that somatisation generates for both patients and doctors, few articles acknowledge that somatisation is an anomaly to biomedical theory or address its challenge to the underlying assumptions of modern medicine. While they recognise that it is a conceptually difficult issue, very few suggest that the disease-based model itself is too narrowly focused for such patients to be adequately theorised – hence the ongoing difficulty for almost all practitioners, despite such helpful articles.

This chapter proposes a revised approach to these patients. As the diagrams are quite complex, we suggest that you sit with these ideas, perhaps remembering patients from your own experience.

A revised consulting model

We propose that medicine needs a revised guide to the content of the medical interview, where the legitimate end point of consulting includes:

- **Disease-based illness:** the patient has a readily identifiable disease that explains the symptoms, or in other words, the traditional biomedical model
- **Illness without disease**: symptoms of unknown origin (SUO), when there is no initial biomedical diagnosis and somatisation is likely.

Illness without disease is usually only an initial diagnosis. This will change over time when further information arises (either from tests or from a second consultation when the patient reports back). How the doctor manages this initial diagnostic puzzle is crucial both to the narrative of illness and to ongoing health outcomes.(11) The differential diagnosis of 'illness without disease' is outlined in Figure 7.2.

FIGURE 7.2 DIFFERENTIAL DIAGNOSIS OF ILLNESS WITHOUT DISEASE

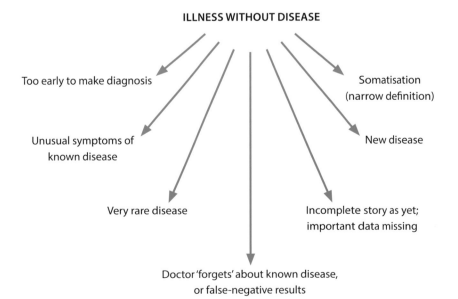

ILLNESS WITHOUT DISEASE

Too early to make diagnosis

Somatisation
(narrow definition)

Unusual symptoms of
known disease

New disease

Very rare disease

Incomplete story as yet;
important data missing

Doctor 'forgets' about known disease,
or false-negative results

On the left side of Figure 7.2, there are many patients who initially may have illness without disease, but who are later identified as having a particular patho-molecular disease (more details provided in Box 7.3). Significantly, however, the 'diagnosis' for many of these patients will be a narrowly defined somatisation (top right).

In brief, then, somatisation needs to be better acknowledged as an end point of the diagnostic process. To achieve this, Figure 7.3 is a revised flow diagram of the medical interview.

Ideally, the doctor is best to keep all possibilities of cause and effect in mind throughout the consultation. This is especially so in primary care, where many symptoms have poor correlation with disease of internal organs.

The doctor's investigation, treatment and plan will follow two broad pathways, which at times can overlap. Once somatisation is accepted as a legitimate end point of consulting, the doctor and patient can then start an interesting journey of discovery about the links between life issues and symptoms.

Notes to Figure 7.3

a. The wavy line between sequence of events and current stressors indicates that there is often a temporal relationship between various stressors and the onset of symptoms, regardless of whether or not there is organ-based pathology.
b. Patterns of how symptoms come and go and are often a clue to important psychosocial factors.
c. 'Disease' here refers to classic single-organ pathology that links directly to the patient's symptoms.
d. As noted above, stress or psychosocial factors can also contribute to severity and flare-ups of 'known disease' and these links should be acknowledged in management.

FIGURE 7.3 THE MEDICAL INTERVIEW – REVISED MODEL

PATIENT'S PROBLEM LIST & EXPLORATION OF PATIENT'S PROBLEMS

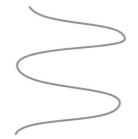

Disease – medical perspective	**Illness – patient's perspective**
Sequence of events[a]	Life events and current stressors
Symptom analysis	Disruption to normal life
Relevant systems review	Loss and dependency
Patterns of symptoms[b]	Emotions, including shame
	Meaning of illness

BACKGROUND INFORMATION – CONTEXT
Past medical history, drug and allergy history
Family history, personal and social history
Review of systems

PHYSICAL EXAMINATION

Initial differential diagnosis for the presenting symptoms

Symptoms of **known** origin:
'**Disease**'-based illness[c]

'Illness without disease': symptoms of **unknown** origin, or no 'disease' identified, at least as yet

Classical pathway or route towards patient management

PHYSICIAN'S INITIAL PLAN OF MANAGEMENT
Investigations, treatment alternatives

Supplementary pathway or route towards patient management

EXPLANATION AND PLANNING WITH PATIENT
What the patient has been told
Plan of action negotiated

Disease-based problem

Differential diagnosis of 'Illness without disease' (Figure 7.2)

(If disease identified)

Somatisation problem

Treatment + psychosocial support =

WHOLE PERSON MANAGEMENT[d]

After Stewart et al.(12) and Silverman et al.(13)

BOX 7.3 DIFFERENTIAL DIAGNOSIS OF ILLNESS WITHOUT DISEASE

Too early in the disease process to show all the symptoms and signs, hence quite difficult to diagnose a known disease. Examples might include influenza, appendicitis, systemic lupus erythematosis, many types of cancer (all in their early stages of development).

Unusual presenting symptoms for a known and particular disease. Examples might be myocardial infarction presenting as back or abdominal pain, meningococcal septicaemia without meningism, back pain as first presentation of cancer. Further examples are side effects from medications or drug interactions.

Rare but known disease. An example might be pituitary tumours, acute intermittent porphyria, or fatigue as presenting symptoms of Addison's disease (all rare in general practice settings). As a variation, tropical diseases are well known but rare in non-tropical countries.

Doctor doesn't know about this disease, has missed key clues, has been misled by false-negative tests, or has temporarily forgotten about it. This category includes doctors confusing dissecting aortic aneurysm (uncommon) with renal colic (quite common) or misdiagnosing an ectopic pregnancy as appendicitis.

Patient's story is as yet incomplete. Although most patients are quite honest about their background, detective work is often required here. This subsection includes the drug-seeking patient who is being dishonest about symptoms in order to gain access to narcotic drugs, the patient being poisoned by someone else, and factitious disease (previously labelled as 'Munchausen's syndrome').

A new disease, not yet known to medical science. As most diseases have now been identified, this set of patients is quite small. HIV infection causing AIDS is a recent example (before the virus was identified).

Symptoms in relation to psychosocial factors or somatisation disorder. This set of patients could be better described as having 'symptoms of known psychosocial origin'. This is quite common and accounts for a large proportion of patients who don't initially have an identifiable disease. A concurrent psychiatric disorder is not required for this problem to be identified.

Somatisation

The word somatisation derives from the Greek word 'soma', meaning the body (as opposed to mind, psyche or soul). To somatise is 'to experience' the body. In other words, these persons feel things in their body, instead of thinking about problems or expressing feelings. The label of somatising illness implies what it is (bodily symptoms in relation to personal or psychosocial distress). On the other hand, the term MUS implies only what it is not: 'not a disease as we understand it'. As we shall explain shortly, the patient can be either aware or unaware of possible links between their psychosocial issues and their symptoms.

There are three main subcategories of somatising illness:
- **Psychosomatic illness** is the most common, where psychological factors contribute to the development and expression of physical symptoms and illness. Irritable bowel syndrome is a good example.
- **Hypochondriasis** is where the person has a fixed belief about a certain body part. One of us (HW) has a patient who is convinced she has rabies. The belief is not verifiable clinically.
- **Conversion disorder** is most often illustrated by the patient who presents with weakness of an arm or leg, but the dysfunction is more symbolic than anatomical. This also used to be known as 'hysterical paralysis'. Pseudo-seizures are another dramatic example.

This framework is a more accurate reflection of the reality of clinical practice. Some patients who start without a diagnosis will eventually acquire one, either as their illness progresses and the diagnosis becomes evident, or as test results become available. However, by having this identified category of illness without disease, the doctor is less compelled to keep hunting for underlying diseases, especially when somatisation is likely. By starting at this point, both doctor and patient are perhaps more open to exploring life issues, rather than embarking on further biomedical searches. The doctor needs to hold both possibilities in mind at all times.

The nature of the physician's *plan of management* in Figure 7.3 will thus be contingent on the nature of the problem. Rather than all patients requiring further biological investigations for symptoms of unknown origin, the doctor can gain more information by enlisting the patient's help in exploring the symptoms over the passage of time. A second or even third consultation may be required for the diagnosis of somatisation to become clear.

Two further issues arise: Can somatisation be diagnosed at the first consultation? And how can doctors make more effective interventions?

Possible diagnosis at the first consultation

As indicated in Figure 7.1, somatisation needs to be considered as part of the differential diagnosis in all new presentations of illness. Experienced practitioners usually observe significant clues in the illness such as atypical symptoms for the relevant organ system and the temporal relationship of life events or stresses to the onset of symptoms.(14)

With only minor changes to the Calgary-Cambridge guides(13) practitioners can quite readily become more skilled at earlier diagnosis. The current guides list useful process skills in eliciting the patient's perspective of illness experience; further questions, however, are required to make the diagnosis of somatisation at the first consultation (Table 7.1).

TABLE 7.1 SUGGESTED REVISIONS TO THE CALGARY-CAMBRIDGE GUIDES (CCG) (PATIENT'S PERSPECTIVE)

	CURRENT GUIDE	FURTHER QUESTIONS: LIFE EVENTS AND CURRENT STRESSORS
CCG SECTION	'Additional skills for understanding the patient's perspective'	*Additional skills for exploring the links between life issues, stressors, and symptoms*
PROCESS SKILL 17	Actively determines and appropriately explores: Patient's **ideas** (i.e. beliefs re cause) Patient's **concerns** (i.e. worries) regarding each problem Patient's **expectations** (i.e., goals, what help the patient had expected for each problem) Effects: how each problem affects the patient's life	***What was going on in your life*** *around the time the symptom or problem started?* *Are your symptoms ever **related** to pressure, responsibility, relationships, stress, personal challenges? (Choose word or descriptor to match the patient's preference)* *Are there any times you **don't** have symptoms, or when they seem to be better?* *Are there any times when you always get symptoms, or are **very likely** to?*

Adapted from Silverman et al.(13)

These additional skills will help the patient to identify the patterns of their symptoms and how they might be related to the ebb and flow of everyday life.(15) Conversely, if the responses to the questions turn out to be entirely negative, then it is reasonable to increase the intensity of the search for organ-based diseases, as illustrated in the vignettes below. These were two patients seen in quick succession, both female and in their early 30s.

VIGNETTE 7.1 FACIAL PAIN AND THE EX-PARTNER

Margaret had endured 18 months of atypical facial pain that had been fully investigated at neurology clinics, including MRI scanning. No diagnosis had been offered and she was using a considerable range of medications. On further questioning as in Box 7.4, her pain seemed to be linked to her relationship with her ex-partner. After years of being together (she had wanted children, he had not been keen), they had split up two years previously. Her pain had started about six months later: this was when she learned her ex-partner was now expecting a baby with his very new girlfriend. She reported later that this single discussion about possible links between her suppressed anger and her facial pain had made a substantial difference.

VIGNETTE 7.2 EXPLORING ALL LEADS

Jane presented with bouts of shortness of breath over a week or so. She recovered over 15 to 30 minutes each time and generally felt quite well. She was in no distress at the time of examination. All answers to questions under 'life events and current issues' were entirely negative. Abdominal examination was difficult due to obesity, but there was an impression of a central mass in the lower abdomen. Because there were no leads in the personal or psychological profile, the doctor was convinced this was a genuine mass, although how it linked to shortness of breath was not clear. Referral to the local emergency department led to an urgent scan. A large uterine fibroid was compressing the inferior vena cava. Her intermittent bouts of shortness of breath were due to small recurring pulmonary emboli.

Being more effective with the somatising patient

As noted earlier, the initial approach of many doctors to the somatising patient is to exclude disease. While this is a necessary aspect of consulting, such a narrowly defined goal does not necessarily help the patient to manage their symptoms. It is rather like to asking what a bird is, and getting the answer that it is not a tree.

To become more effective for these patients, it is helpful for the doctor first to categorise what type of somatisation is occurring. Categorisation is usually based on the patient's ideas about the cause of their symptoms. Blacker, for example, outlines three main groups:

- **Disguisers**, who recognise they have a psychological problem but use their physical symptom as an entry to see the doctor
- **Don't knows,** who are aware of psychosocial issues, but present with somatic symptoms
- **Deniers,** who resist discussion and who often develop chronic somatic disorders.(16)

For many years, our own initial framework has been the **facultative–obligate** spectrum briefly discussed in Chapter 3 (analogous to 'facultative' or 'obligate' anaerobic bacteria). To recap, **facultative** somatisers may present with physical symptoms, but quite readily acknowledge links between their symptoms and their stress or current psychosocial issues. **Obligate** somatisers, on the other hand, find such links very difficult, and generally persist in looking for 'physical' reasons.

Professor Clifton Meador further expands on this framework in his insightful book *Symptoms of Unknown Origin*.(17) Meador, an endocrinologist at Vanderbilt University, USA, spent years trying to understand why some patients had major symptoms but no formal diagnosis (hence the title of his book). His fascinating clinical stories are a powerful example of empirical research: not taking anything for granted and trying to understand the nature of the problem in front of him.

He describes patient after patient with ordinary (or at times quite extraordinary) symptoms unaccounted for by the disease model: 'Each case (as I encountered the person and the facts) began to unravel my rigid views about disease and illness. Eventually I found the biomolecular model of disease applicable only to a narrow segment of patients who seek medical care.'(17)

After extensive investigation and analysis of 78 patients with symptoms of unknown origin – or in our preferred terminology 'symptoms of known psychosocial origin' – he arrived at four main groups (once again, based on how each patient first presented their problem to the doctor):

- **Group 1:** Patients give psychological or social information first, followed by physical symptoms. They *believe* life stress is causing the symptom.

- **Group 2:** The patient initially starts with their physical symptoms, which are then followed by psychological or social information. They *wonder* if life stress can cause such symptoms.
- **Group 3:** The patient gives only physical symptoms in the first interview, in the second interview providing psychological or social information but only if asked directly. They might admit to some life stress but *deny* the possibility of this causing the problems.
- **Group 4:** The patient provides only physical symptoms throughout the first two interviews. Psychological or social information is either ignored or passed over. The patient *firmly denies* any life stress or any possibility of its relationship to any symptom.(17)

Groups 1 and 2 correlate well with 'facultative' somatisation, while Groups 3 and 4 correlate well with 'obligate' somatisation. The doctor needs to be acutely aware of this distinction, because naïvely or enthusiastically attempting to educate patients in Groups 3 and 4 about links between personal life and symptoms can be counterproductive.

Meador also compared the four groups in terms of levels of 'self-awareness', 'connection of self to life', and 'willingness to explore life', as shown in Table 7.2.

TABLE 7.2 GROUPING OF PATIENTS WITH SYMPTOMS WITHOUT MEDICAL DISEASE

	GROUP 1	GROUP 2	GROUP 3	GROUP 4
Level of self-awareness	Aware	Aware	Unaware	Unaware
Level of connection of self to life	Connected	Almost connected	Unconnected	Unconnected
Level of willingness to explore life	Willing (already doing so)	Willing	Willing	Unwilling

From Meador(17)

Management of the somatising patient is thus predicated on which particular group they fall into. Note that the doctor still has a major responsibility to ensure that diseases are not missed, even for Group 1 patients who believe that stress is causing their symptoms.

Because many of these patients find their interactions with doctors fraught with difficulty, all require enhanced listening skills and empathy about their concerns and how the illness is affecting them so far. Gentle and respectful enquiry is required to elicit the patient's level of willingness to explore their own life.

The Calgary-Cambridge guides do not explicitly address ways of *educating* the somatising patient, so we suggest some extra steps, as illustrated in Table 7.3. First, patients are often concerned that having stress-related symptoms implies they are weak or 'not coping'. This is such a significant issue that Mann suggests it needs to be discussed more overtly. This is known as a 'pre-emptive strike' and is best done quite early on in the consultation, even when first exploring the illness experience.(14)

Second, although Group 1 and 2 patients quite readily accept these ideas or even view them as being obvious, many patients benefit from direct explanation of the fact that mind and body are indeed inextricably linked through various anatomical and hormonal pathways. While most people are aware that anxiety and tension cause, for example, an increased heart rate, sweaty palms, loose bowels, or tension headaches, it is helpful to explicitly acknowledge that everyone can develop bodily symptoms when under stress.(11) For facultative somatisers, it may only take one to two consultations to confirm their own ideas or for 'the penny to drop', especially if they are asked to keep a mood/stress/symptom chart over a couple of weeks.(1)

Other methods of helping the patient increase their self-awareness include regular writing about their day-to-day life or about emotionally laden experiences. (18) Learning how to relax and/or meditate can make a difference to the underlying anxiety that is often a significant and hidden feature.(14)

TABLE 7.3 SUGGESTED REVISIONS TO THE CALGARY-CAMBRIDGE GUIDES (CCG) (EXPLANATION AND PLANNING)

	CURRENT GUIDE	SUGGESTIONS FOR THE SOMATISING PATIENT
CCG SECTION	'Additional skills for understanding the patient's perspective'	*Additional skills for exploring the links between life issues, stressors, and symptoms(11)*
PROCESS SKILLS 60, 61	If discussing opinion and significance of problem: **Explains** causation, seriousness, expected outcome, short and long term consequences **Elicits** patient's beliefs, reactions, concerns re opinion.	***Reassures*** *patient that these links do not mean they are 'not coping', despite their symptoms ('pre-emptive strike')* ***Educates*** *on links between stress and bodily symptoms* *'**Normalises**' these links as something that everyone has and can do in times of stress* ***Coaching*** *on relaxation, reflective writing and/or meditation*

Adapted from Silverman et al.(13)

These simple interventions can be quite effective. However, the smaller group of patients within Group 3 or 4 ('obligate' somatisation) is much more difficult to treat, often being quite resistant to education about cause. These patients usually undergo multiple referrals and tests: they are at risk of iatrogenic complications from investigations or invasive treatment such as surgery. Mann sums it up as follows: 'Creative tension needs to be maintained between the patient's conviction that the illness has a physical cause and the doctor's understanding that psychosocial factors are crucial.'(14) The overall goal for these patients is a gradual reattribution of symptoms away from physical causes to more psychological ones, a task made more difficult by the patient's lack of awareness of their own mood and feelings.(3)

Sometimes neither patient nor doctor can see past a biomedical cause for the symptoms. This is known as 'somatic fixation', often increased when doctors continue to search for underlying diseases, ignoring psychological or social elements. Drawing on Grol,(19) Usherwood concludes that 'family doctors clearly have a considerable opportunity to prevent the development of somatic fixation in their day-to-day practice'.(20) Resisting the urge to refer for more tests or to other specialists is often a wise option.

The highly complex patients in Groups 3 and 4 are often identified by an accompanying thick file of notes or by their high rate of attendance. Comparing doctors' experiences with other staff or discussing the case in a peer group can produce a more accurate management plan and reduce the attendant frustration. One of the better methods of review is in a Balint group, where the various possible links can be explored in more depth (see Appendix).

The following vignette is a series of consultations with a young patient, leading eventually to a diagnosis of somatisation. As with all our cases, it is not presented as an exemplar of perfect practice.

VIGNETTE 7.3 EMILY (PART 1)

Emily, aged 19, presented to my out-of-hours clinic with two weeks of lower abdominal pain. She described it as intermittent, dull and associated with some dysuria and frequency. She had no symptoms of bowel upset. She had not been sexually active recently and had no gynaecological symptoms other than some irregular periods. She was unemployed and living in a flat with two friends. She was on no medications, had no allergies and had no medical past history of note. On examination she was not toxic. She was moderately obese, somewhat hirsute, and slightly tender in the suprapubic area. Office-based tests on her urine suggested a urinary tract infection (UTI), while a pregnancy test was negative. I diagnosed a urinary tract infection and suggested oral antibiotics, to which she agreed. I offered a follow-up appointment if her symptoms failed to settle.

Here is the doctor's initial perspective on this consultation.

It was a fairly busy out-of-hours clinic in my small rural practice. Emily did not seem to be particularly unwell, or particularly concerned about her symptoms. It had been, she said, simply more convenient to attend this clinic at this time, just wanting something for the pain. We had a chat about what she had been doing lately ('Not much'). I let that comment go without further elaboration, and asked if there was anything else worrying her, to which she queried her irregular periods, but nothing else.

Even with a positive 'dip test', I had a sense that her symptoms were not quite right for a UTI, but no other diagnosis seemed to fit. I'd excluded pregnancy. I was alone with no nurse to be a chaperone, and as Emily was not sexually active, I decided not to 'go hunting' for a sexually transmitted disease, treating her presumptively for a UTI. I would have liked to have found a biological cause for her pain, but was aware of other possibilities as well. I was aware of feeling slightly irritated that the consultation would have been more appropriate in normal office hours, so I took care not to let that show. We briefly discussed the possibility of polycystic ovary syndrome (PCOS), agreeing we could defer that question till later.

The doctor's reflections on this consultation suggest his awareness of largely functioning in a biomedical mode. He attempted a brief exploration of Emily's thoughts about her symptoms. He was aware of feeling irritated, but remained realistic about what he could achieve. He considered causes other than biological ones for Emily's symptoms, but chose not to explore them further on this occasion.

So what happened next? Let's return to the doctor's narrative.

VIGNETTE 7.3 EMILY (PART 2)

Emily re-presented to the practice about five days later as her pain was unchanged. Her urine test was negative for infection. I reviewed her story and re-examined her but was unable to add anything new. Pelvic examination was normal and I took swabs for culture and an STI check. We discussed her experience of the illness, but apart from the pain making her feel unwell, her life was not significantly disrupted. She was frustrated that the antibiotics hadn't helped, and wanted to know what was going on. While she didn't admit to any recent changes in her life or current stressors, I was wondering about some form of somatisation where her pain was somehow linked to life issues.

We returned to the possibility of PCOS, and concluded with my suggestion that she get a pelvic ultrasound scan and a set of blood tests including hormonal assays. Neither of us was very happy with my inability to provide a definitive (biomedical) diagnosis, but we discussed this quite openly. I didn't get the feeling that she was dissatisfied with me as her doctor, just with not knowing what was happening to her or how to fix it.

Emily's doctor has continued to look for a biomedical explanation of Emily's illness. He has engaged with her illness experience and done an initial screen for psychosocial stress. He is mindful of the doctor–patient relationship, has shared his concerns and frustrations, and has continued to engage with Emily as they consider her problem.

In retrospect, one wonders if the somewhat narrow focus on finding an organ-based disease in the initial consultation had predicated their approach in the second. Perhaps taking for granted her comment of 'not much' was a calculated risk, given the out-of-hours consultation and her readiness for follow-up. However, it now seems more difficult to widen the search; there is perhaps a danger of both parties colluding in a somatic fixation. The narrative continues:

VIGNETTE 7.3 EMILY (PART 3)

Emily's swab results were clear, but four days after the second consultation I received a report from the regional hospital's emergency department. Briefly, Emily had presented with a classical migraine headache. She had been investigated with blood tests and a CT scan of her head (all normal). Her symptoms had settled overnight with pain relief and she had been discharged the following morning with neurology outpatient clinic follow-up.

As I thought about this, the penny finally started to drop. The disparate problems of abdominal pain and migraine seemed most unlikely to have a unifying biological cause, but could be linked as two episodes of somatisation. But what particular issues might be underlying these physical symptoms? I arranged to see her again.

Emily presented just as she had previously: tidily dressed, pleasant and friendly, and not in obvious distress. After initial pleasantries, I broached the issues directly, suggesting that the abdominal pain and the migraine might be related to some sort of ongoing tension, stress, or personal issue, inviting her to tell me about her life.

It turned out that about two months ago, just before her pains started, she had argued fiercely with her father. This was still unresolved. Devoid of supports, she had no one with whom to talk. I asked her to tell me a little of what led to this. What transpired, calmly and (I thought surprisingly) without tears, was a story of childhood physical abuse from her father's former partner. This had lasted until her mid-teens, denied by her father for years until her younger brother corroborated her story, and only ceasing when the perpetrating woman left the family home.

I was the first 'outside' person to hear this rather shocking story. We chatted for a while about mind–body connections and links between stress and symptoms. I suggested specialised counselling would be helpful, an idea she was eager to take up. In terms of suspected PCOS, we agreed to await the results of her pelvic ultrasound scan and serum hormones.

I had been uneasy about Emily's illness since the first consultation, but I now felt that we had made headway and were on the right path.

The iterative nature of primary care medicine appears to be at work in this series of consultations. The doctor wondered if somatisation was a possible cause of Emily's various symptoms and initiated a third consultation to explore this possibility. Perhaps with the benefit of hindsight, the doctor and patient could have explored both options as part of the initial differential diagnosis. A respectful and trusting relationship has enabled Emily to reveal a significant background that might account for her current symptoms. The key to this case was the temporal relationship between her 'falling out' with her father and the onset of abdominal pains, especially as urinary infection was ruled out by a negative culture.

Emily probably started within the bounds of Meador's Group 3 (unaware of links between life and symptoms) but, with some coaching from her doctor, is shifting into Group 2 (willing to explore links). The doctor's task in the long term might be to facilitate further reattribution of symptoms if required, as well as keeping an open mind for other organ-based disease such as PCOS.

Conclusion

Illness without disease is a very common problem in all types of medical practice and needs to be better addressed. Many cases of illness without disease will be somatisation. This is an anomaly to biomedicine. It challenges the traditional framework that underpins current practice, not because the framework is faulty, but because it is incomplete. Identifying somatisation is such an important issue that we contend it warrants being included as one of the main tasks of consulting, as illustrated in Figure 7.4.

As shown in the figure, each patient's symptoms can be identified as biomedical disease, somatisation, or somewhere in between, where intercurrent life stresses

FIGURE 7.4 THE THREE TASKS OF MEDICAL PRACTICE

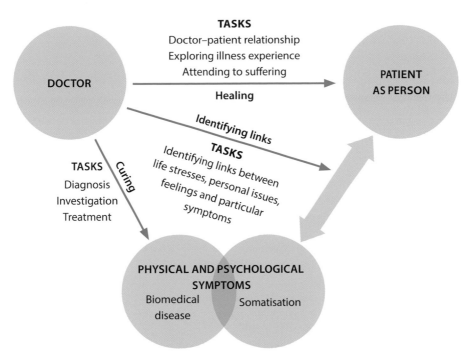

After Hutchinson and Brawer(2)

exacerbate known disease. In our view, somatisation is a legitimate diagnostic end point of consulting, and although serious underlying disease can coexist, diagnosing somatisation is possible in the first consultation. Being open to this possibility can reduce frustration and make clinical practice more satisfying.

SUMMARY POINTS

- All models of consulting need to address 'illness without disease' as an important task of clinical medicine. Somatisation is common and the origin of much suffering. Despite new models of consulting being available, somatisation remains an anomaly to biomedicine, often resulting in a 'heartsink' experience for the doctor.
- Somatisation can be considered early in the consultation process.
- Some patients will be more open to exploration of somatisation (facultative somatisers), while others will be more resistant (obligate somatisers).
- Doctors' somatic fixation is counterproductive to patient recovery and may increase the risks of adverse outcomes.
- Staff, peer group, or Balint discussion about these patients can be very helpful for the attending doctor.
- It is extraordinarily satisfying to help these patients identify links between their symptoms and their lives. This usually results in an easing of the illness and a reduction in health-care costs.

> **BOX 7.4** USEFUL READING ON ILLNESS WITHOUT DISEASE / SOMATISATION
>
> Broom B. *Somatic illness and the patient's other story*. London: Free Association Books, 1997. (A thorough and helpful text for both specialists and general practitioners.)
>
> Meador CK. *Symptoms of unknown origin: a medical odyssey*. Nashville: Vanderbilt University Press, 2005. (One doctor's journey towards better understanding of somatisation, with many insightful clinical stories.)

References

1. Broom B. *Somatic illness and the patient's other story*. London: Free Association Books, 1997.
2. Hutchinson T, Brawer J. The challenge of medical dichotomies and the congruent physician–patient relationship in medicine. In: Hutchinson T, ed. *Whole person care: a new paradigm for the 21st century*. New York: Springer, 2011. pp. 31–44.
3. Morriss R, Dowrick C, Salmon P, Masterton G. Training practices in reattribution for medically unexplained symptoms. *Br J Psychiat* 2007, 191:536–42.
4. Howie J. Diagnosis: the Achilles heel? *J Roy Coll Gen Pract* 1972, 22(118):310–15.
5. Thomas K. The consultation and the therapeutic illusion. *BMJ* 1978, 1(6123):1327–28.
6. Rolfe A. Medically unexplained symptoms. *InnovAiT* 2011, 4(5):250–56.
7. Nimnuan C, Hotopf M, Wessely S. Medically unexplained symptoms: an epidemiological study in seven specialities. *J Psychosomatic Res* 2001, 51(1):361–67.
8. Henningsen P, Zipfel S, Herzog W. Management of functional somatic syndromes. *Lancet* 2007, 369(9565):946–55.
9. Rosendal M, Fink P, Bro F, Olesen F. Somatization, heartsink patients, or functional somatic symptoms? Towards a clinical useful classification in primary health care. *Scand J Prim Health Care* 2005, 23(1):3–10.
10. Hatcher S, Arroll B. Assessment and management of medically unexplained symptoms. *BMJ* 2008, 336:1124–28.
11. Jones R, Barraclough K, Dowrick C. When no diagnostic label is applied. *BMJ* 2010, 340:c2683.
12. Stewart M, Belle Brown J, Weston W, McWhinney I, McWilliam C, Freeman T. *Patient-centered medicine: transforming the clinical method*. 2nd edn. Abingdon: Radcliffe, 2003.
13. Silverman J, Kurtz S, Draper J. *Skills for communicating with patients*. 2nd edn. Oxford: Radcliffe, 2003.
14. Mann B. Generalism: the challenge of functional and somatising illnesses. *NZ Fam Phys* 2007, 34(6):398–401.
15. Mann B, Wilson HJ. A new approach to somatisation in general practice. Forthcoming, 2013.
16. Blacker R. The diagnosis of patients at risk of psychiatric disorders. In: Corney R, ed. *Developing communication and counselling skills in medicine*. London: Routledge, 1991.
17. Meador CK. *Symptoms of unknown origin: a medical odyssey*. Nashville: Vanderbilt University Press, 2005.
18. Pennebaker JW. Telling stories: the health benefits of narrative. *Lit Med* 2000, 19(1):3–18.
19. Grol R, ed. *To heal or to harm: the prevention of somatic fixation in general practice*. London: Royal College of General Practitioners, 1983.
20. Usherwood T. *Understanding the consultation: evidence, theory and practice*. Buckingham: Open University Press, 1999.

Chapter **8**

Doctors' Health and Wellness

CONTENTS

Part 1: Doctors under stress

Introduction

Being a doctor is both rewarding and demanding. As a career, it offers an enormous range of possibilities, including travel, working in different countries and cultures, meeting a wide range of people, and the satisfaction of having made a difference. However, doctoring can also be very challenging, both emotionally and physically.

Generally, doctors appear to have better physical health than their patients, but many have problems with psychological health. Doctors have higher rates of anxiety and depression than the general population, while substance abuse, workaholism, and divorce rates, for example, are the same as or worse than for non-doctors.(1)

Previously, these observations were largely attributed to the stress of doctoring: many sick people needing close attention, limited time to make critical decisions, long hours of work, and so on. However, emerging research is now starting to link these occupational outcomes to the personality profiles of medical students. Perhaps those who choose a medical career are predisposed to certain types of workplace stress.

Similarly, it has long been assumed that doctors can work very long hours under considerable strain, but the quality of their clinical care will remain constant. This is in contrast, for instance, to the aviation industry, where there are stringent codes of practice with respect to hours of continuous work and requirements for rest. This industry has made the link between wellness and workplace performance, but medicine's unwritten expectations of long hours and dedication to others have seemed incontestable.

Yet it does not take too much imagination to acknowledge the difference between two doctors at the extreme ends of a scale that measures wellness. The first doctor is enthusiastic and well rested, feels confident in his knowledge and capacity to interact with patients, can proactively respond to mistakes or complaints with openness and curiosity, can trust others to share medical care, and genuinely believes in each specific treatment as well as in his general efficacy. The second doctor is stressed and anxious, dreads each day at work, dislikes many of his patients, is defensive in response to questions about his quality of care, and is generally burnt out.

The first doctor could be described as having more well-being and resilience than the second. Furthermore, as we shall see shortly, patients attending these very different doctors may have quite different health outcomes. Patients from 'Dr Relaxed-and-Confident' feel adequately heard and understood, will return readily with questions, and are more likely to adhere to treatment. Patients from 'Dr Cynical-and-Depressed', on the other hand, may not feel understood, may be less likely to take their medications as prescribed, might feel reluctant to attend for follow-up, and so on.

It is useful to return to the foundational assumptions of biomedicine that we outlined in Chapter 3. In this understanding of medicine, effectiveness is assumed to be independent of *who* the doctor actually is, how he is feeling at the time and his own health (of lack thereof). The only rule for how to be a doctor appears to be the injunction or imperative to remain detached and observant (Box 8.1). In other words, there is nothing explicitly stated about the *person* of the doctor. It is as if he or she is somehow anonymous, a sort of blank slate. Perhaps the only direction for proper conduct is that the doctor should be a disembodied scientist who absents him or herself from the 'experiment' of doctoring, in order to maintain 'objectivity'.

BOX 8.1 THE ROLE OF THE DOCTOR WITHIN THE 'ASSUMPTIONS' OF BIOMEDICINE

The doctor's effectiveness is independent of gender or beliefs.

The doctor is usually a detached, neutral observer.

From McWhinney(2)

This book attempts to provide a revised understanding of doctoring, as in our experience the reality of practice is quite different. We believe that the basis of modern medical practice is the combination of current biomedical understanding *and* the doctor–patient relationship. Within this relationship, how the doctor behaves and acts *as a person* is extremely important.

This chapter thus focuses on the person of the doctor, teasing out some of the underlying factors that contribute to professional well-being and general resilience. Figure 8.1 illustrates the potential balance within each medical career. On the left side of the fulcrum, various factors can increase a doctor's job satisfaction and general resilience. On the right side, stressors can reduce work performance and efficacy. When stressors increase beyond the individual's capacity for coping, doctors show signs of compassion fatigue and burnout. Other outcomes include marital issues, psychological illness, and addictive behaviour. There may be signs in the workplace of bullying(3) or other 'disruptive' behaviour.(4,5) At this point (often referred to as 'the bottom of the cliff'), doctors may come to the attention of their registration body and be more clearly identified as having professional impairment. Well before that, however, the quality of care from doctors on the right-hand side of the diagram can be compromised. Patients may not do as well as those receiving care from doctors who are more resilient.

FIGURE 8.1 THE BALANCE BETWEEN WELLNESS AND WORK-RELATED STRESS

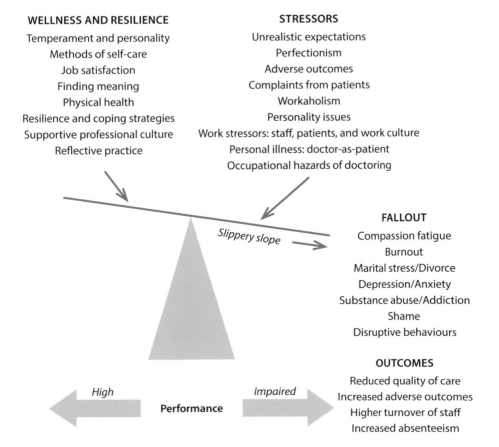

WELLNESS AND RESILIENCE

Temperament and personality
Methods of self-care
Job satisfaction
Finding meaning
Physical health
Resilience and coping strategies
Supportive professional culture
Reflective practice

STRESSORS

Unrealistic expectations
Perfectionism
Adverse outcomes
Complaints from patients
Workaholism
Personality issues
Work stressors: staff, patients, and work culture
Personal illness: doctor-as-patient
Occupational hazards of doctoring

Slippery slope

FALLOUT

Compassion fatigue
Burnout
Marital stress/Divorce
Depression/Anxiety
Substance abuse/Addiction
Shame
Disruptive behaviours

OUTCOMES

Reduced quality of care
Increased adverse outcomes
Higher turnover of staff
Increased absenteeism

High   *Impaired*

Performance

This chapter will explore the issues raised in Figure 8.1 in more detail, starting with statistics on the health of doctors. We also discuss burnout, compassion fatigue and their predisposing factors. Doctor-as-patient is an important issue, as is the link between occupational stress and the quality of medical care. The second half of this chapter explores wellness and how to increase it.

BOX 8.2 DEFINITIONS

Stress occurs when demands or tasks appear to be greater than one's perceived ability to cope or respond. Signs of stress may be cognitive, emotional, physical, or behavioural, and may include preoccupation with issues and details, poor judgement, negative outlook, moodiness, irritability, and inability to relax. Many people develop somatic symptoms in relation to stress, such as headache, insomnia, change in appetite, abdominal pains, skin rashes, and so on. Continued and unresolved stress usually results in illness.(6)

Resilience is the capacity to respond and adapt to significant adversity, trauma, tragedy, threat, or sources of stress. Resilience is best understood as a process, not necessarily as a trait of each individual. It is the result of individuals interacting with their environment and the processes that either promote well-being or protect them against negative risk factors. This coping may result in the individual 'bouncing back' to a previous state of normal functioning, or using the experience of exposure to adversity to perform better than expected (similar to how an inoculation will improve future response to infectious agents).(7)

Well-being now generally refers to psychological health. The term is used more narrowly than overall wellness.

Wellness includes one's general sense of purpose, competence and meaning. 'Wellness goes beyond merely the absence of distress and includes being challenged, thriving, and achieving success in various aspects of personal and professional life.' Wellness includes physical health, psychological well-being, resilience and coping strategies, self-care, and reflective practice.(8)

Doctors' stress and health

Various studies have shown that about 25 to 30 per cent of doctors are significantly stressed, compared to less than 20 per cent of the general population,(9,10). Doctors also appear to be at increased risk of mental ill health, with higher rates of depression, suicide and substance abuse.(11,12) There are significant barriers to doctors accessing health care in the normal way,(13) with the result that unfortunately many doctors self-diagnose and self-treat, rather than having their own doctor who can provide more objective assessment and disease management.

Many young doctors start their career with 'maladaptive' patterns in response to illness. Newly registered doctors in the UK do not usually have their own doctor, preferring instead to ask for 'corridor' advice from colleagues or to self-prescribe.(14) In general, it seems that undergraduate education about self-care and the necessity to have a personal doctor has either been absent or ineffective.

Burnout and compassion fatigue

These are two related but distinct concepts. Burnout is where doctors feel 'at the end of their tether', cynical and inefficient – characteristics that are the opposite of professional engagement (feeling energised, involved and capable). Burnout among doctors is increasing in many Western countries.(15,16) It is generally regarded as having three dimensions: emotional exhaustion (feeling overextended and exhausted by one's work), depersonalisation (lack of feeling or impersonal response to patients), and decreased feelings of personal accomplishment (reduced competence or success in one's work with others).(17)

Doctors' emotional distress from their continued exposure to patient trauma is known as compassion fatigue.(18) This is a form of secondary traumatic stress arising in health professionals because of their persistent close proximity to emotionally and physically traumatised patients. Vicarious traumatisation can lead to stress, poor self-care, and reduction in general well-being.(18) For example, the survivors of major traumatic events such as the World Trade Center attack in 2001 or the Japanese tsunami in 2011 will attend doctors, nurses and counsellors asking for assistance. Their terrible stories of shock and trauma may eventually overwhelm these health professionals, who might suffer from secondary traumatic stress. Stress arises from *knowing about* the traumatising events experienced by these patients.

One does not need to attend major disasters, however, to meet with many patients who have significant suffering. Doctors and other health professionals are commonly interacting with patients who are experiencing life-threatening illness, abuse, serious injury or near-death events. Such patients have often felt intense fear, helplessness or horror. 'Normal' clinical practice can thus be traumatising for many health professionals as well, unless they develop methods of self-care.

Burnout and compassion fatigue are both counterproductive in terms of ideal patient care. In Figure 8.1 these are placed at the bottom of the cliff, as they can lead to doctors requiring unscheduled or enforced time away from work. To a lesser degree, they can also be present but relatively hidden in many other doctors without ever being identified or examined, resulting in reduced job satisfaction and quality of work. A useful tool for measuring the extent or degree of physician burnout is the Maslach Burnout Inventory,(19) typical questions from which are listed in Box 8.3.

On the other hand, however, the concept of 'vicarious resilience' is now emerging, where professionals experience a positive transformation through helping others.(20) This is an aspect of 'positive psychology', which we will discuss shortly.

BOX 8.3 MASLACH BURNOUT INVENTORY:
EMOTIONAL EXHAUSTION DIMENSION (5 QUESTIONS)

I feel emotionally drained from my work.

I feel used up at the end of the workday.

I feel tired when I get up and have to face another day on the job.

I feel that working all day is really a strain for me.

I feel burned out from my work.

Scoring: Never (1); Not very often (2); Sometimes (3); Often (4); Most of the time (5).

Score is the sum of all scores out of 25; the higher the score, the more the degree of emotional exhaustion.

There are further scoring items under the two other dimensions: depersonalisation and reduced personal accomplishment.

From Maslach et al.(19)

Predisposing factors for medical school and workplace stress

It is tempting to attribute the occupational hazards listed above to the stresses of medical work. However, there is increasing evidence that the personal attributes of those who choose a medical career may also increase vulnerability to work-related stress. In other words, doctors may be predisposed to psychological problems in relation to clinical work.

The first longitudinal study to explore these relationships was published in 1972, when Vaillant compared 47 physicians in the US with matched controls (i.e., against other professionals) over a period of 30 years. He found that only doctors with the 'least stable' childhoods and those with problems in 'adolescent adjustment' were vulnerable to occupational hazards such as poor marriages, increased use of drugs and alcohol, and the use of psychotherapy (as a marker of distress).(21)

Since then, further studies have looked at medical students as well as practising doctors, identifying links between childhood experiences and choice of a health professional career.(22) In 1986, Firth found that medical students in the UK had higher rates of stress than other groups in the general population, estimating that rates of 'emotional disturbance' were over 30 per cent.(23) Notably, 'relationships with consultants' were the cause of the 'strongest negative feelings'.

Firth-Cozens identified 'self-criticism' as a strong predictor of subsequent stress and depression.(24) Such traits were more predictive for work-related stress than actual hours of work. Similarly, avoidance of significant issues, denial or 'dismissing events' appears to create more stress in both students and practitioners.(25, 26) We will return to this important observation about coping strategies soon.

McManus et al. tracked over 1600 UK medical students from the start of medical school until about five years after graduation, finding that stress, burnout and job satisfaction correlated with personality traits – such as 'neuroticism' (the tendency to experience more negative than positive emotions) – that they had identified earlier. They linked a greater sense of personal accomplishment with 'deep' (as opposed to 'surface') approaches to learning. Stress was greatest in those with high neuroticism scores, low extraversion scores and low conscientiousness scores. They concluded: 'High perceived workload and poor support are therefore determined as much by the doctors themselves as by specific working conditions'.(27)

These reports hint at possible problems with perfectionism, but it is useful to distinguish between 'adaptive' and 'maladaptive' traits. *Adaptive* perfectionism is related to conscientiousness and striving for achievement, while *maladaptive* is related to excessive concerns about the perceptions of other people (i.e. socially prescribed perfectionism). Enns and others showed, first, that medical students are quite different from arts students and, second, that adaptive perfectionism is correlated with expectations of performance. Maladaptive perfectionism is correlated with distress and negative affect, and also predictive of symptoms of depression later in training.(28)

A possible explanation for these links is as follows. Most medical schools have entry criteria that require detailed study and knowledge recall. Such intense study requires a particular conscientiousness. Furthermore, the sheer volume of information required can mean that students feel they never know quite enough, while the ever-present uncertainty of clinical practice can feel insurmountable and a constant source of stress, especially if one is expecting to gain mastery. With only the 'brightest' students gaining entry, perhaps this particular selection process contributes to the difficulties identified later in the clinical workplace. Box 8.4 contains a 2001 abstract of research on the links between personality, entry to medical school and the 'impaired physician'.(29)

BOX 8.4 PHYSICIAN IMPAIRMENT: A TYPICAL ABSTRACT

'An impaired physician is one unable to fulfil professional or personal responsibilities because of psychiatric illness, alcoholism, or drug dependency. Current estimates are that approximately 15% of physicians will be impaired at some point in their careers. Although physicians may not have higher rates of impairment compared with other professionals, factors in their background, personality, and training may contribute and predispose them to drug abuse and mental illness, particularly depression. Many physicians possess a strong drive for achievement, exceptional conscientiousness, and an ability to deny personal problems. These attributes are advantageous for 'success' in medicine; ironically, however, they may also predispose to impairment. Identifying impairment is often difficult because the manifestations are varied and physicians will typically suppress and deny any suggestion of a problem. Identification is essential because patient well-being may be at stake, and untreated impairment may result in loss of license, health problems, and even death. Fortunately, once identified and treated, physicians often do better in recovery than others and typically can return to a productive career and a satisfying personal and family life.'

From Boisaubin and Levine(29)

Doctors as patients: The personal experience of illness

While information on doctors' health and medical problems is readily accessible, the *illness experience* of doctors is more hidden and complex. A number of research projects have investigated the lived experience of disease when the patient is also a doctor. Such experiences can also shed light on many of the underlying assumptions of medical practice.

In 1985 Hahn used an anthropological and literary approach, analysing 15 personal accounts of illness written mainly by male physicians between 1952 and 1984. 'Between two worlds' is an accurate title for his article, which neatly sums up the challenge of suddenly being on the other end of the stethoscope. For years, these physicians had been fully immersed in their role as doctor, largely within a biomedical framework of objectivity and 'detached concern', if not outright detachment from the illness experience of their patients. Suddenly they found themselves in another world, in which they were uncertain and tentative: 'dependent, anxious, sanctioned in illness only if I was cooperative'. (Geiger(30) quoted in Hahn(31))

While the doctors-as-patients found themselves wanting explanation and reassurance, a consistent pattern in their accounts was that the attending doctors' stance (of emotional distance) seemed alienating. Instead of making connections, their doctors seemed to focus solely on the body part that was damaged or diseased. Sacks, for example, is described by Hahn as being continually dissatisfied: 'He longs for the surgeon's consolation. For the second time, he is severely disappointed by this man. In response to Sacks's stuttering plea, the surgeon answers: "Nonsense, Sacks. Nothing to be worried about. Nothing at all!"' (Sacks(32) quoted in Hahn(31))

The doctor-as-patient has lost his self-identified role as a doctor; he cannot identify with being a patient and he can no longer connect emotionally or existentially with his colleagues. The sick doctor finds himself *between* the diametrically opposed worlds of doctor and of patient. Hahn's findings are quoted in Box 8.5.

BOX 8.5 BETWEEN TWO WORLDS: PHYSICIANS AS PATIENTS

When suffering breaks through, the process of translation – the encounter between two cultures, two languages, and two societies within a single person – is most often not a smooth but rather cataclysmic sequence. The course is not uniform either, but has several shared markers:

1. The damage [to their body] is initially seen as someone else's.
2. It is minimized.
3. It is intellectualized, transformed into a subject for writing and teaching.
4. Physician patients diagnose their own conditions.
5. They may treat or fail to treat themselves, or they may fail to seek treatment by others.
6. They evaluate the diagnoses, prognoses, explanations, treatments, and care given by their colleagues and by others.
7. They mistrust some of their physicians or their physicians' diagnoses, therapeutic prescriptions, or prognoses.
8. They discover a special need for understanding, explanation, support, and sympathy from colleagues, beyond what is strictly "medical."
9. They strive to have non-'crock'-like conditions and to be 'good patients'. [At that time, 'crock' was slang for patients who used their illness to avoid work.]
10. They strenuously avoid passivity, anesthesia, and lack of control.
11. They recall other patients whom they may have misunderstood or who may have had severe side effects with conditions similar to their own.
12. They continue to monitor themselves, medically hypervigilant for signs and symptoms indicating possible changes in their conditions.
13. They reexamine themselves and their histories in the search for aetiology and broader explanation.
14. They reformulate their theory and practice of medicine in the light of their patienthood.

From Hahn(31)

In 1977, McKevitt and Morgan reported remarkably similar findings. They interviewed 64 doctors in the UK about their experience of illness. In 'Illness doesn't belong to us', they observe: 'Whether the illness was physical or psychiatric, many expressed the idea that illness is inappropriate for doctors. This idea is a cultural value among doctors, which is reinforced by the organization of medical work. It discourages doctors from seeking and obtaining appropriate help when they are ill.'(33)

These authors posit that the traditional culture of training and practice has encouraged long hours of study and practice, with relative neglect of one's own needs while performing duties in the service of others. It is little wonder, then, that doctors try to be stoical in the face of illness, often denying the presence of symptoms and/or continuing to work when clearly unwell. Such behaviour is often attributed to loyalty to patients and/or other staff – not wanting to let others down.

Culturally, then, there are significant barriers to doctors acknowledging illness and then being able to receive adequate medical care. In research from New Zealand in 2003, Jaye and Wilson interviewed 26 general practitioners, confirming many of the previous findings noted above.(34) These respondents were also asked to comment on the doctor–patient relationship in cases where their patient is also a doctor. Knowing that such a knowledgeable patient will inevitably test their skills and competence, many GPs approach such consultations with trepidation. Almost invariably, these respondents felt that having consultations with a GP patient is like sitting an exam. Thus, the problem for doctors as patients is twofold: first, they may be ambivalent and conflicted about being in the role of a patient, and second, the doctor they've chosen might be ambivalent or nervous when consulting with them.

This problem is explored at greater length in Klitzman's 2008 book *When doctors become patients*.(35) Klitzman is a psychiatrist and ethicist who interviewed 70 doctors in the US. The motivation for his research came from his own experience of illness in relation to the death of his sister in the World Trade Center on September 11, 2001: 'I thought my training as a psychiatrist would help, but it was quite the opposite. The experience [of depression] forced me to cross the border from provider to patient, and taught me how much I did not know'.(35)

As noted already, sick doctors can find themselves *between* these worlds of doctor and patient: they are now no longer the doctor, but nor can they accept being the patient. Hahn's perceptive analysis includes how this existential crisis or 'liminal zone' is also linked to the resolution of illness: 'many of these physicians are significantly altered, if not transformed, by the events of affliction and/or healing of which they write. When they return to practice, their medical understandings and actions and, more broadly, their lives are substantially altered.'(31)

In Chapter 2, we explored three of the major illness narratives: 'restitution', 'chaos', and 'quest'.(36) In the quest narrative, patients are transformed by their illness, often gaining new meaning in life as part of resolving important questions such as 'Why me?' or 'Why now?' As Hahn points out, many of these illness narratives from doctors are similar: new perspectives on identity and clinical practice start to emerge as part of their recovery. For example, Sacks found that his discipline (neuropsychology) 'had crashed in ruins about me – it retained all of its practical uses and powers, but it had lost all its promises of anything deeper'. (Sacks quoted in Hahn(31)) In response, Sacks resolved to 'reconstruct' his discipline. Likewise Rabin, an endocrinologist who suffered from amyotrophic lateral sclerosis (ALS), called for a better 'response to personal suffering, for solicitation, empathy, and support, to replace the 'deafening silence' [of clinical detachment].'(Rabin(37) quoted in Hahn(31))

Jaye and Wilson also found that most respondents commented on how their personal experience of illness had made a significant impact on their style of medical practice. Many reported being more empathic with patients, especially when the diagnosis remained in doubt and when the dominant issue was one of uncertainty. Some doctors also chose to disclose their own experience of illness to certain patients. While such disclosure is generally frowned on within medical practice, these respondents were careful in its use, noting that it can be helpful for both empathy and reassurance (i.e., that recovery in the future is in fact possible).

These comments point to a possible resolution of the problem of being between two worlds: by acknowledging their own potential for illness and discovering their frailty, these doctors find a way to resolve their existential crisis. Doctors are, after all, just as human as their patients. While this may be blindingly obvious, the intense socialisation into medical culture as part of training and practice means that such acknowledgement can be quite difficult. Our own experiences and observations of doctors as patients are consistent with the published literature. This includes having illness ourselves, doing research into these issues, teaching both under- and post-graduate students on these topics, and attending to other doctors with illness. Some of our personal experiences of being a patient are listed in the following vignette.

VIGNETTE 8.1 DOCTORS AS PATIENTS – PERSONAL EXPERIENCES

HW: I contracted Hepatitis B as a house officer after a needlestick injury in the operating theatre. Rather typically, I was slow in realising I was unwell, then found it difficult to take medical advice about sick leave. I returned to work a bit early and struggled to cope.

Over time, however, and with a few more illnesses, I gradually became more used to being in the sick role, finally realising that I was not immortal and that everyone has their own share of disease. I have had both good and not so-good-encounters with doctors, the worst one being in the emergency department with severe pyelonephritis. The doctor was a young registrar who implied I was making up the illness!

It took some time to find a GP who would treat me the same as any other 'neurotic' patient who could at times both 'over-worry' and 'under-worry' about various symptoms. However, it is now a great relief to be able to trust his judgement, rather than second-guessing myself on both diagnosis and treatment.

It was fascinating to research this subject, noting how colleagues had similar problems in managing their illness, especially in negotiating their treatment with their doctor. In terms of passing on these ideas to students, it has been interesting to realise that early medical students (19- to 21-year-olds) often find it hard to engage with issues that seem (at least to them) to be quite irrelevant. Postgraduate students usually find such discussion very helpful, having already had some encounters with illness themselves. In our teaching, we also discuss how to manage the illness of close family members and medical students.

It has been a steep learning curve, but I now feel much less intimidated when another doctor is my patient. Realising that their attitudes to illness may be complex and ambivalent, I attend quite closely to how they are coping so far. This includes asking who knows about their illness, who is supportive, and how they are making their decisions. Giving simple explanations about their disease is also helpful, as one can never assume their knowledge is either accurate or being applied to themselves. For some of these patients, illness is quite straightforward; for others it is indeed an existential crisis and needs to be handled very carefully.

WC: At the age of 28 I was working in a busy regional hospital as a surgical registrar. One of my consultants was a particularly abusive man who on occasion would quite literally yell at his junior staff (including me) on the ward, in front of nursing staff and patients. About a month after starting this run, I developed a disconcerting painful lump in my throat. Symptoms came on at work and resolved when I went home. I eventually self-diagnosed it as globus hystericus, but did not seek any help.

What I failed to diagnose, however, was my decline into depression. Several months later, and working on a different (but equally stressful) surgical rotation, I recognised that I was struggling to cope and had ceased to enjoy almost any aspect of my work. I approached one of my consultants, asking for time off. At that time, there was little acknowledgement of workplace stress and there were certainly no employee assistance programmes. Given no assistance, I resigned; a surgical career ended. In that era, it seemed the only option.

Gradually I recovered, and I now understand the context and what happened. Hindsight is all very well, and the experience has probably made me a better doctor, but the price paid was high. I am now much more careful with my own health, more mindful of what is stressful to me and much more ready to seek appropriate help when it is needed.

There have been many other research projects on the lived experience of doctors as patients.(13,38–41) It is fascinating that all these projects are remarkably similar to the four discussed above, despite their arising from quite diverse countries and in different decades. Most of them note that doctors' experience of illness is poorly understood and under-researched, and that doctors have difficulty in adjusting to the sick role. All these findings are very similar to the original work from Hahn (Box 8.1), although some also include the issues for the attending doctor. Many comment on the ways in which illness is a salutary experience and can affect professional life and style of practice. All recommend improving the education of medical students about these future challenges and the need to have a personal doctor.

These consistent messages have been in the literature now for 30 to 40 years. Yet it appears that the profession as a whole has been quite slow to acknowledge the importance of such subjective experiences and incorporate them into training. Perhaps each doctor has to reach these conclusions by himself through the painful lived experience of major disease. Forewarning students has proved to be relatively ineffective.

We will touch on these issues again in the final chapter. However, we believe the answer to this puzzling lack of systematic response to work-related stress and doctors' health lies in the ongoing influence of the unstated but powerful assumptions of biomedicine, where the *person* of the doctor is absent.

A possible linking pathway between personality, stress, and quality of care is through the feeling of shame, which we will now explore further.

Shame

Shame is an emotional response characterised by a desire to run away, hide, disappear or withdraw.(42,43) Lazare was the first commentator to draw attention to how difficult it can be for patients to expose themselves, either physically or psychologically, to doctors. Symptoms from the bowel or reproductive tract can be much more than simply embarrassing: patients can feel humiliated on being so exposed. Modern diseases such as HIV or obesity are often seen as moral failings, thus inducing shame.

Doctors can increase or reduce such intense feelings through their awareness of the potential for shame and their manner of interacting with patients.(44)

However, shame can affect doctors as well as patients. While doctors' shame has received little attention so far, it is a potentially important emotion within clinical practice. Davidoff perceptively points out that doctors can feel shame in a variety of situations: when they feel their treatment was not up to standard, when a patient does poorly with treatment (whether or not it is the fault of the doctor), and even if guidelines change, thus casting doubt on previous models of practice. He identifies shame as '"the elephant in the room": something so big and disturbing that we don't even see it, despite the fact that we keep bumping into it'.(45)

In fact, doctors may be particularly vulnerable to shame, having been initially selected as a result of perfectionism, then socialised towards shame-based criticism in medical school (lack of knowledge being implied as a 'shortcoming') and in registrar training (lack of dedication to hard work as a 'moral failing', and so on.)(46) The shame of being exposed as 'not knowing' may be one reason why doctors become reluctant to discuss their work with a mentor or may avoid joining a peer support group.(47)

Shame may also be implicated in doctors' responses to their own illness: admitting to being unwell is somehow 'letting the side down', or showing 'weakness in the face of work requirements'. Apparently such behaviour is reinforced in medical school, where mental health problems are usually concealed.(48)

Stress and quality of care

On two counts, these findings around doctors' health and workplace stress are quite worrying. First, they raise ethical questions about the responsibility of organisations and registration bodies. They are a call to attend more closely to the well-being of doctors and health-care workers as employees. Fortunately, some hospitals are now starting to acknowledge these issues.(49) The findings also raise questions about the duty of medical schools to warn students about, and more effectively prepare them for, the occupational hazards of their chosen career.

Second, do these issues affect patient care? Are patients getting lower quality care? Could they even be harmed if their doctor is stressed, anxious, depressed or burnt out? As we will see in Chapter 11, adverse outcomes from medical care are now being identified in both hospital practice and primary care.(50) However, quality of care is not just about adverse outcomes: poor care also includes problems with communication, low rates of adherence to treatment and lack of follow-up. Doctors themselves have identified the links between stress (fatigue and sleep deprivation, for example) and lowered quality. Many report taking shortcuts, not following procedures, or being irritable or angry with patients as a result of workplace stress.(51)

Di Matteo et al. followed almost 200 physicians over two years, finding links between their job satisfaction and their patients' adherence to treatment.(52) Similarly, Williams and Skinner found that lower job satisfaction was correlated with various parameters of quality, such as poor prescribing profiles and less satisfied patients.(53) In a large and complex series of interventions into 67 hospitals in the 1980s, Jones et al. found that workplace stress correlated significantly with claims for malpractice.

Furthermore, organisational interventions to reduce such stress resulted in lower prescribing errors and lower rates of complaints.(54)

These findings have emerged over the last 30 years or so. First summarised by Firth-Cozens in her benchmark paper in 2001(26), they were updated more recently by Wallace and others in the *Lancet* in 2009.(1) In their seminal article they conclude that the unwell physician has a considerable impact on health system performance: wellness is 'vital to the delivery of high-quality healthcare'. They propose that health systems should routinely measure physician wellness as the 'missing quality indicator' of heath care. Significantly, they also point out that a shift in medical culture is required: both doctors and patients will benefit if there is more attention to the general health of doctors (Figure 8.2).

The left side of the diagram shows three primary factors affecting the doctor: workplace stressors, contextual factors and physician characteristics. These factors contribute to physician outcomes (feelings of stress, burnout, depression, relationship problems, substance abuse, risk of suicide). In turn, these physician outcomes contribute to health-care system outcomes such as lowered productivity and efficiency, suboptimal quality of patient care, reduced patient adherence/satisfaction, and increased risk of medical errors. These links are supported by substantial empirical evidence. The bottom row of the diagram lists various interventions which might theoretically reduce workplace stress and improve patient outcomes.

Having outlined the problems of stress, doctors' ill health, and the impact these problems have on quality of health care, we now take a different approach. How can doctors remain healthy? Or, better still, how can they increase their wellness and develop more resilience to the stressors of modern clinical practice?

Opposite: the links between physician ill health and the health-care system, with potential interventions to improve physician and system outcomes. (Solid lines are empirically supported; broken lines are potential links.) From Wallace et al.(1)

FIGURE 8.2 A MODEL OF PHYSICIAN ILL HEALTH

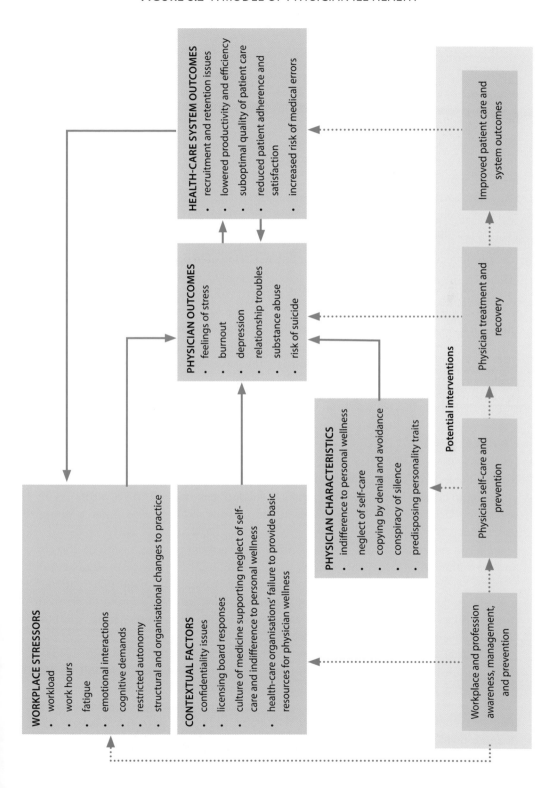

WORKPLACE STRESSORS
- workload
- work hours
- fatigue
- emotional interactions
- cognitive demands
- restricted autonomy
- structural and organisational changes to practice

CONTEXTUAL FACTORS
- confidentiality issues
- licensing board responses
- culture of medicine supporting neglect of self-care and indifference to personal wellness
- health-care organisations' failure to provide basic resources for physician wellness

PHYSICIAN CHARACTERISTICS
- indifference to personal wellness
- neglect of self-care
- copying by denial and avoidance
- conspiracy of silence
- predisposing personality traits

PHYSICIAN OUTCOMES
- feelings of stress
- burnout
- depression
- relationship troubles
- substance abuse
- risk of suicide

HEALTH-CARE SYSTEM OUTCOMES
- recruitment and retention issues
- lowered productivity and efficiency
- suboptimal quality of patient care
- reduced patient adherence and satisfaction
- increased risk of medical errors

Potential interventions

Workplace and profession awareness, management, and prevention

Physician self-care and prevention

Physician treatment and recovery

Improved patient care and system outcomes

Part 2: Health and wellness

The concept of wellness

To summarise thus far, doctors have better physical health and live longer than the rest of the population, but also appear to have worse psychological health in terms of stress, anxiety, fatigue, depression and burnout. There is increasing evidence that doctors' overall health can affect health-care systems and patient care. It is important, then, that doctors learn to look after themselves well. In other words, there needs to be a greater emphasis on doctors' *wellness*.

However, there is currently little focus on wellness as an important aspect of medical training or clinical practice. It is worth returning to the observation made by Shanafelt et al.: 'Wellness goes beyond merely the absence of distress and includes being challenged, thriving, and achieving success in various aspects of personal and professional life.'(8) Thriving in one's personal and professional life includes various overlapping components:

- Physical health
- Psychological health and well-being
- Resilience and coping strategies
- Self-care
- Reflective practice.

We will now discuss these components of wellness in more detail, at times drawing some links between doctor wellness and possible outcomes for patients. Reflective practice will be explored further in Chapter 10.

Physical health

As noted above, doctors have better physical health than the rest of the population (even adjusted for socio-economic status). This is largely because doctors are better at adhering to current lifestyle recommendations relating to use of tobacco, alcohol, safe sexual practices, exercise, dietary habits including fruit and vegetable intake, and use of seat belts.(55)

There are also more subtle research findings about the physical health of doctors and how this links to patient outcomes. For example, if the doctor is eligible and receives screening for a particular condition, there is more likelihood their patients will also get screening (bowel cancer, mammograms, prostate screening, cervical cancer, and so on).(56) Doctors' personal experience and uptake of screening will thus affect the health outcomes of their patients.

In terms of exercise, there is now substantial evidence that 30 minutes a day of moderate intensity physical activity at least five days of the week will confer considerable physical and psychological benefits.(57) Many doctors use physical exercise as one of their main methods of stress reduction. Such doctors are also more likely to recommend physical activity to their patients, hence the possible link between doctor's level of exercise and the health outcomes of their patients.(58)

Psychological health and well-being

Given the consistently presented statistics noted above on stress, anxiety, depression and burnout, the psychological well-being of doctors could do with some improvement. While it is well known that doctors suffer from work-related stress, most organisations (secondary care hospitals and colleges of specialties) do not proactively focus on improving doctors' psychological or emotional well-being.

As we noted in Chapter 4, emotional intelligence or EQ can be distinguished from intellectual intelligence (IQ). EQ is 'the ability to monitor one's own and other's feelings and emotions, to discriminate between them, and to use the information to guide one's thinking and actions'.(59) EQ has five domains: knowing one's own emotions, managing emotions, motivating oneself, recognising emotions in others, and handling relationships.

With respect to the doctor–patient relationship, doctors' actions are often predicated on their subtle (or sometimes not-so-subtle!) emotional responses to various patients. Unless these are acknowledged and understood, medical work can be stressful and taxing, being at the whim of a range of powerful emotions in relation to patient demands or distress. However, most doctors have not received training in how to handle their feelings within clinical practice, unless they have attended counselling courses or have received counselling or psychotherapy themselves.

Two emerging approaches to improving doctors' psychological well-being in the workplace are positive psychology(60) and mindfulness training. These will now be discussed in turn.

Positive psychology

Since World War II, psychological theories have largely been based on the classification of mental distress, which has led to the 'recovery' model: how do people repair the damage from personal and/or psychological trauma? However, this almost exclusive attention on pathological processes has neglected to explore how individuals become fulfilled or how they thrive under normal circumstances. Positive psychology redirects the focus of psychology 'from preoccupation only with repairing the worst things in life to also building positive qualities'.(60) The task is to enhance one's strengths as well as to repair any weaknesses.(61)

This approach has created an understanding of how (a) emotions and (b) personal traits (including optimism) contribute to personal well-being. For example, emotions can be characterised as positive or negative. Positive emotions include gratitude, joy, contentment, love, kindness and compassion, while negative emotions include anger, sadness, hatred, resentment, anxiety, hopelessness, despair and shame. Ideally, individuals experience more of the former than the latter (perhaps a 3:1 ratio). In times of stress, there are relatively more negative emotions. One problem is that positive emotions are generally felt as more fleeting, transitory and ephemeral than negative ones, which usually come with more intensity and power. It is easier to remember instances of being upset than those of being happy.

As we noted in Chapter 5, many doctors are intuitively adept at handling complex and difficult situations, but many patients are emotionally draining and trigger troublesome countertransference (strong reactions towards patients arising from either the patient's or doctor's previous relationships). Positive training for emotions implies that doctors become aware of their own feelings and emotions and can negotiate them more readily.

Positive emotional traits include the capacity for hope, creativity, wisdom, courage, responsibility, perseverance, spirituality and future-mindedness. For example, with optimistic thinking, stressful events or poor outcomes are temporary and particular ('this patient did poorly with antidepressants'). In pessimistic thinking, on the other hand, such events indicate a more general hopelessness ('nothing will work with this patient' or 'antidepressants never work'). Optimism is a particular orientation to the world that confers considerable long-term advantages.(62)

Positive psychology emphasises that these orientations to the world are identifiable and negotiable: by being aware of internal thoughts, it is possible to challenge the assumptions that might underpin them. 'Always' or 'never' can be replaced with 'on this occasion', while words like 'should/ought/must' are a clue to habitual behaviours that may not be productive. Such internal dialogue is a form of cognitive behavioural therapy and can be very helpful in times of work or personal stress.(61)

Positive psychology can thus be a tool for better self-awareness, improved emotional intelligence and increased resilience to workplace demands.

Mindfulness

Mindfulness involves attending closely to both internal and external experiences occurring in the present moment. While originating in Eastern meditation practices, it is now being acknowledged as a powerful method for improving concentration and work performance. It has been shown to reduce stress, increase contentment and peace of mind, and build the capacity for resilience.(63)

Mindfulness training is simply learning to pay close attention to the present experience on a moment-to-moment basis. All models of training emphasise an attitude of non-judgmental acceptance: passing thoughts, sensations and emotions are observed carefully but are not evaluated as good or bad, true or false, or important or trivial. Mindfulness is thus the 'nonjudgmental observation of the ongoing stream of internal and external stimuli as they arise'.(63) Most programmes recommend daily practice for 10 to 20 minutes: effects on stress and capacity for concentration are usually felt within a few weeks.

The medical profession has been somewhat guarded in its response to these claims, perhaps because it seems unlikely that these simple techniques could have such significant outcomes, or because the data did not emerge from traditional biomedical research. Nevertheless, mindfulness is becoming the subject of increasingly intensive study,(64) and the evidence for its effectiveness is quite compelling.(65)

Many doctors are now starting to include mindfulness training as part of their own package of self-care and preventive activities.(66) Medical schools are considering ways to incorporate mindfulness practice for students, given that such training will help them with the well-known stresses of undergraduate training.(67,68) For example, a recent trial in Australia demonstrated significant differences between the mindfulness group and the control group with respect to levels of stress.(69)

The long-term outlook is thus quite positive: these future doctors will have a method for improving their overall wellness; they will be role models for others; and it is likely that they will discuss similar self-care practices with their patients. Box 8.6 summarises a typical review of mindfulness training for doctors.

BOX 8.6 MINDFULNESS-BASED STRESS REDUCTION (MBSR): A REVIEW OF EMPIRICAL STUDIES

'Demands faced by health care professionals include heavy caseloads, limited control over the work environment, long hours, as well as organizational structures and systems in transition. Such conditions have been directly linked to increased stress and symptoms of burnout, which in turn, have adverse consequences for clinicians and the quality of care that is provided to patients. Consequently, there exists an impetus for the development of curriculum aimed at fostering wellness and the necessary self-care skills for clinicians … Empirical evidence indicates that participation in MBSR yields benefits for clinicians in the domains of physical and mental health.'

From Irving et al.(66)

Grounding

A form of mindfulness, grounding particularly involves noticing, accepting and experiencing the physical sensations in the body, while at the same time noticing the surrounding physical world via our physical senses. It is a natural process which recalls us to our physical selves, the present moment and where we happen to be. It promotes centredness, calmness and a sense of balance – outcomes which are especially valuable when busy or stressed.(70) Grounding is a three-step process:

First, notice the physical body by becoming more aware of whatever we may be thinking, feeling, remembering, talking to ourselves about and so on. Second, notice the physical world around us (objects, sounds, etc.) through our five senses (seeing, touching, hearing, smelling, tasting). And finally, notice both the 'inside' (the body) and the 'outside' (the world) at the same time. This combined awareness seems to promote a release of any unbalanced emotional energy – a sort of 'getting earthed' or 'release of electrical discharge'.

The idea is to fully notice and experience what is going on, both internally and externally, in our lives at any moment. It is a simple and effective method of remaining balanced, calm and relaxed, even if our current work or life situation seems chaotic and overwhelming – rather like being in the 'eye of the cyclone'. To get into the habit of grounding, it can be used for brief periods during the day (5–10 seconds every 20 minutes). Then longer sessions can be tried as well (10–20 minutes) every day.(71)

Grounding is also a valuable technique to help practitioners become more emotionally and physically present in their moment-to-moment tasks, such as preparing oneself for interviewing patients and their families, performing a surgical procedure, or before any potentially stressful situation. It is also useful to take a few minutes to ground oneself *after* such situations, literally 'coming back to our senses'.

Resilience and coping strategies

Medicine is inherently stressful, given that much of clinical work is made up of dealing with the major transcendent dimensions of life (birth, suffering, loss of meaning, dying, and so on). Resilience is the capacity to respond and adapt to significant adversity, trauma, tragedy, threat, or sources of stress. Clearly, doctors need to cultivate their personal resilience. For example, the ability to distinguish between positive and negative emotions and the capacity for emotional complexity and ambiguity appear to work as critical buffers against depression after traumatic experiences.(72)

Coping strategies are behavioural and psychological strategies in response to stress. These strategies generally fall into three categories: problem-focused (making a plan of action, ceasing other tasks, enlisting help from others), emotion-focused (seeking emotional support, accepting, turning to religion, using humour), or maladaptive (venting of emotions, ignoring or denying the problem).(73) Linking back to positive psychology, studies show that pessimism as a character trait is associated with maladaptive strategies such as denial of stress and distancing, while optimism is associated with problem-focused coping, finding social support, and emphasising positive aspects of the stressful situation.(74)

Lemaire and Wallace explored the relationship between these various coping strategies and the tendency toward burnout in a large sample of physicians in Canada. (75) The strategies that reflected denial of stress (keeping stress to oneself, concentrating on what to do next) were associated with a higher incidence of emotional exhaustion. Conversely, coping strategies used outside of work (having time off, discussing problems with family) were linked to lower rates of exhaustion.

In other words, the ways in which doctors respond to and cope with stress will have significant implications for job satisfaction and personal well-being. Short-term coping mechanisms are often needed in the heat of the moment, when immediate clinical tasks require setting aside one's personal needs. However, a central theme of this book is that medical practice includes many events and situations that cannot remain unexamined. We advocate exploring the stressors at work through careful retrospective review, identifying and critiquing any stressful or critical event and the responses of those involved. Through such reflection, doctors can more readily bounce back from difficult circumstances and better prepare themselves for future scenarios.

Self-care

While resilience and coping refer to recovery and learning from stressful clinical situations, self-care refers to a range of proactive methods and techniques that maintain and increase one's general wellness. For example, exercise, laughter and meditation have all been shown to increase endorphin levels, which contribute greatly to an overall sense of well-being.

Developing good systems of professional and personal supports are the hallmark of the well-functioning doctor. Ideally, such supports are over and above those gained from family and friends. We recommend focused group work such as peer group(76) or Balint work (see Appendix). One-to-one mentoring(77) and supervision(78) are powerful methods of self-care and professional development and will be discussed in depth in Chapter 10. Similarly, a strong social network and interests outside of medicine are crucial to maintaining a healthy work-life balance.(79)

Boundary issues are important in medical practice, not only to ensure patients' safety and confidentiality, but also for the doctor's well-being. Boundaries that can cause problems include: the division between work and home; treating family and friends; accepting gifts from patients; business or personal relationships with patients; more than one health professional looking after the patient (unless part of formally shared care). Self-care implies that these fluid boundaries should be monitored carefully.

Keeping a personal journal or using other reflective techniques, practising some form of spirituality, education outside of medicine, and personal psychological therapy are all methods to improve self-care.(80) As we emphasise throughout this book, the meaning of medical practice is particularly important.(81) If one's work can resonate with one's goal and philosophy of life, then work can become a source of joy and pleasure, rather than pain and stress.(82)

Given that medical practice has the capacity to be stressful for doctors, resilience and self-care are critical to ongoing wellness. Medical students need to receive focused training in all these components of wellness for their future life and clinical practice.

Conclusion

The self of the doctor is integral to the doctor–patient relationship, which in turn is integral to the delivery of medical care. We have focused on the importance of doctors' wellness and resilience and have discussed some of the current challenges. We hope that by making these issues more explicit, we have shown how doctors' health and clinical competence can be improved so that the 'ambulance at the bottom of the cliff' is not required.

This is not a selfish or doctor-centric approach – we need to preserve and enhance our ability to care for patients, which is the primary task of doctoring. There is more than enough evidence that practising medicine is often stressful, and that this stress can take a toll on us, both as individuals and as a profession. 'Caring for the carers' is essential.

Furthermore, the profession needs to rethink its approach to the sick doctor. At present, doctors have an ambivalent relationship to being in the sick role, and they quite often receive poor-quality care. Future doctors must learn how to seek and receive medical care; they must also learn to provide more effective medical care for their colleagues. The data is already in: there is no need for further research on doctors' health, unless it is to propose and evaluate interventions that improve the outcomes of doctors' illness.

We contend that the person of the doctor is crucially important: this needs more emphasis in both training and practice. Medical culture is often predicated on the idea that 'true objectivity' is both possible and desirable. As a result, the 'self' or 'person' of the doctor has been largely absent or disregarded in the delivery of patient care. The narrowly defined 'doctor-as-scientist' of biomedicine is at odds with the therapeutic doctor–patient relationship that patients require.

SUMMARY POINTS

- The traditional injunction on doctors to be 'clinically detached' is problematic: while at times it might be pragmatic, expedient, and even necessary, it needs to be balanced by thoughtful appreciation of what the doctor brings to medicine, and how medicine is impacting on the doctor.

- Compassion fatigue and burnout are consequences of failing to 'care for the carers'.

- Doctors-as-patients are often caught between two worlds – they may be unable to seek and accept medical care appropriately, and they may not receive the care they need from their colleagues.

- Shame is an important but often hidden emotional response in doctors, a response to both personal illness and perceived failure of treatment or competence.

- Failure to maintain wellness can lead to impaired doctor functioning, both personally and professionally.

- Doctors' wellness is their general sense of purpose, competence and meaning, while resilience is their capacity to respond and adapt to various stressors and setbacks.

- Wellness and resilience are important to counter the stressors associated with medical training and practice.

- The health and wellness of the doctor has a considerable impact on the health of his or her patients.

- Focusing on doctor wellness must become a much higher priority for both students and doctors.

References

1. Wallace JE, Lemaire JB, Ghali WA. Physician wellness: A missing quality indicator. *Lancet* 2009, 374(9702):1714–21.
2. McWhinney I. *Textbook of family medicine*. 3rd edn. Oxford: Oxford University Press, 2009.
3. Kellyn S. Workplace bullying: the silent epidemic. *NZ Med J* 2004, 117:1204.
4. *Guidebook for managing disruptive physician behaviour*. Toronto: College of Physicians and Surgeons of Ontario, 2008.
5. Williams M, Williams B, Speicher M. A systems approach to disruptive behaviour in physicians: a case study. *Fed Bull* 2004, 90(4):120–24.
6. Rahe RH, Veach TL, Tolles RL, Murakami K. The stress and coping inventory: an educational and research instrument. *Stress Health* 2000, 16(4):199–208.
7. Luthar S, Cicchetti D, Becker, B. The construct of resilience: a critical evaluation and guidelines for future work. *Child Develop* 2000, 71(3):543–62.
8. Shanafelt TD, Sloan JA, Habermann TM. The well-being of physicians. *Am J Med* 2003; 114(6):513–19.
9. Appleton K, House A, Dowell A. A survey of job satisfaction, sources of stress and psychological symptoms among general practitioners in Leeds. *Br J Gen Pract* 1998, 48(428):1059–63.
10. Firth-Cozens J. Doctors, their well-being, and their stress. *BMJ* 2003, 326(7391):670.
11. Field R, Haslam D. Do you have your own doctor, doctor? Tackling barriers to health care. *Br J Gen Pract* 2008, 58(552):462–64.

12. Dowell AC, Westcott T, McLeod DK, Hamilton S. A survey of job satisfaction, sources of stress and psychological symptoms among New Zealand health professionals. *NZ Med J* 2001, 114(1145):540–43.

13. Kay M, Mitchell G, Clavarino A, Doust J. Doctors as patients: A systematic review of doctors' health access and the barriers they experience. *Br J Gen Pract* 2008, 58(552):501–08.

14. Baldwin P, Dodd M, Wrate R. Young doctors' health – II. Health and health behaviour. *Soc Sci Med* 1997, 45(1):41–44.

15. Henning MA, Hawken SJ, Hill AG. The quality of life of New Zealand doctors and medical students: what can be done to avoid burnout? *NZ Med J* 2009, 122(1307).

16. Linzer M, Visser MRM, Oort FJ, Smets E, McMurray JE, de Haes HCJM. Predicting and preventing physician burnout: results from the United States and the Netherlands. *Am J Med* 2001, 111(2):170–75.

17. Eckleberry-Hunt J, Lick D, Boura J, Hunt R, Balasubramaniam M, Mulhem E, et al. An exploratory study of resident burnout and wellness. *Acad Med* 2009, 84(2):269-77.

18. Huggard P. Managing compassion fatigue: implications for medical education. PhD Thesis. University of Auckland, 2008.

19. Maslach C, Jackson SE, Leiter MP. *Maslach burnout inventory manual*. Palo Alto, California: Consulting Psychologists Press, 1996.

20. Huggard P, Stamm B, Pearlman L. Physician stress: compassion satisfaction, compassion fatigue and vicarious traumatization. In: Figley C, Huggard P, Rees C, eds. *First do no self-harm*. New York: Oxford University Press (In Press), 2013.

21. Vaillant GE, Sobowale NC, McArthur C. Some psychologic vulnerabilities of physicians. *N Engl J Med* 1972, 287(8):372–75.

22. Elliott DM, Guy JD. Mental health professionals versus non-mental-health professionals: childhood trauma and adult functioning. *Prof Psychol Res Pract* 1993, 24(1):83–90.

23. Firth J. Levels and sources of stress in medical students. *BMJ* 1986, 292(6529):1177.

24. Firth-Cozens J. Individual and organizational predictors of depression in general practitioners. *Br J Gen Pract* 1998, 48(435):1647–51.

25. Koeske GF, Kirk SA, Koeske RD. Coping with job stress: which strategies work best? *J Occup Organ Psychol* 1993, 66:319–35.

26. Firth-Cozens J. Interventions to improve physicians' well-being and patient care. *Soc Sci Med* 2001, 52(2):215–22.

27. McManus IC, Keeling A, Paice E. Stress, burnout and doctors' attitudes to work are determined by personality and learning style: a twelve year longitudinal study of UK medical graduates. *BMC Med* 2004, 2(1):29.

28. Enns MW, Cox BJ, Sareen J, Freeman P. Adaptive and maladaptive perfectionism in medical students: a longitudinal investigation. *Med Educ* 2001, 35(11):1034–42.

29. Boisaubin EV, Levine RE. Identifying and assisting the impaired physician. *Am J Med Sci* 2001, 322(1):31–36.

30. Geiger H. The causes of dehumanization in health care and prospects for humanization. In: Howard J, Strauss A, eds. *Humanizing health care*. New York: Wiley, 1975. pp. 57–102.

31. Hahn RA. Between two worlds: physicians as patients. *Med Anthr Quart* 1985, 16(4):87–98.

32. Sacks O. *A leg to stand on*. New York: Summit Books,1984.

33. McKevitt C, Morgan M. Illness doesn't belong to us. *J Roy Soc Med* 1997, 90(9):491–95.

34. Jaye C, Wilson HJ. When general practitioners become patients. *Health: Interdisc J Social Study Health Illness Med* 2003, 7(2):201–25.

35. Klitzman R. *When doctors become patients*. New York: Oxford University Press, 2008.

36. Frank A. *The wounded storyteller: body, illness, and ethics*. Chicago: University of Chicago Press, 1995.

37. Rabin D, Rabin PL, Rabin R. Compounding the ordeal of ALS. *N Engl J Med* 1982, 307(8):506–09.
38. Richards J. The health and health practices of doctors and their families. *NZ Med J* 1999, 112(1084):96.
39. Fox F, Harris M, Taylor G, Rodham K, Sutton J, Robinson B, et al. What happens when doctors are patients? Qualitative study of GPs. *Br J Gen Pract* 2009, 59(568):811–18.
40. Noble S, Marie AN, Finlay I. Challenges faced by palliative care physicians when caring for doctors with advanced cancer. *Pall Med* 2008, 22(1):71–76.
41. Tyssen R. The physician–patient relationship when the patient is a physician. *J Nor Med Assoc* 2001, 121(30):3533–35.
42. Lewis M. *Shame: the exposed self*. New York: The Free Press, 1995.
43. Jacoby M. *Shame and the origins of self-esteem*. London: Routledge, 1994.
44. Lazare A. Shame and humiliation in the medical encounter. *Arch Int Med* 1987, 147(9):1653–58.
45. Davidoff F. Shame: the elephant in the room. *Qual Saf Health Care* 2002, 11(1):2–3.
46. Sinclair S. Making doctors: an institutional apprenticeship. New York: Berg Publishers, 1997.
47. Cunningham W, Wilson HJ. Shame, guilt and the medical practitioner. *NZ Med J* 2003, 116(1183).
48. Chew-Graham CA, Rogers A, Yassin N. 'I wouldn't want it on my CV or their records': Medical students' experiences of help-seeking for mental health problems. *Med Educ* 2003, 37(10):873–80.
49. Rees D, Cooper CL. Occupational stress in health service workers in the UK. *Stress Med* 1992, 8(2):79–90.
50. Kohn L, Corrigan J, Donaldson M. *To err is human: building a safer health system*. Washington, DC: National Academy Press, 1999.
51. Firth-Cozens J, Greenhalgh J. Doctors' perceptions of the links between stress and lowered clinical care. *Soc Sci Med* 1997, 44(7):1017–22.
52. DiMatteo MR, Sherbourne CD, Hays RD, Ordway L, Kravitz RL, McGlynn EA, et al. Physicians' characteristics influence patients' adherence to medical treatment: results from the medical outcomes study. *Health Psychol* 1993, 12(2):93–102.
53. Williams ES, Skinner AC. Outcomes of physician job satisfaction: a narrative review, implications, and directions for future research. *Health Care Man Rev* 2003, 28(2):119–40.
54. Jones JW, Barge BN, Steffy BD, Fay LM, Kunz LK, Wuebker LJ. Stress and medical malpractice: organizational risk assessment and intervention. *J Appl Psychol* 1988, 73(4):727–35.
55. Frank E, Rothenberg R, Lewis C, Belodoff BF. Correlates of physicians' prevention-related practices: findings from the Women Physicians' Health Study. *Arch Fam Med* 2000, 9(4):359.
56. Frank E. Physician health and patient care. *JAMA* 2004, 291(5):637.
57. Blair SN, Church TS. The fitness, obesity, and health equation. *JAMA* 2004, 292(10):1232–34.
58. Lobelo F, Duperly J, Frank E. Physical activity habits of doctors and medical students influence their counselling practices. *Br J Sport Med* 2009, 43(2):89–92.
59. Salovey P, Mayer JD. Emotional intelligence. *Imagin Cognit Person* 1990, 9:185–211.
60. Seligman MEP, Csikszentmihalyi M. Positive psychology: an introduction. *Am Psychol* 2000, 55(1):5–14.
61. Fredrickson BL. The role of positive emotions in positive psychology: the broaden-and-build theory of positive emotions. *Am Psychol* 2001, 56(3):218–26.
62. Peterson C. The future of optimism. *Am Psychol* 2000, 55(1):44–55.
63. Baer RA. Mindfulness training as a clinical intervention: a conceptual and empirical review. *Clin Psychol Sci Pract* 2003, 10(2):125–43.
64. Hölzel BK, Carmody J, Vangel M, Congleton C, Yerramsetti SM, Gard T, et al. Mindfulness practice leads to increases in regional brain gray matter density. *Psychiat Res Neuro* 2011, 191(1):36–43.

65. Grossman P, Niemann L, Schmidt S, Walach H. Mindfulness-based stress reduction and health benefits: a meta-analysis. *J Psychosomatic Res* 2004, 57(1):35–43.

66. Irving JA, Dobkin PL, Park J. Cultivating mindfulness in health care professionals: a review of empirical studies of mindfulness-based stress reduction (MBSR). *Compl Ther Clin Pract* 2009, 15(2):61–66.

67. Hassad C, de Lisle S, Sullivan G, Pier C. Enhancing the health of medical students: outcomes of an integrated mindfulness and lifestyle programme. *Advs Health Sci Educ Theory Pract* 2009, 14(3):387–98.

68. Adams-Hillard P, Basaviah P, Osterberg L. Medical student wellness: an essential role for mentors. *Med Sci Educ* 2011, 21(2). In Press.

69. Warnecke E, Quinn S, Ogden K, Towle N, Nelson MR. A randomised controlled trial of the effects of mindfulness practice on medical student stress levels. *Med Educ* 2011, 45(4):381–88.

70. Mellor K. *Urban mystic: discovering the transcendent through everyday life*. New York: Strategic Book Publications, 2009.

71. Davis M. Methods for enhancing relaxation. In: O'Hagan J, Richards J, eds. *In sickness and in health: a handbook for medical practitioners, other health practitioners, their partners and families*. Wellington: Doctors Health Advisory Service, 1997.

72. Luthar SS, Cicchetti D, Becker B. The construct of resilience: a critical evaluation and guidelines for future work. *Child Develop* 2000, 71(3):543–62.

73. Carver CS, Scheier MF, Weintraub JK. Assessing coping strategies: a theoretically based approach. *J Pers Soc Psychol* 1989, 56(2):267–83.

74. Scheier MF, Weintraub JK, Carver CS. Coping with stress: divergent strategies of optimists and pessimists. *J Pers Soc Psychol* 1986, 51(6):1257.

75. Lemaire J, Wallace J. Not all coping strategies are created equal: a mixed methods study exploring physicians' self-reported coping strategies. *BMC Health Serv Res* 2010, 10(1):208.

76. Watson A. *The peer group movement: what goes into making a successful peer group?* Wellington: Royal New Zealand College of General Practitioners, 1997.

77. Freeman R. *Mentoring in general practice*. Oxford: Butterworth-Heinemann, 1998.

78. Wilson HJ. Supervision and the culture of general practice. Masters thesis. Dunedin, NZ: University of Otago, 1999.

79. Sisley R, Henning MA, Hawken SJ, Moir F. A conceptual model of workplace stress: the issue of accumulation and recovery and the health professional. *NZ J Employ Relat* 2010, 28(2):3–15.

80. Moir F. *Improving the health of our doctors: good mental health and well-being*. Auckland: University of Auckland, 2010.

81. Remen RN. Practicing a medicine of the whole person: an opportunity for healing. *Hemat Oncol Clin N Am* 2008, 22(4):767–73.

82. Garfinkel PE, Bagby RM, Schuller DR, Williams CC, Dickens SE, Dorian B. Predictors of success and satisfaction in the practice of psychiatry: a preliminary follow-up study. *Can J Psychiat* 2001, 46(9):835–40.

Chapter 9

The Culture of Medicine

CONTENTS

Introduction

The previous chapter identified characteristics of doctors and workplace stressors that impact on quality of care. This chapter considers the 'culture' of medicine: the set of attitudes, values, goals and practices that characterise an institution, organisation, or group. This concept is usually applied to whole societies or nations, while 'small' cultures are local groups or organisations that develop their own cultural norms. Biomedicine is one such culture. Individual doctors are part of, and contribute to, the 'culture' of medical practice. (1, 2)

Exploring this topic is by no means straightforward. It is much easier to observe the culture of *others* (overseas visitors, foreign countries) than it is to see our own. In particular, medicine has long attempted to portray itself as having 'no culture', as being somehow removed from the usual social forces and structures that apply to other sectors of society. As Taylor notes, '[m]edical knowledge is understood to be not merely "cultural" knowledge but *real* knowledge.'(3) As we mentioned in

Chapter 3, 'real' here refers to objective or materialist knowledge, apprehended and acknowledged through empirical study. Personal, family, and social influences are traditionally excluded, and the culture of medicine itself remains unexamined.

Being embedded within a culture makes it more difficult to see its customs dispassionately or become aware of the ways in which they influence one's day-to-day work. Such analysis is the domain of medical anthropology, a division of social science, but few of the insights gained from anthropological research have made their way into the usual discourse of medicine. O'Boyle observes: 'The biomedical model of disease is so pervasive that we often fail to see it as such, but view it as reality. Questioning this model is like asking whether a goldfish knows it is in water.'(4) There is much to be gained in looking at how biomedicine is taught, practised, perpetuated and 'continually reconstructed'.(5) While doctors do not need to become anthropologists, having some basic knowledge of this field is helpful when examining a work environment.

This chapter explores current trends in the culture of biomedicine, looking at variations between subcultures, the ways in which students become 'acculturated' into medicine, and differences between supportive and unsupportive communities of practice. The 'self' of the doctor is intrinsically linked to the environment and culture of the doctor's work. We start by reiterating the biomedical emphasis of both research and practice.

Trends in biomedical culture

The profession of medicine has undergone profound changes in the last hundred years. To mark the turn of the twenty-first century, the *New England Journal of Medicine* listed what the editors considered to be the 'most important medical developments' in the last thousand years (Box 9.1).

BOX 9.1 THE MOST IMPORTANT MEDICAL DEVELOPMENTS OF THE PAST MILLENNIUM

1. Elucidation of human anatomy and physiology
2. Discovery of cells and their substructures
3. Elucidation of the chemistry of life
4. Application of statistics to medicine
5. Development of anaesthesia
6. Discovery of the relation of microbes to disease
7. Elucidation of inheritance and genetics
8. Knowledge of the immune system
9. Development of body imaging
10. Discovery of antimicrobial agents
11. Development of molecular pharmacology.

From Angell et al.(6)

Significantly, however, this list does not include major advances in the understanding of psychological, cultural, or socio-economic influences on physical and personal health. Instead, the developments can all be located under quite a narrowly defined biological framework: the idea that diseases and treatments must be explicable in physical terms. This particular (and current) understanding of 'medicine', then, is profoundly biomedical.[1]

Biomedicine itself continues to evolve, in part due to the ever-increasing influence of science on society. Burri and Dumit have identified this trend as the 'scientification of biomedicine'.(1) Recent developments in biotechnology, genomics, bioinformatics and imaging technology are providing more sophisticated investigatory and treatment techniques, transforming hospitals into so-called 'biomedical platforms', where the process of medical care is predicated by technology. The trend towards practice guidelines based solely on narrowly defined randomised trials has also been critiqued as 'the over-rationalisation' of biomedicine.(7)

Burri and Dumit further propose that society is becoming ever more 'biomedicalised', where many aspects of normal life are now becoming defined as *medical* problems. The body is 'constructed, seen and talked about' in a more biomedical way: cosmetic surgery and lifestyle drugs are now a 'normal' feature of modern life, partly reflecting the scientification of biomedicine noted above.(1)

While the modern doctor incorporates these trends within biomedicine (that is, being conversant and skilled with technological innovations and modern pharmacology), there are aspects of biomedical culture that seem relatively stable. This leads to what is known as 'cultural analysis'.

Cultural analysis

One recent tool for analysing and comparing different cultures is Hofstede's 'cultural dimensions'.(8) Although these particular dimensions have been contested, they provide a useful starting point for comparing societies and subcultures (Box 9.2).

BOX 9.2 HOFSTEDE'S DIMENSIONS OF CULTURE

Power distance

This dimension is the underlying degree of hierarchical structure, defined as 'the extent to which the less powerful members of institutions and organizations expect and accept that power is distributed unequally'. This dimension can range from small to large, commonly referred to as a flat or steep hierarchical culture. Cultures with small power distance will stress equality between individuals and de-emphasise rank or level of authority.

---

1 As we indicated in the Introduction, we very much welcome the advances that biomedicine has provided. These are based on scientific principles in order to find effective treatment (rather than continuing the use of leeches, arsenic, or other traditional remedies). The comments above are intended to illustrate how the underlying principles of biomedicine are taken for granted within medical culture: they are not a criticism of those advances.

BOX 9.2 CONTINUED

Uncertainty avoidance

This dimension is defined as 'the extent to which the members of a culture feel threatened by ambiguous or unknown situations (from weak to strong)'. This dimension reveals how individuals within a culture respond to the problem of uncertainty (which usually causes anxiety). In high uncertainty avoidance, people reduce their uncertainty and anxiety by adopting certain behaviours, such as keeping to established practices or guidelines and avoiding experimental ideas. Hofstede found that most high uncertainty avoidant cultures also had high power distance, such as dependence on authority.

Individualism and collectivism

In individualistic cultures the basic social unit is the *individual*, whereas in collectivist cultures the basic unit is the *group*. Individualism describes a society in which the ties between individuals are loose: everyone is expected to look after him- or herself alone, plus his or her immediate family. Its opposite, collectivism, describes a society in which people from birth onwards are integrated into strong, cohesive in-groups which, throughout people's lifetime, continue to protect them in exchange for unquestioning loyalty. The USA, UK and Australia are highly individualistic societies, whereas Latin American and Asian cultures are more collectivist.

High and low masculinity

'High masculine' cultures value achievement, control and social power in addition to well-defined gender roles. In 'low masculine' cultures, cooperation is valued and achievement should not come at the expense of others: gender roles are also less distinct or more overlapping. Japan is the most masculine culture identified by Hofstede, while Scandinavian countries were among the lowest. Attitudes toward science are reflected in this dimension. High masculine cultures value proactive problem solving and view science as the key to addressing many problems. Low masculine cultures are more willing to tolerate problems and ambiguity while multiple solutions are weighed for their possible benefits and disadvantages.

Adapted from Hofstede and Hofstede(9) and Dysart-Gale(10)

Applying these dimensions to medical culture can provide perceptive insights. Like an army, medical culture is characterised by quite a rigid hierarchy.(11) As we hinted in Chapter 3, this traditional model of power and interpersonal relations emerged from a combination of factors in the nineteenth century.(12) Hierarchical relationships are a useful strategy to reduce the anxiety associated with uncertainty, as doubt or unknown outcomes are better tolerated through reliance on the authority of those with more status and power. The negative corollary, however, is that junior staff are largely unable to question the behaviours or decisions made by their seniors.

Medical culture scores quite high on the 'masculinity' dimension, where achievement, control and social power are considered more important than mutual cooperation. Similarly, those higher up the food chain have considerable power and control, not only over medical decisions, but also over their interactions with juniors, who find they are largely required to accept these power differentials. At worst, this culture then lends itself to disrespectful behaviour towards juniors, without fear of challenge or recrimination. For example, bullying within training or in medical practice has been identified as a pervasive and ongoing problem that seems quite difficult to stop or prevent.(13)

Despite the general trend in Western society towards individualism, medical culture appears to be located at the collectivist end of the spectrum, where individualism is secondary to group loyalty. As an illustration, 'whistle-blowers' are not well tolerated in medicine: this probably arises from a perceived failure to be loyal to the ideals and reputation of the group.(14, 15) Whistle-blowers may also be exposing the profession to potential shame. Similarly, interpersonal conflict in medical practice is largely avoided: doctors are often strangely reluctant to give direct feedback to colleagues who are not doing well or who have made a technical error.

In summary, medical culture appears to be more collectivist than individualist, with high power distance, high masculinity, and high levels of uncertainty avoidance. Interestingly, this particular set of interpersonal relations has not been problematised in the academic literature. The absence of critical articles about medical hierarchy, for instance, illustrates how these particular underlying dimensions are quite pervasive, how members of the community are highly acculturated into these social mores, and how difficult it is to question the 'rules' that guide our day-to-day behaviours and actions.

Subcultures of medicine

While these comments refer to biomedical culture generally, there are considerable local variations. Hospital practice is now quite different from primary care in focus, goals and work culture. Even within hospital practice, there is considerable difference in the work culture between general physicians, obstetricians, surgeons, and so on.(16) The culture of specialist training also varies considerably. Most schemes expect high levels of commitment and duty to service, often requiring trainees to put their personal needs aside for many years.

The capacity to tolerate uncertainty has been noted as a feature of general practice, where undifferentiated disease is common. There is perhaps less emphasis on power and control: a low masculine culture and a flatter hierarchy might be more attractive for female graduates.(17) Similarly, GPs often think of themselves as 'cultural brokers', negotiating between the world of the patient (background, ideas, personal culture) and the world of biomedicine (understanding disease, requirements for surgery or medications, and so on). GPs often negotiate between primary care and hospital practice, with its (necessarily) different focus on technical tasks and procedures. Some GPs visit their own patients when they are in hospital, helping their later transition back into primary care.

What, then, of undergraduate training? How do students learn the rules and expectations of the culture they are now entering? In a similar way, novice monks would need to learn the particular rules and behaviours for their monastery and profession. The next section looks at undergraduate acculturation into medical ways of thinking and being.

Acculturation into medicine

While much of medical training is exciting and exhilarating, becoming a doctor is a complex and potentially difficult process. Students commonly enter training with two underlying ideas: that medicine is a science; and that learning medicine will help them to help others.

Lock and Scheper-Hughes have identified various routines that characterise each particular subculture.(18) In medical training, students have to learn to comply with these routines, even if they appear quite strange initially. Similarly, there are many social rituals in medicine that reaffirm medicine's dominant values and the dimensions of culture noted above. Behaviour in ward rounds and operating theatres, for example, has been identified as important reinforcing rituals within medical practice.(19)

As students have already developed their own identity before they enter medical school, learning to become a doctor is a secondary socialisation process.(20) While this is a complex process, most students receive no explicit teaching on professional identity formation. Hilton and Slotnik describe three contributing factors that will eventually transform students' thinking about themselves and their world. These are: learning from, and reflecting on, clinical experience; role modelling,(21) where students are exposed to the behaviour of teachers and peers; and the institutional environment that will both foster and inhibit their emerging identities.(22)

This process of *how* students move from being 'lay people' with limited medical knowledge or skills to the role of 'doctor' has been the subject of considerable research. In their now-classic 1961 study into the socialisation of medical students, Becker and others identified some of the characteristics that medical students tend to adopt during their training. We believe these observations remain true today. One is the acquisition of a point of view and terminology of a technical kind, which allows students to think about patients and disease in quite new and different ways: 'They look upon death and disabling disease, not with the horror and sense of tragedy the layman finds appropriate, but as problems in medical responsibility.'(23)

Becker writes of a 'transformation of identity' that helps medical students to *separate* themselves from their patients. Hafferty also identifies how students' first exposures to death and dying act as 'rites of passage', effectively distancing them from their previous lay identities and enabling a more 'medical' persona. In this way, students' encounters with dying patients can help them acquire medicine's dominant value of 'detachment' and provide some separation from lay values of concern and affectivity.(24)

Hafferty suggests that students are initially engulfed by their learning tasks as basic science students and are thus effectively distanced from their more caring roles. Early in their course, then, many students believe their very survival in training depends on accumulating sufficient scientific facts and finding general principles that explain particular observations.(24) Students may then surmise that the correct stance is to be observant, detached, and objective about one's findings and conclusions.

Other researchers (for example, Konner(25) and Sinclair(26)) have also explored this socialisation process. Medical students learn to acquire codes of behaviour – such as prioritising biomedical data over psychosocial information – within medico-cultural institutions. They adopt hierarchical systems of knowledge (evidence over anecdote), hierarchical roles (senior doctors over juniors, doctors over other professionals), and the capacity for distancing, as noted above. And they learn to conform to the cultural expectations that govern interpersonal relationships.

Learning to be a doctor requires some reconciliation between two broad ideas: doctor as scientist, and doctor as helper. Learning to participate in medicine will necessarily involve an ongoing tension between these two major tasks.

Student observations of clinical training

Medical student writing can theoretically reveal the tension between 'letting go of old' and 'acquiring new' behaviours. In the last 30 or so years, written accounts from medical students around the world have been used to illustrate how this reconciliation can be quite problematic, providing an interesting window into the culture of medicine. In 1993, Branch et al. first discussed 'critical incident reports' written by junior students. These reports are short narratives about meaningful clinical events which are then read and discussed with other students and faculty. From reviewing over 100 reports, they concluded that students were struggling with 'a deep-seated conflict – maintaining empathy for patients while becoming acculturated to medicine'.(27)

Examples of these reports include students being shocked at the behaviour of senior doctors (e.g., an argument between a surgeon and his obese patient who required – but did not receive – surgery); rudeness and derisive behaviour towards patients; and sexist behaviour towards nurses. Other students reported their struggle not to identify 'too closely' with patients of their own age, feeling overwhelmed by failed cardiopulmonary resuscitation, or feeling remorse that their capacity for empathy was being reduced (also known as 'emotional blunting' (28)). Such blunting seems to be an almost inevitable outcome of the necessity to acquire and maintain a certain degree of distance from various patients or situations that could overload the student's capacity for clear thought and action.(29)

In our university, undergraduate students in their last three years of training write 'Thought Provoking Episode Reports': structured reflection on professional issues arising from day-to-day learning experiences.(30) We have reviewed over 1000 TPERs since 1999.(31)

For example, a student describes the interaction between a registrar and an elderly woman. During the physical examination, the registrar rather abruptly tells her she has a cancerous tumour, then walks off, leaving the student with the patient. 'I wanted to do serious bodily harm to my registrar for betraying my admiration for him for his callous treatment of a terrified old lady … but I felt powerless to do or say anything, I was also furious with myself, for my lack of knowledge to answer her questions … and worst of all for not knowing what to say to her.'

A significant sociocultural process here has effectively silenced this student. He realises the elderly woman has been callously treated, but he is caught in a bind between his personal knowledge ('this is not how we treat vulnerable old people') and the prevailing professional milieu ('the registrar has higher status and as such is unquestionable'). He is furious but unable to act because he has been rendered impotent by the discourse of medical training, which says he has no power or speaking rights.

These accounts correlate closely with recent research from Murison and others from John Hopkins School of Medicine in the US. Their survey of graduating students identified three clusters of major formative events: 'inspiring experiences' (especially finding a positive role model), 'mortality-related experiences', and 'negative experiences related to the learning environment'.(32) These clusters are consistent with the underlying tension noted above: between helping people through empathic connection, and the required stance of distance and objectivity.

Inspiring experiences usually describe a role model who is 'scientific' but who is also capable of authentic and empathic relationships with patients. Mortality-related experiences are often very powerful ones, where students lament the perceived lack of response or anguish from other health professionals after a death, worrying that they too 'might end up like that'. 'Negative experiences' in the learning environment include instances of disrespectful behaviour towards patients or students, including overt cases of bullying.(33, 34)

In terms of the socialisation process in becoming a doctor, such negative experiences can be devastating. Students' naïve expectations of the caring profession they are aspiring to join are now being contested. How do they reconcile their ambitions to help others, if this is how they are expected to behave? While fortunately most role modelling is positive, it is likely that many students are profoundly affected by the dissonance between their ideals about medical practice and their observations of clinical reality. Students are often critical of poor role modelling, perhaps as part of the inherent tension between 'discipline' (learning to conform) and 'dissent' (feeling uncomfortable with required tasks) that characterise entry into any new culture.(18)

In summary, these accounts illustrate a particularly difficult transition for students as they enter the medical profession. The existential problem is how to continue to engage as a caring person, while also acquiring the necessary 'objective' clinical detachment. Fortunately, there is a solution to these complex – and at times negative learning experiences, and that is through reflective practice. Facilitated reflection as part of experiential learning is crucially important if students are to reconcile their wide variety of learning events with their emerging professional identity. Methods of reflective practice include writing, peer discussion and mentoring, which we will discuss in the next chapter.

The next section explores a 'worked example' of the intersection between individual and medical cultures: the reactions of doctors to complaints.

Complaints and medical culture

We will discuss adverse outcomes of medical care in more depth in Chapter 11. In the meantime, analysis of doctors' reactions to complaints provides useful insight into the self of the doctor and the culture of medicine.

Doctors often feel a complaint is an indication of professional or personal failure. Many doctors have a high investment in their role as a doctor, making little differentiation between their own self and their workplace role. Complaints, then, can feel like an assault or threat to one's sense of self, and have the potential to trigger substantial guilt and shame.(35, 36) After an adverse outcome or on receipt of a complaint, the doctor usually searches for where he or she went 'wrong': what they did not know, or what was the error in diagnosis or management. Many doctors make highly critical and internalised judgements about their own competence and identity.(37)

Doctors appear to have both emotional and intellectual responses to complaints: these responses emerge concurrently. The intellectual response is based on a biomedical appraisal of the circumstances, while emotional responses are frequently reported to be disproportionate to the degree of accuracy of the complaint.(38) For example, a complaint about a minor medical omission, or about having been a bit offhand, may be quite devastating for the doctor. Conversely, a complaint following a serious adverse outcome may barely trigger an emotional response. These responses often occur in private and are often not shared with trusted colleagues or spouses.

Complaints have an impact on the person of the doctor both immediately after they are received and in the long term, although the impact usually softens over time. (39) Significant emotional responses include feelings of anger, depression, and loss of enjoyment in the practice of medicine. Doctors report feelings of reduced trust of patients and of reduced goodwill towards them. These findings are significant: if the doctor is emotionally damaged from a complaint, their ability to bring their whole self to consultations for the benefit of future patients is reduced. More recent research has indicated that doctors' emotional recovery from these events is highly variable.(40)

In terms of future practice, other responses that may impact on patient care after a complaint is received include reduced confidence in clinical judgement and reduced ability to tolerate uncertainty.(41) Instead of the complaint triggering a thoughtful review of individual competencies within complex medical systems, some doctors lose confidence and become quite apprehensive and guarded in their practice.(42) This can lead to the practice of what is known as 'defensive medicine' (see Chapter 11).

In brief, doctors' personal and emotional responses to errors and/or complaints are highly significant, but the potential impact of these responses on the well-being of the doctor and their clinical work has been recognised only in the last decade or so. Their responses indicate a considerable fragility of doctors within the culture of medicine. The doctor may be isolated, might not feel safe enough to discuss errors or complaints with others, and is usually unsupported in an environment where perfection is expected and mistakes are seen as a moral failing. The personality of doctors, their training, and the culture of medicine all contribute to these overall outcomes.

We continue this chapter by further exploring variations in the work culture of clinical practice.

Supportive and unsupportive working environments

Significant variations can be identified and examined within different communities of clinical practice.(43) It is helpful to compare two highly polarised working environments – one supportive, the other unsupportive (Box 9.3).

BOX 9.3 THE CULTURE OF CLINICAL ENVIRONMENTS

Unsupportive working environment	Supportive working environment
You're expected to know verything	It is OK to not know everything
Questions indicate 'poor knowledge' or not coping	The motto is: 'There is no such thing as a stupid question'
Hierarchy-centred	Patient- or learner-centred
'Keep your mouth shut, don't rock the boat'	Can express views freely, can challenge others' ideas
Time pressure, everyone is always very 'busy'	Time to discuss work, time to reflect on work
Atmosphere is tense, 'walking on egg-shells'	Relaxed but focused environment
Very serious, no laughter	Regular laughter
High staff turnover, always seem to be working with new nurses, doctors, other staff	Staff very stable with a long history of working together, many respectful nurse–doctor relationships, can trust each other's assessments
Contribution of other professional groups less valued	Nurses, receptionists respected as providing important contributions in patient care
Focus on disease and medical details exclusively	A further focus on persons, their supports and social contexts
Patients who are not doing well are blamed for being 'difficult' or 'non-compliant'	Regular team review of 'difficult' patients and how to understand them
No one makes decisions or takes initiative; wait instead for orders from above	People take initiative in the service of the patient
Not OK to ask others for help	OK to ask for help
Mistakes not discussed, seen as indication of 'failure'	Mistakes seen as an opportunity for learning about systems and risks to patient safety
Inability to help patients is not discussed	Despite best efforts, suffering is acknowledged as unavoidable, i.e. staff have realistic goals
Leaders are 'the boss' all the time, micro-management of small tasks	Leaders trust other staff, can delegate tasks effectively
'Lone Ranger' environment, individuals work separately	Team environment with shared goals
Shame-based culture	Learning-based culture
No professional supports in place	Staff have wide variety of professional supports, e.g. mentoring, peer groups, Balint groups
Limited range of non-professional activities	Staff have wide variety of personal activities away from medicine
High power distance or hierarchical structure; juniors are unable to debate or question decision-making	Lower power distance / flatter hierarchy; juniors can raise questions about decisions and how they are made
Achievement, control and social power highly valued (high masculinity)	Cooperation and relationships more valued (lower masculinity)
Guidelines and rules followed rigidly (low tolerance of uncertainty)	Guidelines less rigid (higher tolerance of uncertainty)

This table also illustrates the connections between support, reflection, and learning. In a supportive environment, reflection and learning take place as part of regular and normal clinical enquiry without hierarchical barriers. As we saw in Chapter 8, these more supportive cultures will enhance patient outcomes, largely because individual doctors will be less stressed and they will be able to work well with each other. Vignette 9.1 includes examples from our own experience at both ends of the spectrum.

VIGNETTE 9.1 EXPERIENCES OF MEDICAL CULTURE

WC: My early training experience of general practice was in one of the best learning cultures of my medical training. My GP teacher cared about his patients, his colleagues in the practice, his staff, his patients, and me! I had seen caring for others in previous work environments but never as a complete package.

His patients trusted him, not because he was a superb diagnostician or because he was more therapeutically perceptive than other doctors were, but because he genuinely cared about their well-being. His staff trusted him because he demonstrated this caring, shared his uncertainties when they arose and valued their opinions.

Hospital-based specialists did not intimidate him: they were simply colleagues who had a different skill-set to access for the benefit of his patients. Similarly, I was a colleague who was still learning in this particular field. My lack of knowledge did not make me a lesser person, just less expert as a GP. He did not dismiss my questions born of ignorance as being too stupid, and the learning environment that this attitude created was fantastic.

In short, the culture of his practice was based on support and caring. It was novel to me, and it worked! As a GP and teacher myself now, I try to support this sort of culture in my own practice, modelled on that experience.

HW: I have experienced some of the best and worst of medical cultures. Many medical workplaces are welcoming, respectful and energised, but in some others I have felt guarded and on edge. Perhaps my worst experience was during my Diploma of Obstetrics in the early 1980s in Auckland, NZ. This was at National Women's Hospital, found later to have been conducting the infamous observational trial of untreated cervical cancer.(44)

This hospital was run on a 'bully system', initiated from the professors at the top. While many staff were individually good to work with, the prevalent culture was one of poor teamwork and criticism of others. Paediatric and obstetric staff seemed at times to be at loggerheads in their approach to shared care of mothers and their babies, while the rigid hierarchical structure meant that junior staff and nurses were not treated respectfully. On arriving each day at the hospital gates, I often developed abdominal pain, which usually disappeared in the evenings on return home. I was unaware of the unethical research going on, but it was no surprise when the scandal broke in the public media later.(45)

Fortunately, things have changed considerably. From the professional horror that the above scandal evoked, there is now more awareness of ethical issues in clinical research and the influence of culture on patient outcomes.

Culture and professionalism

The final aspect of medical culture that we will discuss is that of professionalism. Doctors are members of the medical profession and as such are expected to embody certain behaviours. Societal expectations of a profession, and of doctors within it, can change over time. The question then arises: who is responsible for monitoring and regulating the actions of doctors – the profession itself, or society? First, however, what does 'professionalism' actually mean?

A 'profession' is an abstract term that identifies a particular group, then describes that group's role and function. There is a loosely defined social contract or relationship between a profession and society, which is always in negotiation and changing over time. The word 'profession' comes from the ancient notion 'to profess', in which a group claims to hold knowledge or skill in some particular area.(46) Being *expert* is not the same as being *professional*. A painter may 'expertly' paint a building, but successfully completing a task does not in itself indicate professionalism, merely expertise. Teachers, lawyers, clergy and doctors are considered professionals, as they have particular tasks and characteristics over and above being an expert.

Sociologists, and more recently doctors, have considered professionalism from differing vantage points. Three major theoretical approaches we will discuss are 'structural-functional', 'values-based', and 'civic'. In the **structural-functional model**, a profession has characteristics including a particular body of knowledge or skills, self-regulation of training and standards, and special privileges or rights that other members of society would not usually have.(47) In this historical model, the profession is also expected to be dedicated to public service. Individual professionals are expected to 'subordinate personal financial gains to the higher value of responsibility to the patient and to public interests.'(48) The profession is awarded a monopoly over specialised knowledge and skills. In return for this autonomy, society expects the knowledge to be used altruistically.

However, the tacit contract between the profession and society may break down in various ways. The profession could monopolise trade in a particular area, while members of the profession could excessively reward themselves for work that only this profession is permitted to perform. There was criticism of the structural-functional model of professionalism because of such issues in the 1960s and 1970s.(49) In response to these societal misgivings, the idea of **values-based professionalism** developed.

In this model, particular values are expected to be acknowledged and upheld by individual professionals and the profession as a whole. To be a member of their profession, doctors are expected to conform to its technical and ethical standards, exhibit particular types of behaviour in the workplace, and respect patients' human worth. This means a sense of trustworthiness and protection of values, non-exploitation, commitment, protection of confidentiality, compassion, integrity and interprofessional respect.(50)

Human experimentation in Nazi Germany is a well-documented example of a lack of professionalism and intraprofessional regulation. Those experiments were performed by doctors, apparently supported (or at least, not prevented) by the wider profession.(51) Another historic example was the misuse of psychiatry in the USSR. (52) These situations illustrate a failure of internal regulation by the profession, as well as a breakdown in the contract or relationship between the profession and society.

More recently, **civic professionalism** has developed in response to 'managed care', a method of health-care delivery in the US. There is a perceived mismatch between the profession's managerial approach and the actual needs of patients and communities, especially in disadvantaged areas.(53) Civic professionalism attempts to highlight the obligation of the profession to care for financially disadvantaged sectors of society, protect core health values, and remain accountable to public need.(54) This is a call for a more effective and functional medical–societal alliance.(55)

In all models of professionalism, there is an implied issue of regulation: who is responsible for acting when a doctor behaves 'unprofessionally' – the profession or society? Paul helpfully distinguishes between an *internal* morality of medicine ('values, norms, and rules that are intrinsic to the profession'), and an *external* morality (controls imposed from society on the profession to regulate doctors' behaviour).(56)

A recent example of these tensions is the 'unfortunate experiment' on women with cervical cancer in New Zealand. Internal and traditional values were illustrated by doctors who raised concerns about research ethics (the 'whistle-blowers'). Paul noted 'trustworthiness [of the medical profession] is enhanced by the self-respect accompanying ownership of professional standards', whereas the societal response was for more external regulation of ethical behaviour.(56)

The idea that the medical profession is in relationship with society is inherent in all these perspectives on professionalism. It is the profession's responsibility to monitor doctors' competence and performance. The profession also needs to monitor and comment on specific activities of doctors, such as the role of the doctor in political interrogations.(57) The culture of medicine is thus intricately related to professional mores and practices.

Conclusion

It is helpful to critically review one's own culture, noting the underlying expectations or social rules. Observations of student acculturation into medicine are useful, as they highlight students' difficulties in developing a coherent professional identity. Such observations also help to identify the hidden dimensions of medical culture and the ongoing tension between objectivity and caring.

While this chapter has identified many problems within medical culture, we are also mindful that when the culture is supportive, medical work can be exhilarating and rewarding.

SUMMARY POINTS

- Medical culture is the prevailing set of rules, expectations of behaviour, and social discourse that guides doctors' actions and interpersonal ways of relating.

- While biomedical rules remain quite homogeneous, subcultures or individual communities of clinical practice vary considerably.

- Students need to be provided with adequate coaching and mentoring if they are to successfully develop their own professional identity.

- Our responsibility as a profession is to recognise the importance of having a healthy, well-supported and resilient workforce set within a supportive medical culture.

References

1. Burri RV, Dumit J, eds. *Biomedicine as culture: instrumental practices, technoscientific knowledge, and new modes of life*. New York: Routledge, 2007.
2. Rhodes LA. Studying biomedicine as a cultural system. *Med Anthr* 1990:160–73.
3. Taylor JS. Confronting 'culture' in medicine's 'culture of no culture'. *Acad Med* 2003, 78(6):555–59.
4. O'Boyle CA, Waldron D. Quality of life issues in palliative medicine. *J Neurol* 1997, 244:S18–25.
5. Lock M, Gordon D, eds. *Biomedicine examined*. Dordrecht: Kluwer Academic Publishers, 1988.
6. Angell M, Kassirer JP, Relman AS. Looking back on the millennium in medicine [Editorial]. *N Engl J Med* 2000, 342(1):42–49.
7. Timmermans S, Berg M. *The gold standard: the challenge of evidence-based medicine and standardization in health care*. Philadelphia: Temple University Press, 2003.
8. Hofstede G, Bond MH. Hofstede's culture dimensions: an independent validation using Rokeach's value survey. *J Cross-Cult Psychol* 1984, 15(4):417–33.
9. Hofstede G, Hofstede G. *Cultures and organizations: software of the mind*. 2nd edn. New York: McGraw-Hill, 2005.
10. Dysart-Gale D. Cultural sensitivity beyond ethnicity: a universal precautions model. *Int J Allied Health Sci Pract* 2006, 4(1).
11. Kushner T, Thomasma D, eds. *Ward ethics: dilemmas for medical students and doctors in training*. Cambridge: Cambridge University Press, 2001.
12. Porter R. *The greatest benefit to mankind: a medical history of humanity*. New York: Norton, 1997.
13. Paice E, Aitken M, Houghton A, Firth-Cozens J. Bullying among doctors in training: cross sectional questionnaire survey. *BMJ* 2004, 329(7467):658.
14. Rhodes R, Strain JJ. Whistleblowing in academic medicine. *J Med Ethics* 2004, 30(1):35–39.
15. Near JP, Miceli MP. Retaliation against whistle blowers: predictors and effects. *J Appl Psychol* 1986, 71(1):137–45.
16. Katz P. *The scalpel's edge: the culture of surgeons*. Needham Heights, MA: Allyn and Bacon, 1999.
17. Kilminster S, Downes J, Gough B, Murdoch-Eaton D, Roberts T. Women in medicine – is there a problem? A literature review of the changing gender composition, structures and occupational cultures in medicine. *Med Educ* 2007, 41(1):39–49.
18. Lock M, Scheper-Hughes N. A critical-interpretive approach in medical anthropology: rituals and routines of discipline and dissent. In: Sargent C, Johnson T, eds. *Medical anthropology: contemporary theory and method*. Westport, CT: Praeger, 1996.
19. Fox NJ. Space, sterility and surgery: circuits of hygiene in the operating theatre. *Soc Sci Med* 1997, 45(5):649–57.

20. Cruess R, Cruess S, Steinert Y. *Teaching medical professionalism*. New York: Cambridge University Press, 2009.
21. Brosnan C, Turner B. *Handbook of the sociology of medical education*. London: Routledge, 2009.
22. Hilton SR, Slotnick HB. Proto-professionalism: how professionalisation occurs across the continuum of medical education. *Med Educ* 2005, 39(1):58–65.
23. Becker HS, Geer B, Hughes EC, Strauss AL. *Boys in white: student culture in medical school*. Piscataway: Transaction Books, 1977.
24. Hafferty FW. *Into the valley: death and the socialization of medical students*. New Haven: Yale University Press, 1991.
25. Konner M. *Becoming a doctor: a journey of initiation in medical school*. New York: Penguin Books, 1988.
26. Sinclair S. *Making doctors: an institutional apprenticeship*. New York: Berg Publishers, 1997.
27. Branch W, Pels RJ, Lawrence RS, Arky R. Becoming a doctor: critical-incident reports from third-year medical students. *N Engl J Med* 1993, 329:1130–32.
28. Bellini LM, Shea JA. Mood change and empathy decline persist during three years of internal medicine training. *Acad Med* 2005, 80(2):164–67.
29. Hojat M, Vergare M, Maxwell K. The devil is in the third year: a longitudinal study of erosion of empathy in medical school. *Acad Med* 2009, 84:1182–91.
30. Wilson HJ, Egan T, Friend R. Teaching professional development in undergraduate medical education. *Med Educ* 2003, 37(5):482–83.
31. Wilson HJ, Ayers K. Using significant event analysis in dental and medical education. *J Dent Educ* 2004, 68(4):446–50.
32. Murinson BB, Klick B, Haythornthwaite JA, Shochet R, Levine RB, Wright SM. Formative experiences of emerging physicians: gauging the impact of events that occur during medical school. *Acad Med* 2010, 85(8):1331.
33. Lempp H, Seale C. The hidden curriculum in undergraduate medical education: qualitative study of medical students' perceptions of teaching. *BMJ* 2004, 329(7468):770–73.
34. Paice E, Heard S, Moss F. How important are role models in making good doctors? *BMJ* 2002, 325(7366):707–10.
35. Firth-Cozens J. Doctors, their well-being, and their stress. *BMJ* 2003, 326(7391):670.
36. Wu AW. Medical error: the second victim. *BMJ* 2000, 320(7237):726.
37. Cunningham W, Dovey S. The effect on medical practice of disciplinary complaints: potentially negative for patient care. *NZ Med J* 2000, 113(1121):464–67.
38. Christensen JF, Levinson W, Dunn PM. The heart of darkness. *J Gen Int Med* 1992, 7(4):424–31.
39. Cunningham W. The immediate and long-term impact on New Zealand doctors who receive patient complaints. *NZ Med J* 2004, 117:1198.
40. Scott SD, Hirschinger LE, Cox KR, McCoig M, Brandt J, Hall LW. The natural history of recovery for the healthcare provider 'second victim' after adverse patient events. *BMJ* 2009, 18(5):325–30.
41. Cunningham W, Dovey S. Defensive changes in medical practice and the complaints process: a qualitative study of New Zealand doctors. *NZ Med J* 2006, 119:1244.
42. Wu AW, Folkman S, McPhee SJ, Lo B. Do house officers learn from their mistakes? *BMJ* 2003, 12(3):221–26.
43. Wenger E. *Communities of practice: learning, meaning, and identity*. Cambridge: Cambridge University Press, 1999.
44. Cartwright SR, Mackay EV. *The report of the committee of inquiry into allegations concerning the treatment of cervical cancer at National Women's Hospital and other related matters*. Wellington, NZ: Government Printing Office, 1988.
45. Coney S. *The unfortunate experiment*. Auckland: Penguin, 1988.

46. Richard L, Sylvia R, Sharon E. Professionalism and medicine's social contract. *J Bone Joint Surg* 2000, 82(8):1189–94.
47. Parsons T. The professions and social structure. *Social Forces* 1939, 17(4):457–67.
48. Oreopoulos D. Is medical professionalism still relevant? *Perit Dialysis Internat* 2003, 23(6):523–27.
49. Freidson E. *Professionalism reborn: theory, prophecy, and policy*. Chicago: University of Chicago Press, 1994.
50. Freidson E. *Professional dominance: the social structure of medical care*. New Brunswick: Transaction Publishers, 2006.
51. Alexander L. Medical science under dictatorship. *N Engl J Med* 1949, 241(2):39–47.
52. Bloch S. The political misuse of psychiatry in the Soviet Union. *Psychiat Ethic* 1991, 24:493–515.
53. Relman AS. Medical professionalism in a commercialized health care market. *JAMA* 2007, 298(22):2668–74.
54. Rothman DJ. Medical professionalism – focusing on the real issues. *N Engl J Med* 2000, 342(17):1284–86.
55. Cohen JJ, Cruess S, Davidson C. Alliance between society and medicine. *JAMA* 2007, 298(6):670–73.
56. Paul C. Internal and external morality of medicine: lessons from New Zealand. *BMJ* 2000, 320(7233):499.
57. Bloche MG, Marks JH. Doctors and interrogators at Guantanamo Bay. *N Engl J Med* 2005, 353(1):6–8.

Chapter 10

Reflective Practice

CONTENTS

Part 1: Reflection

Introduction

We have already mentioned the word 'reflection' in several previous chapters, suggesting it is a helpful method for exploring the assumptions of medicine and problems in the doctor–patient relationship. It also contributes to self-care and emerging professional identity. By reflection, we mean taking the time to review and analyse the work of doctoring. This chapter provides more details about the role and outcomes of reflection in clinical practice. Reflective skills can be learned, and the outcomes of putting them into action can be considerable for both doctors and their patients. In our postgraduate courses it has been fascinating both to watch experienced clinicians learn to use these reflective techniques and to see what happens with their patients when they do.

Epstein talks about the capacity of doctors to 'question, expand and contextualise their own knowledge continuously.'(1) The goal of reflection is to 'develop not only one's knowledge and skills, but also habits of mind that promote informed flexibility, ongoing learning, and humility'. In the past, reflection was neither discussed nor taught formally. Now, it is becoming a professional requirement: all health professionals, not just doctors, have to demonstrate that they are using some method of reviewing their work as part of their continuing professional development.

There has been growing criticism of the effectiveness of older models of continuing medical education (CME), traditionally based on formal didactic teaching and narrowly focused academic knowledge.(2) Davis et al., for example, draw on a number of well-conducted trials to show that 'didactic sessions do not appear to be effective in changing physician performance'. Instead, the data showed 'evidence that interactive CME sessions that enhance participant activity and provide the opportunity to practice skills can effect change in professional practice and, on occasion, health care outcomes'.(3)

Brigley et al. expand on this theme, suggesting that continuing education for medical professionals needs to be based on a reflective model. As they put it, 'continuing professional development, which draws on learning by reflective practice ... emphasises self-directed learning, professional self-awareness, learning developed in context, multidisciplinary and multilevel collaboration, the learning needs of individuals and their organizations, and an inquiry-based concept of professionalism.'(4)

The literature on reflection has increased enormously in the last 20 years. At times taking a lead from nursing, this subject is becoming well theorised in the medical literature. Undergraduate medical students are now provided with regular structured reflective activities.(5) Students also receive feedback on their capacity for reflection,(6) which is often incorporated into summative assessment through portfolios,(7, 8) 'significant event analysis'(9) or other essays that require reflection on learning and/or clinical experiences.(10) Reflection must be integrated with experiential learning if students are to develop their professional identity.(11)

Having studied effectively for entry to medical school, most doctors have the ability to identify areas of weakness and plan for further revision. However, there is a difference between reflection on one's knowledge in preparation for written examinations, and reflection on clinical practice; it is this latter aspect that we focus on now. Mulling over clinical situations or simply chatting about one's day with friends, colleagues or spouse is a helpful start to reflection, but it is not necessarily very focused or effective.

Reflection can be difficult, even painful, so it is often avoided. At times there are subtle pressures on students and doctors *not* to look very closely at specific situations, as doing so might raise uncomfortable questions. Reflection in those situations can be subversive, destabilising, even a 'political act'.

On the other hand, reflection can make medicine much more enjoyable, provide more job satisfaction, and give more meaning to one's work. It can make the difference between repeating one's style of work over and over again, or each year of work building on the last, providing the basis for interesting and stimulating learning. In brief, we believe that reflection is a clinical tool, just like doing an accurate cardiovascular examination or knowing which investigation to use. Reflection is also supportive and sustaining for the doctor as a health professional.

We will now turn to some vignettes which illustrate general concepts. This leads to a discussion of various types of reflective techniques and activities that can be used for specific purposes. Journals of medical indemnity providers often include short clinical stories like those below.

VIGNETTE 10.1 JUST A SORE THROAT

A 59-year-old female smoker attended her GP with a two-week history of sore throat and hoarse voice. The doctor diagnosed a viral respiratory infection and provided paracetamol. Over the next two to three months the patient had four further consultations, variably describing similar symptoms. On each occasion she was diagnosed with a throat infection and/or tonsillitis and given antibiotics.

She then saw a different doctor with a further sore throat. The history was now of four to five months, and hard immobile lymph nodes were found in the neck. The patient was referred urgently to an Ear Nose and Throat specialist, where laryngeal cancer with secondary lymph gland enlargement was diagnosed. A complaint was made about the first doctor for 'delay in diagnosis'.

Briefly then, the first doctor had attributed each of the recurring upper respiratory symptoms to infectious causes, perhaps forgetting about other diagnoses. The cognitive error might have been 'availability bias' and/or 'premature closure' where the diagnosis each time was influenced by the previous and readily available one.(12) We will return to this story shortly.

VIGNETTE 10.2 BREAKING BAD NEWS

A 65-year-old female patient was admitted to hospital after vomiting up blood. On further questioning, she also mentioned she had suffered a previous bout of abdominal pains and had been generally unwell for some months. An MRI revealed a large cancer in the pancreas. The news of this cancer was broken to the patient during the ward round the next day. However, the patient felt disappointed and unsupported about how this was done ('It was abrupt, no time for discussion, family not present, no treatment offered', and so on). The family made a complaint to the hospital about her 'quality of care'.

It is possible, of course, that the patient and family were 'shooting the messenger', or in other words, becoming angry at the person who was informing them of the bad news. However, there did seem to be a problem. The medical team appeared to be unaware of the immediate effect of this news on the patient. One wonders why this might be so. Was it a problem of fatigue, a workload issue, or difficulty in responding to her apparent distress? One could also consider the use of a routine ward round for such a major disclosure, wondering about other venues or arrangements for doing so.

VIGNETTE 10.3 THE NEW REGISTRAR

The third case is a 28-year-old registrar on a medical ward. There had been some mutterings of discontent from his colleagues and he was called to see the Chief Medical Officer about being 'continually rude, dismissive of others' opinions and excessively critical of their patient care'. It seemed that this doctor was unaware of his effect on others in the team, or if he was aware, was not able to act on it.

The common theme in these three cases seems to be the absence of thinking carefully about the *work of doctoring*. Either this can be in the actual moment while the patient is present, or later, at the end of the day, when things have settled down. Reflective practice is designed to increase the capacity to be fully present for each particular clinical moment.

What is reflection?

A commonly used definition is that proposed by Schon: 'Reflection involves thoughtfully considering one's own experiences in applying knowledge to practice, while being coached by professionals within the discipline.'(13) This is different to ordinary thinking: it is purposeful, intentional, structured, and focused. It requires time and effort, it is aimed at producing better clinical outcomes, and it is a skill that can be learned. Our own definition is slightly different and broader, leading to three outcomes:

Reflective practice is an approach to health professional work where structured reflective activities such as writing or mentoring are used regularly to enhance learning, clinical efficacy, and professional resilience.

'Reflection-in-action' and 'reflection-on-action'

Schon helpfully distinguishes between two different, but related, types of reflection. (13) **Reflection-*in*-action** means taking a pause in the moment to think about what is happening. With reference to the vignettes above, such thinking could be: 'Why does this patient get so many so sore throats?' 'How is this patient taking this bad news so far?' 'How I am getting on with others?'

Reflection-*on*-action occurs later: 'How did my day go today, what sticks in my mind? Was there something not quite right that I need to think about more carefully?' Usually, the unsatisfactory or unresolved issues spring to mind. The task then is to have a method of more structured reflection, over and above simply chatting or mulling things over.

Neighbour's model of consultation includes a final task of 'housekeeping': a quick review of what has happened.(14) This reflection-*on*-action encourages the doctor to be aware of his emotional responses within each consultation, making those feelings overt rather than shelving them away. Practising reflection-*on*-action leads to more effective reflection-*in*-action. 'Pausing' a consultation, for example by doing a brief summary or looking something up, helps to get one's breath back in order to review what is actually happening in the room. This is reflection-*in*-action.

Reflection in the moment or answering the question 'What is happening here right now?' brings both content and process issues to fuller consciousness, enabling the doctor to identify any doubts or warning bells. It is often helpful to acknowledge, and then act on, one's intuition.

The experiential learning cycle

The concept of reflective practice links with that of experiential learning. To briefly summarise, experiential learning is learning through the transformation of experience. (15) This theory proposes four processes in developing a high degree of competence: participating in particular experiences; reflecting on what happened; building theory to support practice; and experimenting further to develop competence and confidence. This outline applies just as much to sporting situations as it does to learning communication skills or how to perform a clinical examination (Figure 10.1).

FIGURE 10.1 THE EXPERIENTIAL LEARNING CYCLE

New ways of behaving
(increasing confidence
and competence)

Experience

Planning and
incorporating
new ideas

Review and reflect
(What is going on here?
What is this all about?)

Understanding background
issues (building theory)

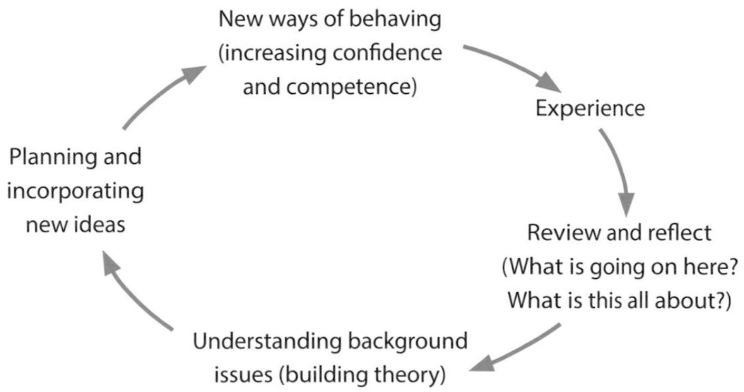

Adapted from Kolb(15)

In this understanding of learning, the learner engages with each step of the cycle (e.g. learning to be a doctor, flying an aeroplane, playing golf, inserting intravenous lines, consulting with patients, and so on), transforming their current and future experiences. Practical learning is more than knowing facts. Learning includes changing behaviours (such as clinical technique) and attitudes, as well as accumulating a body of knowledge (theories and facts). Learning is 'constructed' by learners, being relevant to their own current needs and values, especially those they perceive to be important. In the practice of medicine, with its wealth of clinical experience, reflection is integral to the process of learning because it enables those experiences to contribute to the learner's emerging professional identity.

Effective learning is best attained by engaging in all four of the processes described above. When learning feels difficult, it is likely that one or more of them has been omitted. Learning consultation skills, for instance, is helped by later review or reflecting-on-action. Here is an example.

VIGNETTE 10.4 THE BAR MANAGER

A 23-year-old bar manager attended his GP with urinary frequency and dysuria. The GP considered a couple of diagnostic possibilities and did an STD check and urinalysis, telling the patient that the likely diagnosis was chlamydia, for which there is oral treatment. However the patient insisted on getting an injection. The GP maintained that unless the swab result came back as gonorrhoea, an injection is not usually required.

That night, the GP went to a friend's place for a meal. She managed to find a couple of private moments to chat with a colleague about the case, since she was puzzled as to why a patient would want a painful injection rather than tablets. On chatting, she realised that she knew very little about her patient, but had simply assumed that he was single and that STDs were an occupational hazard. As they talked, she wondered whether this patient's request for an injection might have been a sort of 'punishment' for his 'crime' of unprotected sex.

During a follow-up consultation with the patient later, the GP was more curious, asking some naïve questions of the patient about his life and the impact of these symptoms. It turned out that the patient was from a large religious family. He felt guilty, but was also afraid of becoming infertile from having an STD. With more open and frank discussion, the patient's fears were addressed more fully.

This short scenario illustrates the benefit of simply chatting about medical issues of the day with a colleague. Reflection-on-action often increases the capacity for thinking in the moment during later consultations. The reflection here was relatively unstructured, but it was still quite effective. In an informal way, doctors are doing this all the time with their colleagues. We contend that more structured methods of reflection are required when such chats are not quite sufficient.

Before we list these more structured methods, it is helpful to acknowledge that there are many 'barriers' to reflective practice. These barriers need to be identified and worked through if one is to try these techniques or, in the longer term, to include regular reflective activities as part of one's working life.

Barriers to reflection

Thinking back to the assumptions of biomedicine outlined in Chapter 3, the first barrier is that reflection is not 'in the rules' or part of the 'culture' of medicine. If doctors are scientists, and scientists are supposed to be 'detached observers', then there is no need to reflect on one's interpersonal interactions with patients. Scientists are not 'part of the picture': they are on the outside, looking in.

The second barrier is medicine's focus on *content*, as compared to *process*. In the 'Breaking bad news' vignette, for example, the content is *what* was discussed: cancer of the pancreas, various treatment options, and so on. The process is *how* it was discussed: the choice of venue and controlling for privacy, introductions from the team, eliciting the patient's current understanding, breaking the news, and so on. The problem in the ward round seemed to be less about the actual diagnosis and possible treatments (which were not in doubt). Instead, the problem seemed to be *how* the team conveyed that news and *how* they responded to the patient's reaction to that news.

Speaking broadly, medicine has been rather slow to pick up on the importance of process, no doubt due to the heavy emphasis in the last hundred or so years on improving biomedical content and knowledge. Reflection, on the other hand, helps to elicit the issues around process that are less readily apparent. Most students and doctors think about their work a great deal, as they have considerable investment in being a good doctor and in developing a sense of competence and satisfaction. They attend conferences, workshops and ongoing medical education activities, but most of this work is orientated around the content of clinical medicine and the latest diagnostic and treatment techniques. When it comes to the less well-defined process of interpersonal issues with patients or colleagues, methods of reflection and improvement are less organised and accessible.

Third, most role models in medical school and early clinical years do not demonstrate how doctors might reflect on their practice.(16) For example, reviewing the more difficult consultations at the end of a ward round would highlight a focus on the interpersonal aspects of medical care.(17) The absence of explicit reflection within role modelling is a significant barrier to further uptake by future students and doctors.

The fourth barrier is that reflection can be uncomfortable. It can raise feelings and issues that are difficult to live with. Reflection might identify things about ourselves that we would rather not know, or things that would be difficult to change. So intuitively it is often put off until later. This is known as procrastination.

The final barrier to reflection is the issue of shame.[1] Shame is a difficult problem in medicine, because by definition it is hidden and not discussed.(18) Lempp and Seale, for example, have noted how undergraduate students describe a 'hierarchical and competitive atmosphere … in which haphazard instruction and teaching by humiliation occur, especially during the clinical training years'.(19) Sinclair also points out: 'Teaching by humiliation can only work if the failure to give the right answer is seen as a personal moral failing.'(20) In other words, students can learn to

---

1 See also Chapters 3 and 8.

internalise any lack of knowledge as a personal deficit, rather than as something they could simply look up later.

Perhaps the emphasis in medicine on always 'getting it right' or 'training for certitude'(21) causes a particular learning injury which then acts as an ongoing barrier to reflection. From the fear of further humiliation, doctors are less likely to raise their own doubts about their practice or ask another person for advice. In a previous publication, we have already identified shame as a potential barrier to one-to-one mentoring or supervision.(22)

These are significant barriers that need to be identified and acknowledged if medical culture is to become more reflective.

Depth of reflection

Three commonly observed levels of reflection are **description**, **analysis**, and **evaluation** (or implications). In **descriptive** writing, for example, events – including the people involved and their roles – are described simply and factually. Ideas are linked by time or the sequence of events, rather than by their inherent meaning.(23)

Analysis identifies the main topics or issues arising from the story. Points on which further reflection might occur are identified but not discussed in depth. Usually, these points are common professional issues such as confidentiality, communication between professionals, death and dying, adverse events, hierarchy, and so on. Feelings and emotions might be mentioned, but with limited acknowledgement of their influence in the situation. Interpretations are often couched in rather simplistic terms (black and white, good versus bad), without further nuances being considered.

The third and deeper form of reflection is known as **evaluation**. This level of reflection includes mulling over various possible angles on a particular incident, wondering about motives and background influences, and being open to a range of possibilities and multiple perspectives without simplistic judgement. Such deliberations include consideration of the influence of the wider context and background. Self-questioning and the effect of the incident on oneself is discussed, including feelings and responses to those feelings. Professional insights are identified, including the implications for future learning, work, or even for the profession as a whole. Often, the *meaning* of the event or clinical situation is clarified for the writer, including any shifts in understanding from a prior stance to a modified one.

Al-Shehri, for example, classified GPs who wrote about their clinical work as descriptive, analytical, and evaluative.(24) Descriptive GPs 'wrote about their experience without any ownership of that experience or its implications'; nor did they discuss what 'those events meant for them'. Analytical GPs elaborated more on their experiences and noted the underlying topics at hand, but did not include the implications for them professionally. Evaluative GPs included discussion about what these events actually meant for them or for the profession, including imaginative conjecture on the various motives and backgrounds of people involved.

For each level of writing, Al-Shehri provided feedback that was designed to help that GP progress to a deeper level, concluding that it was both possible and helpful to increase GPs' level of reflection about clinical practice. Similarly, it is possible to grade and coach medical students into greater depths of reflection on learning.(25)

Perspective transformation

Deeper reflection is necessary in situations that don't fit the usual pattern, such as an adverse outcome arising from a routine procedure or strong unexpected feelings emerging within a consultation. Evaluative reflection on such occasions has also been referred to as 'premise' reflection, since the process of examining and exploring an experience or issue of concern can alter one's underlying ideas, concepts, or even sense of self.(26) This outcome is known as perspective transformation.

According to Mezirow, premise reflection means 'the critique of *assumptions* about the content or process of problem solving': 'The critique of premises or presuppositions pertains to problem *posing*, as distinct to problem *solving*. Problem posing involves making a taken-for-granted situation problematic, raising questions regarding its validity.'(27) [Our emphasis]

For example, the 'heartsink' experience is an excellent trigger for premise reflection. Here, the expectation of the doctor's efficacy is being challenged by the patient, who is somehow not behaving as expected. Rather than blaming the patient, premise reflection can identify the hidden rules or assumptions that have created this tension.

A second example is the doctor-as-patient. As we have seen, doctors can react rather poorly to their own illness, often presenting late to others for medical help. However, illness also comes with considerable potential for learning about the lived experience or nature of illness. Suddenly, the world of the patient is accessible and familiar. Many pathographies (personal accounts of illness by doctors) illustrate an extraordinary perspective transformation, impacting on how the doctor works in the future, as well as their capacity for understanding and empathy with patients. There is now a bridge between the world of the patient and the world of the doctor.

A third example of perspective transformation is the insightful clinical work by the US endocrinologist Clifton Meador, who identified many patients who did not fit the disease model – patients with 'undiagnosable' persisting symptoms. Rather than taking for granted the assumptions that underpin much of modern clinical practice, Meador reflected deeply on these unexpected illness patterns.(28) Just as Alexander Fleming noticed the rings of bacterial inhibition on his agar plates, Meador noted what was different and unexpected, and then explored why. This is the true scientist at work: not taking observations for granted; not forcing the patient into pre-identified categories; but coming up with an alternative explanatory theory. His book is an excellent example of perspective transformation through reflection on clinical experience.

A final example is drawn from our own teaching practice: we provide our postgraduate GPs with seminal articles on medical practice, many of which are acknowledged in this book. Through both iterative discussion about those challenging concepts and reflective writing about their own clinical work, GPs revise their understanding of general practice and their role within it. Many mention their increased resilience and better appreciation of their professional identity as a result.

Part 2: Methods of reflection

Various methods of structured reflection are available to doctors. Ideally, students in medical school will learn to use some of these techniques so they can more readily utilise them within specialty training programmes and clinical practice.

Reflective writing

Writing is a good entry into building reflective skills. Writing about particularly difficult work or clinical situations can be traced back to Flanagan's original work on 'critical incidents' in airline safety, which has now been transferred to many industrial and health professional contexts.(29) In medicine, this seminal work has led to Significant Incident Analysis(9) as a method of learning for undergraduate medical students, as well as for analysis of adverse outcomes of medical care.(30) There is a well-developed academic literature in the nursing profession on the value of reflection for clinical practice and much of this is based on reflective writing. There is no reason why doctors cannot follow this lead.

It is helpful to use a simple structure for writing down one's ideas and thoughts. Feelings such as disappointment, fear or embarrassment can be a barrier to reviewing particular events, so having a formal writing structure helps bypass any procrastination. Box 10.1 outlines two approaches which can be used as triggers for writing and subsequent reflection.

BOX 10.1 REFLECTIVE WRITING FRAMEWORKS

Johns and Freshwater(31)
- Background of/to the incident – time, place, location
- Details of what happened
- What were your thoughts and concerns at the time?
- What did you find most demanding about the incident?
- Which aspects of the incident do you consider most important for reflection?

Smith and Russell(32)
- Describe the events as you understood them
- Describe your feelings about the event
- What have you learned from this event?
- Given a similar situation, how would you now behave?

The writing task is to fill in the blanks under each point as honestly as possible. Sometimes it takes two or even three passes over the written material before the underlying major issues and implications begin to emerge or to make sense. It is not necessary to show the writing to anyone else, though of course that may be helpful. Writing about particular patients or incidents can be done as one-off exercises or incorporated into an ongoing record of work and learning as discussed below.

Logs, diaries and journals

A log is simply a list of events. In medicine, logs can keep track of the various types of patients that are seen, the hours worked, or even include rating scales on the difficulty of the day. Logs contain useful overall data as the basis for further analysis and reflection.

Diaries are like a stream of consciousness, a private record of significant events on a daily or regular basis. They usually include personal ideas and thoughts. Looking over the entries later can provide a fascinating insight into how experiences and values have changed (or not) after a passage of time.

Journals are a more comprehensive collection of writing about events, thoughts and feelings, sometimes based on a particular structure. They usually include deliberate analysis of specific events as well as various reflective tasks. Bolton talks of the learning journal as the 'cornerstone of reflective practice'.(33) The usefulness of journals (or any other reflective technique) will depend on the writer's depth of reflection.

In our postgraduate courses, we introduce reflection with the 'free writing' method (Box 10.2). Workshops for aspiring writers or health professionals often start with similar exercises.(33)

BOX 10.2 FREE WRITING METHOD

Step 1

Choose any clinical incident that has stayed with you for more than a few days. You may or may not have discussed it with others. It may be recent, or date from months or even years ago.

Divide a piece of writing paper into three columns, with the central column being the largest. In this central column, write an unedited narrative of the situation you have chosen. There are only two rules:

1. *Once you begin writing, continue to do so without stopping and without regard to spelling, grammar, or sentence structure. Just let your pen do the writing about the event and see where it takes you.*

2. *No one else is allowed to read what you have written, as this is completely private and personal. Write until you come to a natural stop, anywhere from 5 to 15 minutes.*

Step 2

Pause for a few minutes, then review what you have written. In the left-hand column, identify the topics and issues you were writing about (a word or two is sufficient). Go through your narrative a couple of times doing this sort of review. Read through all these annotations again as an overview.

Step 3

Then, in the right-hand column, note down any wider issues that emerge from your narrative and analysis. What does this situation mean for you? What might you do now? How would you approach similar situations in the future? Are there any changes you might make? And so on: write down whatever arises from your review.

Our postgraduate students often report how much they surprise themselves with what arises. Sometimes a clinical situation or event emerges from their writing that they had forgotten about. This writing can be very helpful, especially if they have wrestled internally for years about a particular patient or event. Given the research on personal disclosure, this result is not so surprising, as just getting significant events onto paper facilitates closure.(34) Free writing in this way is useful after a long day, after a stressful event, before going on holiday, before starting work again, and so on.

Reflective writing can also be combined with group work.(35, 36) Registrars in general practice, for example, are usually required to participate in various reflective activities about the process of their learning to become a GP. Various writing techniques could be usefully added.

In brief, writing is an effective, inexpensive and readily available reflective tool. Doctors can be coached into further depths of reflection. Generally speaking, the deeper one goes, the greater the benefit gained.

Other methods of reflection usually involve talking rather than writing, and this can be done with just one other person or in groups.

Specific insightful questions

Reflective discussion or writing can be triggered through the use of carefully chosen questions about a clinical issue or specific incident, with the aim of becoming more thoughtful about the doctor–patient relationship. Dobie uses these regularly in her work with family medicine residents: 'In a variety of settings, we ask students and residents to identify something they have received through a particular relationship with a patient, specifying that it be something they are carrying into their life outside of medicine.'(37) Questions include:

- What were your expectations going into this clinical situation?
- What do/did you need from this encounter?
- What did you learn about yourself?
- What were you feeling during the encounter?
- What gift did you receive from this relationship? / What will you take away from this relationship and into your personal life?

Over and above any necessary discussion about the technical aspects of the case or clinical management, these questions are designed to increase the self-awareness of the doctor. Tutors, preceptors or colleagues can ask such questions or, alternatively, doctors can find some quiet time to ask themselves.

Peer groups

Within secondary care, doctors often meet with their colleagues in formal settings to discuss cases (for example, in obstetrics, cardiology, neurology, etc.) where group consensus about patient management is important. Doctors also meet in other organised forums such as morbidity and mortality (M & M) meetings. However, it is only in general practice that peer groups have been developed. These groups encourage a wider range of discussion than simple discussion of clinical cases. However, apart from Watson's review(38) there are very few academic articles on the role and function of peer groups for doctors.

In New Zealand, peer groups have been taken up with enthusiasm in the last 30 or so years. GPs receive reaccreditation points for attendance. Groups meet regularly to discuss interesting or problematic cases, audit each other's work, share journal reviews, hear from visiting speakers, discuss resource issues, and so on.

As a form of reflection-on-action, peer groups have a number of key advantages. Topics are based on the needs of the participants, utilising the combined resources of those who have experienced similar issues and/or 'difficult' cases. The financial cost of peer groups is minimal, as participants take turns at leadership and use their own premises for meetings.

Balint groups

A Balint group is a small group of health professionals which meets regularly to discuss clinical cases, the focus being on psychological aspects of practice, especially the doctor–patient relationship. The term derives from Dr Michael Balint, a Hungarian-born psychiatrist and psychoanalyst who, together with his wife Enid, developed such groups in London in the 1950s and 1960s.(39) Their initial focus was on helping GPs develop skills in managing their therapeutic relationships,(40) although the method is now being used by psychotherapists as well. What differentiates Balint groups from peer groups is that Balint groups are based exclusively on clinical cases and are usually led by trained and paid leaders.

Balint groups could be described as a group method of reflection-on-action through the use of clinical stories, with the specific focus being on process issues and the doctor–patient relationship. As a group, the task is to speculate and brainstorm about the patient under discussion and their relationship with their doctor. The group usually picks up on the minimal clues offered within the short presentation, both about the patient and about the therapeutic relationship, and is often able to provoke new ideas which help the presenting doctor see the case in a new light. Over time, such wondering and speculating become increasingly intuitive.

A major outcome of Balint work appears to be better empathy with both patients and colleagues.(41) Balint members report an increased capacity for sitting with the unknown and for considering a wider range of possible causes for someone's illness behaviour. As a method, Balint groups also appear to increase doctors' resilience to the stresses of medical work.(42) There are further notes on the Balint method and professional outcomes in the Appendix.

Mentoring

While peer groups and Balint groups are *group* methods of encouraging reflection and providing support, there are two main methods of encouraging reflection through one-to-one relationships. These are mentoring and supervision.

Mentoring usually refers to regular one-to-one meetings between colleagues who are in the same profession. The model is used quite frequently in business and other professions, where a younger practitioner seeks out a more experienced one for advice and practical wisdom. This method of professional review and support for doctors became popular in the UK as a way of coping with the well-documented stress that followed the 1990 to 1991 National Health Service (NHS) reforms in the UK.(43, 44)

Mentoring is an intensive relationship, in which one person is designated mentor to help develop competence and effectiveness in the other (sometimes called the 'mentee'). The focus is on the overall work of being a doctor. Clinical details about patients usually enlighten and inform this process. The mentor's task is to create a safe and trusting environment within which the mentee can learn and develop professionally. It is an excellent method for deepening the mentee's awareness of himself and his effect on others. The emphasis on educational processes means that ultimately patients will benefit.

Ideally, mentoring is not problem solving, although that may happen as an outcome of the iterative discussions. Mentoring is also not an opportunity for the mentor to do clinical practice via the mentee, although mentoring can contribute towards quality control.

Mutuality versus functional difference

One particular issue that needs to be considered is the difference in roles between mentor or mentee, also known as 'mutuality versus functional difference.' As mentees, doctors usually seek mutuality, collegiality, and a friendly, non-threatening session, while the doctor who is designated to be mentor needs to maintain a 'difference of function'. She has a responsibility to help the mentee improve the quality of their professional care. Just as doctors need to retain their objectivity with their patients, mentors need to maintain their perspective of distance.(45)

Although the relationship is between colleagues, it is ideally not intended to become too mutual. The mentor who has difficulty in challenging, asserting, confronting, and sustaining functional difference when necessary may let the mentee down. The session might become an hour of friendly chat. It is the task of mentoring to help the mentee look at his/her behaviour. This can only be done by attending to mutuality first. Confrontation without mutuality will be destructive. Similarly, friendship without objectivity will be ineffective.

There are useful parallels when a doctor presents himself to a colleague *as a patient*. The consulting doctor must attend to the illness experience and be watchful of the doctor–patient relationship. She must also reserve the right to make her independent medical assessment of this patient (quite apart from the patient's own diagnosis and treatments so far).

Because of these role differences, would-be mentors generally require specific training. The benefits of successful mentoring are listed in Box 10.3.

BOX 10.3 BENEFITS OF MENTORING

Successful mentoring relationships will help doctors (and students) to:

- feel supported generally in their work
- feel legitimated and validated in their learning
- become more aware of their own responses to various situations
- learn how to respect others and to acknowledge differences
- become better able to sit with the feeling of not knowing what to do
- increase their capacity for empathy with patients, be able to sit with their suffering
- have less anxiety about work generally
- have less urgency to use a fix-it approach
- learn about boundaries and responsibilities
- challenge colleagues, patients, institutions where necessary
- learn how to be in a professional relationship with the patient
- become more authentic in their learning, their work and in themselves as persons.

Supervision

While mentoring is generally with a colleague, supervision refers to one-to-one meetings with a psychotherapist or psychologist, the focus being more on the interpersonal relationship than on technical or medical issues. Supervision is an integral part of the work structure in other health professions, such as social work, psychotherapy and counselling. These health professionals discuss their clients/patients on a regular basis with their supervisor and also talk about their work generally or their role in their particular organisation. The best example in medicine is psychiatry, where most training registrars and qualified psychiatrists have regular supervision to discuss their specific interactions with patients and their general caseload.

Wilson did extensive research on GPs' experience of one-to-one supervision in the 1990s, carrying out both in-depth interviews and focus groups.(46) While supervision remains uncommon, the respondent GPs gave it strong endorsement. Using psychotherapists as their supervisor (in preference to other doctors) allowed more in-depth discussion of the doctor–patient relationship and their own professional responses to 'heartsink' experiences such as the somatising patient.(47)

Initial barriers to GPs starting supervision included lack of awareness of this method, time constraints, cost, and the fear of being exposed as incompetent. Over time, however, GPs reported that these barriers tended to melt away as they became more comfortable with the structure and as their familiarity with supervision increased. As Wilson notes, supervision became a valuable and necessary part of their work structure:

> General practice supervision is a powerful method of professional maintenance and development, involving a structured and intensive one-to-one relationship between

a GP and a psychologist or psychotherapist. Some GPs use the supervisor to develop psychotherapy skills in general practice. By holding and validating the GP in his or her work, the supervisor provides a safe place for professional reflection and challenge. Supervision assists GPs to resolve personal and professional work-related issues, it helps GPs become more aware of their own 'self' in the work environment, and it provides insight into the doctor–patient relationship.(48)

The structure of mentoring and supervision

Both of these methods of reflection and professional development are based on one-to-one relationships. Briefly, the patient consults with his/her doctor (the 'medical system'), then the doctor discusses that patient with the mentor or supervisor (the 'supervisory system'). There are six identifiable points of focus within these two systems (Figure 10.2).

FIGURE 10.2 THE SYSTEM OF SUPERVISION

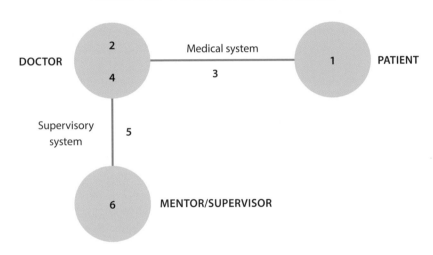

Adapted from Williams(49) and Wilson(46)

Explanation: points of focus

1. The patient's medical state and his/her illness experiences, as narrated by the doctor, with the focus on the **patient**.
2. The doctor's medical and counselling activities: what the doctor did with and for the patient; theory, practice and treatment. The focus is on the **doctor**.
3. Doctor–patient relationship, exploring the interaction between the patient and doctor, and the dynamics of their relationship. The focus is on the **patient and doctor.**
4. The doctor's functional state. Here the supervisor focuses on the immediate state of the doctor in the supervision session. This would include his/her emotional state, as well as the state of his or her career so far and professional development. The focus is still with the **doctor**.

5. The supervision process between supervisor and doctor: what goes on between doctor and supervisor, including projections and transferences. The focus is on the **supervisor and doctor**.
6. The supervisor's experience: here the supervisor brings his or her own immediate feelings or hunches into conscious awareness, sometimes unlocking unexpressed parts of the doctor's narrative or the doctor's state. The focus is now on the **supervisor**.

This conceptual diagram helps the mentor or supervisor to identify their point of focus during a supervision session. The diagram also helps to illustrate the difference between mentoring and supervision. In mentoring, the mentor (who is another doctor) has special focus on Points 1, 2 and 4. The mentor considers the work of the doctor (mentee) using the clinical details of the patient's circumstances and the doctor's responses (Points 1 and 2), and is mindful of the doctor's functional state (point 4) as it pertains to that doctor's ability to deliver appropriate care. The importance of the doctor–patient relationship is not overlooked, but it is not the primary focus. Mentoring is helpful for junior doctors starting in their chosen discipline.

In supervision, the supervisor (who is not a doctor) has a particular focus on Points 1, 3 and 4. The supervisor considers the responses of the doctor towards the patient that contribute to or inhibit the doctor–patient relationship. The doctor's functional state (Point 4) is the focus of the supervisory interaction, as this is the point where the supervisee may have less insight. Often, the doctor's relationship with the particular patient (Point 3) is the reason the doctor needs help. A supervisory relationship would have been useful in the earlier examples from Vignettes 10.2 and 10.3, of the doctor who struggled with his colleagues and the patient who complained about the breaking of bad news (though a mentor may have been equally comfortable addressing this issue).

The model helpfully illustrates the potential for 'parallel process' between the medical and supervisory systems. This is where interpersonal or thematic processes between doctor and patient are unconsciously (and sometimes inevitably) played out between the doctor and supervisor.(50) This can also occur in group work such as in peer or Balint groups. Identifying and discussing these parallels is often the key to unlocking the issues in the case. Parallel process was illustrated in the seminal work of Doehrman in the 1970s,(51) when she interviewed patients, their doctors and their supervisors over considerable lengths of time.

In brief, then, mentoring and supervision are one-to-one methods of reflective practice. Long considered essential aspects of other health professional work, they are now being taken up by doctors who wish to become more thoughtful about professional relationships and their roles within medical work.

Consultation analysis

Writing out or recording a consultation is a powerful method of reflection. Cassell, for example, audiotaped 800 consecutive consultations in the 1980s. These were transcribed and analysed, so that he could note what he said to each patient and how they responded. The outcome of his analysis was a much greater understanding of suffering and both the interactions between doctor and patient.(52)

This is an example of 'interpersonal process recall', where the consultation is analysed in depth, including the minute-to-minute thoughts and feelings of the doctor. Many colleges of general practice now require evidence that trainees have completed such exercises to a satisfactory standard, in order to demonstrate their capacity for reflection on their consulting and their development of self-awareness.(53)

A teacher or preceptor is often involved in process recall, as many students and doctors overestimate their interviewing competence, while others underestimate. This process of structured reflection and feedback usually increases the accuracy of their self-assessment.

Reflection as a clinical tool

In the past, reflection might have seemed a bit irrelevant to clinical practice, but there is now an emerging recognition that reflection can impact on clinical outcomes. Often the clinical issue or problem is a deficiency less based in knowledge or skills than in knowing how to respond to complex situations where there is no easy answer. For example, the diagnosis may be quite clear, but there is no available treatment – or perhaps there are some treatments, but the patient is not keen to try any of them, and so on. In such instances, the issue is more about how the doctor and the patient are working together.

In our postgraduate courses for GPs, we include a variety of reflective techniques. Over the course of the year, doctors use these with their most difficult, complex and frustrating patients. They can choose any method (for example, creative writing, consultation analysis, one-to-one review with a colleague, group discussion in peer group or Balint group, mentoring or supervision), as long as they record what they did and how it worked. They then discuss the outcomes for themselves and their patient in a follow-up essay. Here are two examples that illustrate the outcomes of these reflective processes.

VIGNETTE 10.5 THE ANGRY PATIENT

Jane, a 45-year-old woman who was doing poorly after a moderate head injury, was troubled with headaches, lack of concentration and poor work attendance. She had been referred to physiotherapy and occupational therapy but was not attending. She seemed angry and frustrated with her ongoing symptoms and the GP was finding it very difficult just to be in the same room as her.

The GP then rather perceptively asked this patient to write about her own experiences as a person with a head injury. As it turned out, he received more than he had bargained for, because once this patient started writing, she also wrote about significant family issues that had predated the injury and, to a large extent, were the real reasons behind her ongoing distress. Once the GP read this story and listened more carefully to the patient, things changed. The patient felt heard and understood by her doctor: she started back into rehabilitation, and all the anger and frustration began to be resolved.

The resolution here seemed to be in the doctor–patient relationship. This patient now had a doctor who could listen attentively without becoming defensive.

VIGNETTE 10.6 SOMATISATION

Mary was a 56-year-old patient with distressing diarrhoea over two years, which had been fully investigated. Her GP had thought it was some sort of irritable bowel, but it was resistant to all forms of intervention, including seeing a psychologist. This GP's heart really sank when Mary turned up with a new symptom, in this case quite severe headaches: the GP intuitively felt that once again a formal diagnosis would be difficult to find.

The GP did some reflective writing using the free writing method above, then also met with the patient's psychologist. These two interventions seemed to help him to gain a better understanding of this patient and his own responses to her so far.

At the next consultation he asked: 'What was happening in your life at the time this new symptom first started?' Mary then disclosed a longstanding unresolved personal loss that had started at the same time as the diarrhoea, as well as a further recent loss that had reinforced the original grief. Over the next few weeks, Mary started to make the links between what had been happening in her life and her symptoms. She engaged more fully with her psychologist, the diarrhoea resolved after two years, while her headaches relented as well.

As we noted in Chapter 7, the timing question used above is very useful, but it was the combination of the earlier reflection and more attentive listening that seemed to make the difference with this 'heartsink' experience.

Reflection, resilience and wellness

As we will see in the next chapter, the outcomes of medical care are related not only to the doctor's technical competence, but also to teamwork and the culture of that particular community of medical practice. In the three clinical stories at the beginning of this chapter, for example, patients were at risk of adverse outcomes, arguably because those doctors were not constantly reviewing their work. Reflective practice helps to broaden the focus of the clinical gaze to include both the context of health-care delivery and the role of the doctor. In this way, reflection contributes to patient safety.

Reflection is also a method of finding meaning. As we noted in Chapter 4 on the doctor–patient relationship, doctors look for and find a significant sense of purpose and meaning through their therapeutic interactions with their patients. Any of the methods listed above will help them explore the nuances of connection and relationship, reconnecting them back to their original purpose in doing medicine. Thus doctors become more resilient to the stresses of clinical work.

Such reflective skills act as a self-care mechanism. In the past, doctors have not been very skilled in looking after themselves: building a style of reflective practice can help considerably. This was demonstrated in recent research by Stevenson et al. in Australia, who explored practitioners' experiences of working in high-needs populations – situations where work stressors are high and there is usually a high turnover of staff. The 'resilient' practitioners they encountered had respect for patients, a sense of control, and the ability to reflect deeply on their work.(54) These are significant findings with respect to developing resilience and models of 'pro-social' career choice.

Reflective techniques are also very useful in times of transition. There are many such points within a medical career: when graduating, when starting as a resident or registrar in training, when starting in one's own practice. Each new step gives rise to the possibility of developing 'impostor syndrome', where the doctor feels 'everyone else knows what is going on and what to do, but I don't'. As this is quite common, the trick is to find some way to work through these feelings and lack of confidence. Whatever method is used, formal reflection on the transition is usually quite helpful.

Conclusion

The literature on the health of doctors is clear: there needs to be greater emphasis on reducing doctor stress and increasing wellness. Reflection is one of the better methods for achieving these aims. There are many barriers to the use of reflection in medical practice, but once students or doctors have identified and worked through them, reflection can be surprisingly powerful. We advocate reflection as a key aspect of learning and clinical practice.

Reflection allows doctors to transform experience into learning. Without it, there is a risk that lower quality medical care will remain unexamined. Doctors can choose from a range of reflective tools that best suit their needs and those of their patients, rather than using one type exclusively. Deriving a sense of meaning from practising medicine and developing resilience to the stresses and strains of day-to-day practice are important goals. These are readily achievable with reflective activities that enhance learning and professional identity.

SUMMARY POINTS

- Reflecting on one's performance is not necessarily an innate skill.
- Observing and monitoring one's clinical competence is an integral part of professional practice.
- Reflective practice is a philosophy or style of clinical practice, where reflection is used to enhance clinical efficacy and professional resilience.
- Reflective practice could reduce the rate of adverse outcomes and complaints.
- Reflection can take place during clinical situations or later in retrospect. It can be informal or highly structured.
- Experiential learning is enhanced through reflection. Insights become more available and the meaning of the work more apparent.
- Medical students can be coached towards effective reflection.
- Tutors can be coached towards identifying and coaching authentic reflection.
- Learning reflective techniques as an undergraduate may lead to a more reflective style of work in clinical practice.
- Reflection can lead to changes in conceptual understanding of clinical practice and of oneself.

References

1.   Epstein RM. Reflection, perception and the acquisition of wisdom. *Med Educ* 2008, 42:1048–50.
2.   Haynes RB, Davis D, McGibbon A, Tugwell P. A critical appraisal of the efficacy of CME. *JAMA* 1984, 251:61–64.
3.   Davis D, O'Brien MA, Freemantle N, Wolf FM, Mazmanian P, Taylor-Vaisey A. Impact of formal continuing medical education: do conferences, workshops, rounds, and other traditional continuing education activities change physician behavior or health care outcomes? *JAMA* 1999, 282(9):867–74.
4.   Brigley S, Young Y, Littlejohns P, McEwen J. Continuing education for medical professionals: a reflective model. *Postgrad Med J* 1997, 73:23–26.
5.   Sandars J. The use of reflection in medical education: AMEE Guide No. 44. *Med Teach* 2009, 31(8):685–95.
6.   Mann K, Gordon J, MacLeod A. Reflection and reflective practice in health professions education: a systematic review. *Adv Health Sci Educ* 2009, 14(4):595–621.
7.   Driessen EW, Van Tartwijk J, Overeem K, Vermunt JD, Van Der Vleuten CPM. Conditions for successful reflective use of portfolios in undergraduate medical education. *Med Educ* 2005, 39(12):1230–35.
8.   Dannefer EF, Henson LC. The portfolio approach to competency-based assessment at the Cleveland Clinic Lerner College of Medicine. *Acad Med* 2007, 82(5):493–502.
9.   Henderson E, Berlin A, Freeman G, Fuller J. Twelve tips for promoting significant event analysis to enhance reflection in undergraduate medical students. *Med Teach* 2002, 24(2):121–24.
10.   Branch Jr WT, Paranjape A. Feedback and reflection: teaching methods for clinical settings. *Acad Med* 2002, 77:1185–88.
11.   Hilton SR, Slotnick HB. Proto-professionalism: how professionalisation occurs across the continuum of medical education. *Med Educ* 2005, 39(1):58–65.
12.   Groopman JE. *How doctors think*. Boston: Houghton Mifflin, 2007.
13.   Schon DA. *Educating the reflective practitioner: toward a new design for teaching and learning in the professions*. San Francisco: Jossey-Bass, 1996.
14.   Neighbour R. *The inner consultation: how to develop an effective and intuitive consulting style*. Oxford: Radcliffe, 2005.
15.   Kolb DA. *Experiential learning: experience as the source of learning and development*. New Jersey: Prentice-Hall, 1984.
16.   Paice E, Heard S, Moss F. How important are role models in making good doctors? *BMJ* 2002, 325(7366):707–10.
17.   Egnew TR, Wilson HJ. Role modeling the doctor–patient relationship in the clinical curriculum. *Fam Med* 2011, 43(2):99–105.
18.   Davidoff F. Shame: the elephant in the room. *Qual Safe Health Care* 2002, 11(1):2–3.
19.   Lempp H, Seale C. The hidden curriculum in undergraduate medical education: qualitative study of medical students' perceptions of teaching. *BMJ* 2004, 329(7468):770–73.
20.   Sinclair S. *Making doctors: an institutional apprenticeship*. New York: Berg Publishers, 1997.
21.   Esmail A. Clinical perspectives on patient safety. In: Walshe K, Boaden RJ, eds. *Patient safety: research into practice*. Maidenhead: Open University Press, 2006. pp. 9–18.
22.   Cunningham W, Wilson HJ. Shame, guilt and the medical practitioner. *NZ Med J* 2003, 116(1183).
23.   Moon JA. *Critical thinking: an exploration of theory and practice*. London: Routledge, 2008.
24.   Al-Shehri A. Learning by reflection in general practice: a study report. *Educ Gen Pract* 1995, 7:237–48.
25.   Wald HS, Borkan J, Taylor J, Anthony D, Reis SP. Fostering and evaluating reflective capacity in medical education: developing the REFLECT rubric for assessing reflective writing. *Acad Med* 2012, 87(1):41–50.

26. Kember D, Jones, A, Loke A, McKay, J, et al. Determining the level of reflective thinking from students' written journals using a coding scheme based on the work of Mezirow. *Internat J Lifelong Educ* 1999, 18(1):18–30.

27. Mezirow J. *Transformative dimensions of adult learning*. San Francisco: Jossey-Bass, 1991.

28. Meador CK. *Symptoms of unknown origin: a medical odyssey*. Nashville: Vanderbilt University Press, 2005.

29. Flanagan JC. The critical incident technique. *Psychol Bull* 1954, 51(4):327–58.

30. Cote CJ, Notterman DA, Karl HW, Weinberg JA, McCloskey C. Adverse sedation events in pediatrics: a critical incident analysis of contributing factors. *Pediatr* 2000, 105(4):805–14.

31. Johns C, Freshwater D. *Transforming nursing through reflective practice*. Oxford: Wiley-Blackwell, 2005.

32. Smith A, Russell J. Using critical learning incidents in nurse education. *Nurse Educ Today* 1991, 11(4):284–91.

33. Bolton G. *Reflective practice: writing and professional development*. London: Sage Publications, 2001.

34. Pennebaker JW. Telling stories: the health benefits of narrative. *Lit Med* 2000, 19(1):3–18.

35. Charon R. *Narrative medicine: honoring the stories of illness*. New York: Oxford University Press, 2006.

36. Riley-Doucet C, Wilson S. A three step method of self reflection using reflective journal writing. *J Adv Nurs* 1997, 25(5):964–68.

37. Dobie S. Viewpoint: Reflections on a well-traveled path: self-awareness, mindful practice, and relationship-centered care as foundations for medical education. *Acad Med* 2007, 82(4):422–27.

38. Watson A. *The peer group movement: what goes into making a successful peer group?* Wellington: Royal New Zealand College of General Practitioners, 1997.

39. Balint M. *The doctor, his patient, and the illness*. London: Pitman, 1957.

40. Elder A, Samuel O, eds. *'While I'm here, doctor': a study of change in the doctor–patient relationship*. London: Tavistock, 1987.

41. Kjelmand D. Balint training makes GPs thrive better in their job. *Pat Educ Couns* 2004, 55:230–35.

42. Benson J, Magraith K. Compassion fatigue and burnout: the role of Balint groups. *Austral Fam Phys* 2005, 34(6):497–98.

43. Sutherland VJ, Cooper CL. Job stress, satisfaction, and mental health among general practitioners before and after introduction of new contract. *BMJ* 1992, 304(6841):1545–48.

44. Freeman R. *Mentoring in general practice*. Oxford: Butterworth-Heinemann, 1998.

45. Sweet G. *The advantage of being useless: the Tao and the counsellor*. Palmerston North, NZ: Dunmore Press, 1989.

46. Wilson HJ. Supervision and the culture of general practice. Masters thesis. Dunedin, NZ: University of Otago, 1999.

47. Wilson HJ. Reflecting on the 'difficult' patient. *NZ Med J* 2005, 118(1212).

48. Wilson HJ. Self-care for GPs: the role of supervision. *NZ Fam Phys* 2000, 27(5):51–57.

49. Williams A. *Visual and active supervision*. New York: Norton, 1995.

50. Williams A. Parallel process in a course on counseling supervision. *Couns Educ Supervision* 1987, 26(4):245–55.

51. Doehrman MJ. Parallel processes in supervision and psychotherapy. *Bull Menninger Clin* 1976, 40:1–87.

52. Cassell EJ. *Talking with patients. Vol. 1: The theory of doctor-patient communication*. Cambridge: MIT Press, 1985.

53. Boon H, Stewart M. Patient–physician communication assessment instruments: 1986 to 1996 in review. *Pat Educ Couns* 1998, 35(3):161–76.

54. Stevenson AD, Phillips C, Anderson K. Resilience among doctors who work in challenging areas: a qualitative study. *Br J Gen Pract* 2011, 61(588):e404–e410.

Chapter 11

Adverse Outcomes and Patient Safety

CONTENTS

Introduction

Biomedicine has been a major advance in the delivery of health care. Most of the time, clinical practice is 'as expected': the patient presents with symptoms, doctors diagnose the problem, and there is an effective form of treatment or disease modification.

This chapter raises a quite different perspective because at times there are unexpected, unintended, or even negative consequences of health care, where the patient is actually made worse in some way. Although the profession is now discussing these 'adverse outcomes' of medical care more openly, such incidents are extremely disturbing for both patient and doctor.

The profession has been aware of the potential for adverse outcomes for millennia: think of Hippocrates' invocation 'first, do no harm'. Nevertheless, this subject has remained rather taboo in clinical practice, even if the effect on individual doctors who are party to an adverse event can be quite profound.

An interesting historical example was Semmelweiss in nineteenth-century Austria. He proposed that new mothers were dying after childbirth because doctors were 'carrying' something from their postmortem dissections back into maternity care.(1) We now know about bacteria causing puerperal sepsis, but Semmelweiss was ridiculed by his colleagues and it was a long time before his ideas were accepted. This was not simply because microbes were yet to be discovered, but also because doctors at the time could not accept that they might be implicated. There were two issues blocking further understanding: the lack of an acceptable explanatory model (transmission of streptococcal infection), and the inability of the profession to see itself as part of the problem (inadequate hygiene).

Similar delays have arisen in another area of practice: talking to patients about death and dying. Kübler-Ross's influential work was first published in 1972,(2) but it was not until many years later that the profession began to talk more openly with patients about cancer, prognosis and dying. And while this is now expected practice, it is still very difficult for many doctors to actually broach these subjects with their patients. The problem of adverse outcomes is much the same, as these are difficult subjects to introduce and teach.

We are not suggesting that medical standards are poor, as in general the quality of health care in the Western world is high. Instead, adverse events can happen to the patients of highly competent doctors who have the latest knowledge and up-to-date skills. They are usually unexpected events involving patients of good doctors and it is important to figure out why they occur.

Historically, then, the profession has tended to avoid or even deny the issue of adverse outcomes. As Reason says, '[d]octors have been given very little training in understanding, anticipating, detecting, preventing, and responding to errors'.(3)

This chapter is an introduction to the general concept of adverse outcomes (now known as patient safety), focusing on the implication of these events for doctors. Our intention is to demystify a difficult area in clinical practice. Short examples of adverse events within our own careers are described in Vignette 11.1.

VIGNETTE 11.1 ADVERSE OUTCOMES – PERSONAL EXPERIENCES

1. *As a house surgeon in the early 1980s, I remember standing beside a patient who was on the operating table having a bronchoscopy. In those days, pulse oximetry was not being used routinely, although this patient had quite severe aortic incompetence. I found myself taking his pulse, knowing something was going wrong, but unable to articulate what that was (in all likelihood, episodes of anoxia). And a few minutes later he arrested. Despite resuscitation, he died shortly after. This was a completely unexpected death from minor surgery. (HW)*

2. *An orthopaedic surgeon at that same hospital had a high rate of post-operative infections. Everyone knew about this but no one mentioned it. I went to the*

superintendent at the time to helpfully point this out, but was told quite clearly not to raise questions about another doctor's competence. (HW)

3. *As a GP locum, I had two consultations with a 25-year-old woman with irregular vaginal bleeding. In the second consultation she was accompanied by her husband (the second 'red flag' that I had missed). My notes read 'obviously dysfunctional uterine bleeding' and I still remember my rather glib reassurance that they could go on holiday. I heard from their GP later that she had ruptured her ectopic pregnancy while travelling and required emergency surgery. (HW)*

4. *We have met many doctors over the years who have revealed their own longstanding trauma from bearing witness to patients who have been harmed, rather than helped, by medicine. Many of them stood alongside the patient, feeling unable to stop the impending train wreck. By association, they have had recurrent feelings of guilt and remorse ever since. (HW and WC)*

Our considerable experience of these issues is not unique: all doctors are involved in, or have been affected by, adverse outcomes. This chapter provides a brief history of the emerging discipline of patient safety and the background of clinical uncertainty in medical practice; it also covers the inevitability of adverse outcomes, doctor fragility in relation to them as well as to patient complaints, and current initiatives in medical practice and medical education.

These are complex issues, and you may need to sit with them or withhold judgement as you read this chapter. Many of the points require thinking about the culture of medicine, including the social norms and expectations found within training and practice.

Current definitions

Before discussing these issues, it is helpful to provide some key definitions.

Adverse event

A harmful and undesired effect resulting from medication or other intervention such as surgery.

Patient safety

'The avoidance, prevention, and amelioration of adverse outcomes or injuries stemming from the process of healthcare.'(4) *Or:*
'A discipline in the health-care sector that applies safety science methods towards the goal of achieving a trustworthy system of health-care delivery ... an attribute of health-care systems that minimizes the incidence and impact of adverse events and maximizes recovery from such events.' (5)

The goal of the discipline of patient safety is to create what is known as a 'safety culture' for each particular community of practice, such as an operating theatre, a general practice, or a medical ward.

Taxonomies of error

There is an extensive literature on the taxonomies of error and adverse events.(6) In industrial settings, initial taxonomies emerged as tools to analyse and prevent worker injury. For example, the 'domino' model included the social environment, any fault of various persons, unsafe acts, the accident, and the resulting harm. Organisational safety models posit that unsafe acts by human operators are linked to various organisational factors. Unless there are adequate defences, an unsafe act can penetrate the system and an adverse outcome may result.(7) As health-care systems are now increasingly complex, many factors contribute to adverse outcomes.(8) Examples are included in Box 11.1.

BOX 11.1 COMMON ERRORS LEADING TO ADVERSE OUTCOMES

Diagnostic error: Mistaking dissecting aortic aneurysm for renal colic, or bacterial septicaemia for influenza.

Medication error: Incorrect drug, incorrect site or dose, drug interactions.

Treatment error: Surgical damage to a ureter when doing a hysterectomy, or perforating the uterus when doing a dilatation and curettage.

Systemic error: Incorrect labels on patient specimens, wrong-side surgery, misplaced laboratory reports.

Communication error: Essential details missed in handovers from one team to another.

In Australia, it has been calculated that medical error causes 18,000 unnecessary or premature deaths and more than 50,000 disabled patients per year. In the US, the celebrated Harvard Medical Practice Study estimated that annual deaths from medical error were between 44,000 and 98,000 and that there are up to 1,000,000 excess injuries per year.(9) In New Zealand, the 1998 Davis study reviewed the data from 6000 hospital records and found that the proportion of hospital admissions associated with an adverse event was 12.9 per cent and that '15% of those were associated with permanent disability or death'. Of 850 events, one third (315) were considered to be preventable.(10)

A brief history: the emerging discipline of patient safety

The unintended outcomes of health care used to be labelled as 'iatrogenic disease'. 'Iatro' is Greek for physician and 'genic' means to generate, hence 'doctor-generated disease'. However, this label implies that adverse events are only attributable to the doctor, so the responsibility and blame is carried by a single practitioner. This approach reduced the need to examine other contributing factors.

In the second half of the twentieth century, many doctors raised concerns about adverse outcomes. For example, in 1984 Hilfiker publicly acknowledged that he had inadvertently terminated a live and very much wanted baby, thinking he was doing a dilatation and curettage for a miscarriage.(11) Some responses by his colleagues were positive, noting his courage and honesty, while one correspondent was scathingly critical: 'This neurotic piece has no place in the *New England Journal of Medicine.*'(12)

These responses nicely encapsulate a divided profession. Some saw errors as opportunities for learning, recognising that doctors need support and specific training for the complexity and dangers of modern practice, while others were keen that the profession did not discuss these issues at all.

In 2009, Wears and Vincent from the US commented on the slowness of the profession's response to the increasing rate of adverse outcomes in the 1960s, 1970s and 1980s: 'The fact that thousands, probably millions, of people were being harmed unnecessarily and vast amounts of money being wasted seemed to have escaped everyone's attention. From our current understanding, this seems a curious state of affairs; it is as if an epidemic were raging across the country without anybody noticing or troubling to investigate'.(13)

Fortunately, things have changed since then. The profession has borrowed ideas and concepts from other disciplines and is now developing a revised approach to health care. This approach acknowledges the extent of unintended consequences and how they might be prevented.

Micro- and macro-ergonomics

What made the profession's collective attitude of denial change to more appropriate academic and clinical engagement? First, the public was increasingly aware of these unexpected outcomes and demanded increased safety.[1] This was perhaps reflected in the increasingly litigious climate in the US in response to perceived error.

Medicine also gained ideas and inspiration from other high-risk industries, including insights from the study of 'human performance'. This discipline looks at human fallibility within a range of complex situations such as flying aeroplanes, operating nuclear power plants, or running aircraft carriers – situations where planners need to prepare for worst possible events, such as planes crashing or nuclear meltdowns.

The airline industry has been a useful model. For example, flying an aeroplane in the 1940s was quite dangerous, as crashes often occurred during landing. This was usually attributed to pilot error. Aeroplanes at that time had two very similar levers in the cockpit: one to lower the flaps so the plane could land, and the other to raise the wheels. When plane manufacturers changed the style and orientation of those levers, the crash rate was immediately reduced, as the pilot could no longer confuse them at a critical time. Labelled 'pilot error' because of inattention, these crashes were instead an issue of cockpit design. This is an example of **micro-ergonomics**: the interface between the human operator and their tools or controls. The original cockpit design was identified as an 'error trap' where mistakes happened regularly.

The first medical field to start using these ideas was anaesthesia. It used to be

---

1 There are some fascinating parallels with Semmelweiss – childbearing women at that time started to avoid teaching hospitals, preferring instead to have childbirth in smaller facilities run by local nuns.

possible to make incorrect connections between gas cylinders and the patient's ventilation tube, as a result of which many patients died. Mostly this was blamed on the anaesthetist for being inattentive or unprofessional. Fortunately, in the 1970s an engineer named Jeffrey Cooper carried out extensive research on the design of the anaesthetic machine, in the context of the habits and procedures of the operating theatre. He published his groundbreaking findings in 1978, concluding that many factors contributed to anaesthetic mishaps at that time: these included inadequate experience and supervision, lack of familiarity with the equipment, poor communication between team members, haste, inattention, fatigue, and ambiguously designed machines.(14)

Since then, and under the guidance of Dr Ellison Pierce from the American Society of Anaesthesiologists,(15) the anaesthetic trolley has been reconfigured. It is now physically impossible to connect up the wrong tube or make many other micro-ergonomic mistakes. Because of this detailed analysis, error traps have been identified and anaesthesia has become considerably safer. However, this increase in safety would never have been achieved if the profession had relied solely on better training and improvements in the competence of individual doctors. Anaesthesia necessarily involves a complex interface between the doctor, several machines, and a patient, who is usually unconscious and unable to fend for him or herself.

Human fallibility

James Reason is a professor of psychology in the UK and leading researcher on human and organisational contributions to accidents and errors. He has extensively researched how complex systems appear to break down.(16) The outcome has been a better understanding of the gap between intentions and actions, or in other words, human fallibility. For example, many drivers are quite careful about cyclists when driving, but sometimes after parking they forget to check if there is a cyclist approaching before opening the car door. The outcome of this minor inattention can be injury to the cyclist, or even death. Another example of human fallibility is the difficulty in remembering and copying numbers or other numerical data.

The implication of this research for medicine is an increasing appreciation that doctors simply cannot get it right all of the time. This seems obvious now, but it represents a profound change in understanding. Doctors are just as fallible as anyone else, and being in the act of doctoring does not stop us from completely forgetting about particular conditions (such as in Vignette 11.1) or making a numerical mistake with drug doses. This is why working in teams and double-checking medications is a helpful safeguard against human fallibility.

The 'Swiss cheese' model of medical error

The next historical development in a better approach to adverse outcomes was the concept of **macro-ergonomics**, focusing on all the wider interlinked systems, rather than on just the individual operator. This focus was useful in analysing major industrial accidents in the 1970s, such as the nuclear meltdown at Three Mile Island. It was also the start of what is known as 'systems thinking'. This leads to 'root cause analysis', a method of analysing all the contributing factors that lead to each disastrous outcome.

Reason introduced the medical profession to the 'Swiss cheese' model as a method of understanding systemic error (Figure 11.1). The model identifies latent conditions that contribute to an error-producing situation. These latent factors enable harm to occur, through a combination of failure of prevention and a final unsafe act.

FIGURE 11.1 MEDICAL ERROR – THE 'SWISS CHEESE' MODEL

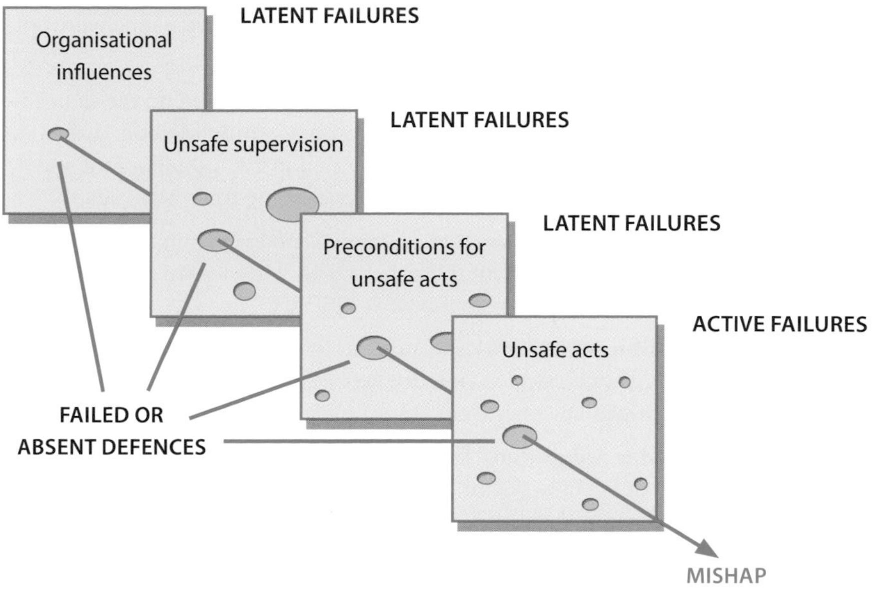

Adapted from Reason(17)

A worked example: Intrathecal vincristine

To illustrate this model of error, Reason analysed the recurring deaths of patients from incorrect administration of vincristine. In some cancer protocols, patients receive this drug intravenously, as well as another drug called methotrexate intrathecally. However, if medical staff confuse the two and inject vincristine into the intrathecal space, then the patient will usually die a very painful death within a few days.

Reason performed a detailed root cause analysis of one of these deaths, identifying all the interpersonal and prescribing systems involved. He concluded that this adverse outcome was a classic error trap. The Swiss cheese model helps to avoid an exclusive focus on the doctor who gave the wrongly sited injection.(18) It is a useful aid in analysing why an adverse event occurred, as well as how it can be prevented in the future. Box 11.2 is Reason's root cause analysis with respect to a vincristine death.

BOX 11.2 ROOT CAUSE ANALYSIS: FACTORS CONTRIBUTING
TO A VINCRISTINE DEATH[2]

Administrative and procedural matters: The cancer protocol for combined use
of vincristine and methotrexate is explicit about different day administration,
packaging and handling from the pharmacy, and a prohibition of use on the same
ward trolley. However, all these protocols were bypassed, staff were unaware of
hospital policy about drug administration, and ampules of vincristine were not
accompanied by warnings about intrathecal use.

Indicators and barriers that failed: Both drugs were prescribed on the same
prescription, handwritten notes indicated the route of administration, drug
labelling was in small font, warnings were provided in even smaller font and
partially obscured, and there was similar drug packaging for both drugs.

Failures of supervision and instruction: There was no induction and training of
new staff or specific warnings about the potential hazards within this particular
cancer protocol.

Communication failures and 'workarounds': Roles and responsibilities of new
staff were not clear, it was common practice for both drugs to arrive on the ward
on the same day, various key staff were absent for personal reasons.

Collective knowledge failures and false assumptions: Staff were unclear about
the responsibilities of the new doctor and the role of supervising procedures, the
nurse (falsely) assumed that the doctors would do the drug checking and that
they were experienced in intrathecal administration.

Adapted from Reason(18)

It is quite shocking to realise that there have been over 70 reported cases of this
error in the last 30 to 40 years, and that in all likelihood there have been many more
cases that were not reported.(19) The implication is that despite all the publicity about
vincristine, no amount of narrowly focused medical training has been able to prevent
this disaster happening time and time again.

Reason's step-by-step review is a superb example of root cause analysis,
generating ideas for the prevention of similar events in the future. Questions might be:
What are the potential errors in the system when a patient is prescribed this particular
cancer protocol? Are medical and nursing staff on the ward aware of these and do they
know how to guard against them for each particular patient? The focus needs to be on
systems, teams, and how to avoid latent error.

Several doctors in the UK have been prosecuted for manslaughter after a vincristine
death.(20) However, in a more recent case, the injecting doctor was acquitted. This
decision marked a shift towards a better understanding of the contribution of micro-
and macro-ergonomic factors in causation.

---

2   The case has now been dramatised by the World Health Organization as a teaching and learning
    tool for hospitals, doctors, and medical students. See 'Learning From Error' at: http://www.who.
    int/patientsafety/education/en/

'To Err is Human'
We complete this abbreviated history of patient safety with a pivotal moment in 1999, the publication of the landmark US Institute of Medicine report *To err is human: building a safer health system,* which provided the major stimulus for a revised approach to medical care.(21)

The report has three significant foci: high-profile cases that illustrate the absence of safeguards in medicine (wrong leg amputation, deaths during anaesthesia for minor surgery, deaths from incorrect dosage or site of drugs); the increasing numbers of such events; and the potential insights for medicine from the psychology of human fallibility, now referred to as 'human factors'. It also offers suggestions for prevention, including better acknowledgement of organisational and other factors that set up the unwitting physician for the final 'unsafe' act.

Since then, the concept of patient safety has gained considerable momentum. National bodies now provide funding for research as well as guidelines for clinical practice. Examples are the Agency for Healthcare Research and Quality (USA), the National Patient Safety Agency in the UK, the Australian Patient Safety Foundation, and the Health Quality and Safety Commission in New Zealand.

By the end of the twentieth century, then, the profession had made a start in addressing the emerging concept of patient safety. Human fallibility is now being more realistically acknowledged within medical practice, as is the concept of medicine as a complex social system where micro- and macro-ergonomic factors contribute to patient outcomes. A further concept that relates to adverse outcomes and patient safety is the ubiquitous issue of uncertainty within medical practice.

Uncertainty in medicine
Both doctors and patients find uncertainty in medicine a difficult concept. Professor Renée Fox, an American sociologist with an interest in medical training and ethics, accurately identified three areas of uncertainty in clinical practice.(22)
1. The limitations and gaps in current medical knowledge. While medical knowledge is increasing exponentially, it is hard to envisage a situation where medical science knows all there is about particular conditions.
2. How medical knowledge will actually apply to each individual patient. While research trials provide statistical trends for conditions and treatments, population data does not predict the outcome for a particular patient.
3. The difficulty, especially for students, in distinguishing between personal ignorance on the one hand, and the limitations in knowledge on the other. This is an ongoing problem for more experienced practitioners as well.

Translating these general principles to clinical practice, doctors face the following areas of uncertainty on a day-to-day basis:

Diagnostic uncertainty: A child with a high fever might possibly have meningitis. This diagnostic challenge is even more difficult if there is a major outbreak of influenza in the community at the same time. Similarly, patients with major problems such as heart attacks or cancer do not always present to their doctor with typical symptoms suggesting those diagnoses.

Disease uncertainty: While the statistics for groups of patients are well known (for example, the chances of stroke after years of high blood pressure), it is impossible to know which particular patient will eventually succumb.

Treatment uncertainty: The latest and best medications can give some patients severe side effects and perhaps even kill them, but doctors have no way of knowing in advance which patients will be affected. These are idiosyncratic responses to normal treatments.

To summarise this chapter so far, we have identified human fallibility, the inherent uncertainty in medicine, and the increasingly complex nature of modern medical practice since World War II (many players, complex procedures, powerful drugs, and so on). As Figure 11.2 illustrates, three factors combine and contribute to a wide range of error traps in clinical practice which, if not identified and prevented, can result in adverse outcomes or, at best, a 'near miss'. Traditional medical training has not taught students how such factors can combine in these ways.

FIGURE 11.2 ERROR TRAPS AND ADVERSE OUTCOMES – CONTRIBUTING FACTORS

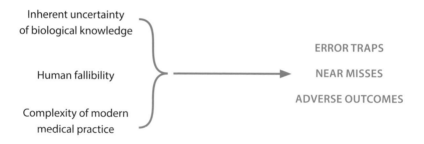

We now wish to explore the profession's usual responses to uncertainty – responses which appear to be increasingly inadequate.

The response to uncertainty

Medical students have particular difficulties with the inherent uncertainty of clinical practice. Perhaps learning vast amounts of medical facts about the body and disease gives an initial impression that medical science will be knowable and absolute. However, students quickly realise that the complexity of medical knowledge means absolute certainty will be unobtainable. To live with this realisation, Fox suggests that medical students acquire various coping mechanisms, as otherwise the task of learning medicine and becoming competent would feel quite overwhelming.(22)

For example, Guenter and Fowler suggest that learners 'tend to avoid situations that will reveal [their] uncertainty, or when avoiding it is impossible, [they] might either disguise it or reposition it as someone else's problem'.(23) As a result, the learner 'expends a great deal of effort maintaining a "cloak of competence" … as a sort of survival technique'.

Along the same lines, Esmail, a GP in the UK, describes the way students develop the coping mechanism of 'certitude': a feeling of certainty, assurance, or confidence about what is going wrong, learning not to show any doubt or hesitancy. This psychological defence against uncertainty is both modelled and reinforced by the doctors they learn from.(24) Reason describes medical school in similar terms: 'Healthcare professionals, particularly doctors, are raised in a culture of trained perfectibility. After a long, arduous, and expensive education, they are expected to get it right. Errors equate to incompetence, and fallible doctors are frequently stigmatised and marginalised.'(3)

Such ideas led Dr Richard Smith, a former editor of the *BMJ*, to formulate his theory of the 'bogus contract' between doctors and society.(25) He posits that doctors are often acutely aware of the limitations of what they can do, whereas patients have more inflated ideas about the power of medicine (Box 11.3).

BOX 11.3 THE 'BOGUS CONTRACT' BETWEEN DOCTORS AND THEIR PATIENTS

The patient's view:
- Modern medicine can do remarkable things.
- You, the doctor, can see inside me and know what's wrong.
- You know everything it's necessary to know.
- You can solve my problems.
- So we give you high status and a good salary.

The doctor's view:
- Modern medicine has limited powers.
- Worse, it's dangerous.
- We can't begin to solve all problems.
- I don't know everything.
- There is a fine balance between doing good and harm.
- I'd better keep quiet about all this so as not to disappoint my patients and lose my status.

Adapted from Smith(25)

Given this mindset of doctors (always having to give the impression of knowing, and not being transparent about the dangers of medicine), a major problem arises when things do go wrong. Adverse outcomes become personalised as the fault of the doctor, who now gets blamed. Students and doctors can internalise the medical outcome as a personal failure.

As the doctor and anthropologist Dr Simon Sinclair noted, students start to absorb this dominant ethos very early in their training. Certitude means students are supposed to 'know' the answers to questions from their teachers. He suggests that failure 'may be felt as deeply wounding to [students'] own personal sense of identity and moral purpose'.(26)

We can now upgrade Figure 11.2 to include doctors' responses to the uncertainties of clinical practice. This has been the profession's approach in the attempt to minimise error.

FIGURE 11.3 TRADITIONAL RESPONSES TO UNCERTAINTY

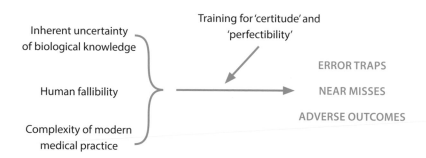

Instead of being proactive about potential adverse outcomes within each clinical situation, medical training has focused rather narrowly on *improving knowledge* as a method of reducing uncertainty, rather than understanding human fallibility within the complexity of modern practice. Given that the factors on the left are ultimately unresolvable, the overall problem of adverse outcomes becomes clear. Traditional responses to uncertainty are insufficient to identify error traps or prevent adverse outcomes. The focus has been misplaced.

We are not the first to propose that clinical certainty and perfection by doctors are unachievable goals.(24, 27) The problems of uncertainty and human fallibility need to be acknowledged, introduced and discussed quite early within medical school curricula as a precursor to clinical practice. Adverse outcomes need to become a starting point for learning, rather than a trigger for denial and shame. We will return to Figure 11.3 near the end of this chapter.

Wu's perceptive comments about doctors' responses to adverse outcomes and their training culture serve to summarise this chapter so far.(28) Links to preceding points are noted in brackets.

> Strangely, there is no place for mistakes in modern medicine. Society has entrusted physicians with the burden of understanding and dealing with illness. Although it is often said, 'doctors are only human', technological wonders, the apparent precision of laboratory tests and innovations that present tangible images of illness have in fact created an expectation of perfection. Patients, who have an understandable need to consider their doctors infallible, have colluded with doctors to deny the existence of error. [The 'bogus contract']

> Hospitals react to every error as an anomaly, for which the solution is to ferret out and blame an individual, with a promise that 'it will never happen again'. Paradoxically, this approach has diverted attention from the kind of systematic improvements that could decrease errors. Many errors are built into existing routines and devices, setting up the unwitting physician and patient for disaster. [Reason's 'error traps']

And, although patients are the first and obvious victims of medical mistakes, doctors are wounded by the same errors: they are the second victims.(28)

With Wu's insights in mind, we now turn to the effect of adverse outcomes and complaints on the *person* of the doctor.

'Second victims'

Wu uses a very curious phrase: 'the second victims.' It seems to run quite counter to the traditional image of the competent and powerful doctor, in control, fighting disease, saving lives, and so on. Box 11.4 contains a few short stories about doctors and their responses to adverse outcomes or to other similar situations. These doctors had not been trained in a patient safety approach to clinical practice.

BOX 11.4 DOCTORS' RESPONSES TO ADVERSE OUTCOMES

1. 'You killed that patient.' This was a comment from a registrar to a new house surgeon after their mutual patient had died. The house surgeon then gave up clinical medicine. *[Both doctors' responses seem problematic]*
2. We know of a doctor who was quite unable to open a letter from the Medical Council, from extreme fear that it was about disciplinary action.
3. We have seen many examples of intensely troubled responses from doctors to spurious or quite inconsequential complaints from a patient. These doctors' fury and anger seemed quite out of proportion to the validity of the complaint.
4. We know of several instances of doctors altering the medical notes after an adverse outcome or receiving a complaint.

These brief examples illustrate a sort of curious fragility. Certain types of professional challenge seem to incite strong and powerful emotions in doctors, which drive behaviours in unusual ways – ways that are less than professional, and certainly not what is expected of professionals with many years of training. It is not very helpful to say that they *shouldn't* behave like this: as a profession, we need to try to understand *why* they do.

Such stories could also be contrasted with aviation, where there are similar concerns about the safety of passengers and crew. In the professional culture of the airline industry, however, pilots who speak up about near misses usually receive professional credit and commendation. This is quite different from the culture of medicine where whistle-blowers (see page 167) have not been welcome.(29) Instead, those drawing attention to adverse outcomes are often given a very difficult time.(30) As Bolsin et al. recently asked, 'How can it be that selfless and ethically sound behaviour [i.e. whistle-blowing] continues to be punished by the medical establishment?'(31)

To provide an answer to this question, we once again draw on work from outside the profession – in this case, from Jungian analysis. This framework may also help to explain the profession's historical delay in addressing these issues.

Jungian analysis

In Jungian terms, the 'shadow' is the opposite of one's outward intention or demeanor, usually referring to negative feelings or behaviours. Jung maintained that the more these negative aspects of personhood are denied rather than acknowledged and incorporated, then the more they are 'liable to burst out in a moment of unawareness, thwarting our most well-meant intentions'. According to Jung, the shadow is 'the thing a person has no wish to be'.(32)

As we noted in Chapter 1, Jung also pointed out that doctors are in an 'archetypal role', a variant of the traditional 'healer' in society, and certainly not a role to be taken lightly. Inevitably, the *person* of the doctor is involved, as there are deep, archaic, even atavistic impulses in the choice of becoming a health professional where the goal is helping others.

There is a major problem when the healer inadvertently injures the patient. The doctor wants to be helpful, but now realises that he or she has created sickness. This can create a profound injunction or challenge to this deep-seated archetypal role. We posit a further explanation, then, for the profession's failure to act when increasing numbers of patients are being harmed by modern medicine. Adverse outcomes are the 'shadow' of helping patients and, collectively, the profession has been disavowing or denying this potential risk.

It is also no coincidence that the profession required help from the outside to initiate questions about patient safety. Those who were not fully acculturated into medicine could perhaps identify the problems more clearly. The profession's blindness was incurable from within.

With respect to Bolsin's question (Why are whistle-blowers so ostracised and punished?), adverse outcomes are the unacknowledged 'shadow' of the genuine intention of clinical practice (to help people in their distress). Unless the possibilities of harming patients are more openly considered and owned, then negative outcomes can generate a collective denial which includes 'shooting the messenger' – in this case, the whistle-blower who raises concerns about quality of care.

Doctors' responses to complaints and/or adverse outcomes

Box 11.4 also illustrates the ways complaints from patients can generate quite idiosyncratic reactions from the doctors involved. Receiving a complaint could be considered an adverse outcome of practice, at least from the doctor's point of view. Doctors are generally well intentioned and believe they are doing their best for their patients. A complaint, like an adverse outcome, is usually unexpected and not part of the unvoiced or tacit contract between doctor and patient.

Existing complaints systems, where a patient or family member officially raises concerns about an outcome of medical care, have a number of purposes. These include acting as a voice for patients, maintaining trust between society and the medical profession, and providing the opportunity for reconciliation and closure between doctor and complainant. However, the relationship between quality of medical care and patient complaints is complex. Adverse outcomes don't usually generate a complaint, while complaints can arise even if the standard of care has been exemplary.(33, 34) It is important to realise that both events can generate similar responses within the doctor.

In brief, complaints are not necessarily a reliable indicator of the quality of practice. However, given the historical reluctance of the profession to address the issue of adverse outcomes and the profession's usual response to whistle-blowers, the complaints system has often been the first (and sometimes only) trigger to initiate an enquiry into a particular area of clinical practice. In other words, in the absence of a systematic approach to patient safety, the complaints system has become the default method of ensuring better standards of care.

Most current doctors have been given very little training in understanding, anticipating, detecting, preventing, and responding to errors.(3) The emerging evidence is that many doctors respond poorly to such situations and become the 'second victim'.(28) Instead of the complaint triggering a thoughtful review of individual competencies within complex medical systems, some doctors lose confidence and become quite defensive in their practice.(35)

In Chapter 6, we discussed how complaints can have two main impacts: on the person of the doctor and on their future work. Another possible outcome is that doctors start to practise what is known as 'defensive' medicine.

Defensive medicine

This term describes changes to a doctor's practice in response to a complaint or when trying to avoid one: 'Deviations, induced by a threat of liability, from what the physician believes is, and what is generally regarded as, sound medical practice'.(36) Clinical decisions are thus predicated on a desire to avoid medical liability or malpractice suits, rather than the usual risk-benefit analysis.(37)

There are two directions in which practice can change – defensive medicine may be either 'positive' or 'negative'.(38) Positive defensive medicine or 'assurance behaviour' is when doctors increase their testing or services, not because of increased benefit for the patient, but to be *seen to be* reducing the risk of 'missing something'. The doctor believes such actions will reduce the risk of receiving a further complaint or increase their ability to defend one. Negative defensive medicine or 'avoidance behaviour' refers to withdrawal of medical services. Doctors stop providing care to particular types of patients in order to reduce their ongoing liability and risk.

Cunningham and Dovey found that assurance behaviour is linked to perceived reduction in confidence, reduced ability to make decisions and patient pressure. (39) Doctors increase their referrals and admissions to hospital, increase their use of investigations (to cover themselves against uncommon or unlikely diagnoses), attempt to pre-emptively identify problem patients, excessively document and consent, and alter their consulting times. Analysis of these responses showed that changes are based on a disease-centred model of practice. Such doctors tend to exclude the person of the patient and rely on narrowly defined biomedical rules to defend criticism in the event of further adverse outcomes or complaints.(39)

In contrast, avoidance behaviour is characterised by ceasing clinical practice in fields such as obstetrics, intensive care or psychiatry, shifting from rural to urban practice, or avoiding patients with particular conditions. These responses are idiosyncratic to the individual doctor. They are related to the context of clinical practice and the specifics of the complaint. The downside of negative defensive medicine is that the needs of certain patients and communities are excluded in an ill-founded attempt to reduce liability.

In New Zealand, doctors are protected against lawsuits through the Accident Compensation Corporation, which provides indemnity against personal liability. However, doctors' responses to complaints in New Zealand are very similar to those practising in tort-based legal systems (dominated by legal liability for adverse outcomes). Evidence from the US, the UK and Australia indicate that positive defensive medicine such as increased referrals, test ordering, and prescribing are also responses to litigation.(35) These common findings from disparate cultures (vis-à-vis complaint and litigation procedures) suggest that these doctors' responses arise more from internalised mechanisms, than from externalised modifiers of behaviour.

Is there an explanation, then, as to why doctors around the world change their practice in ways that are counterproductive for the medical care of individuals and communities? One idea is that *shame* is a possible link between biomedicine, complaints and defensive practice.(40)

Shame

Shame was introduced in Chapter 8 as an important but hidden concept within medical practice.(41, 42) Complaints or adverse outcomes can feel like an assault or threat to one's sense of self, thus triggering shame. The doctor often believes the complaint is an indication of medical failure. Many doctors receive and examine complaints in secret, often making highly critical and internalised judgements about their own competence and sense of self. Judged by themselves to have failed, doctors can internalise this failure and experience shame.(43)

After an adverse outcome or on receipt of a complaint, there is often a rather simplistic search for where they went wrong. They might question what they did not know or whether they had made an error in diagnosis or management, appraising their practice using the biomedical paradigm. Arguably, the shame response drives the observable changes in attitude towards patients as well as changes in practising behaviour towards defensive medicine.(43, 44) This is why we contend that defensive medicine is less driven by external litigious environments than by these internal responses arising within the doctor.

On being shamed, some doctors change their way of practising, viewing medical practice as a dichotomy of right or wrong. Defensive medicine indicates that doctors have learned poorly from the experience, altering their practice in a way that fails doctors, patients and the communities they serve. If complaints are to be used as a 'window of opportunity' to improve health services,(45) it is essential that the profession and society recognise the current maladaptive learning processes that can characterise some doctors' responses to complaints and adverse outcomes. The issue is one of resilience and wellness, set within the culture of medical practice.

Learning from complaints and adverse outcomes

The key to effective learning after complaints is to minimise the induction of these internalised shame responses. Doctors need to engage in appropriate reflective processes that allow them to explore not only the biomedical issues involved, but also their own responses and the implications of the event for the care and ongoing well-being of their patients.

If the doctor's responses are explored in a safe, caring and non-judgmental environment, the complaint can be reframed as an opportunity towards improved practice (if that is needed) and to provide help for the patient who may have suffered harm. A start to addressing these issues has been successfully made in New Zealand, with a counselling service that is freely available to doctors.(46)

Patient safety innovations in current practice

This chapter has lamented the absence of a patient safety approach to clinical practice, but there are now some significant advances. One of the most high-profile ideas is the **Surgical Safety Checklist**. This international innovation has been led by Dr Atul Gawande and others from around the world.(47) During each operation, there are three built-in pauses, where everyone identifies their role in the theatre team, which then carefully runs through a list of checking points (Box 11.5).

BOX 11.5 THE SURGICAL SAFETY CHECKLIST

Three pauses:

1. Sign in (before anaesthesia)
2. Time out (before skin incision)
3. Sign out (before completion)

Details of 2. 'Time out'

Before skin incision, the entire team (nurses, surgeons, anaesthesia professionals, and any others participating in the care of the patient) orally:

- Confirms that all team members have been introduced by name and role.
- Confirms the patient's identity, surgical site, and procedure.
- Reviews the anticipated critical events.
    - Surgeon reviews critical and unexpected steps, operative duration, and anticipated blood loss.
    - Anaesthesia staff review concerns specific to the patient.
    - Nursing staff review confirmation of sterility, equipment availability, and other concerns.
- Confirms that prophylactic antibiotics have been administered at least 60 min before incision is made or that antibiotics are not indicated.
- Confirms that all essential imaging results for the correct patient are displayed in the operating room.

Adapted from Haynes et al.(48)

Initial research showed that these checks had almost halved the death rate from complications during surgery.(48) While it is remarkable that a slight change in culture can have such a significant clinical effect, the uptake of this innovation was at times resisted by medical staff. Gawande posits a number of reasons for this resistance, including professional defensiveness. For example, introducing such changes might imply someone's surgical practice had previously been deficient.(47)

The Surgical Safety Checklist appears to be effective because of its influence on 'culture', in this case on the habits, relationships and expectations of staff within each operating theatre. We noted in Chapter 9 that culture is the set of attitudes, values, goals and practices that characterise an institution, organisation, or group. Medical culture itself has been the subject of many books and dissertations, although largely within other disciplines such as anthropology and sociology.

With respect to patient safety, particular attitudes and approaches to safety are now being identified through the lens of culture: 'Organizations with a positive safety culture are characterised by communications founded on mutual trust, by shared perceptions of the importance of safety, and by confidence in the efficacy of preventive measures.'(49) These ideas are quite different from traditional perceptions of a doctor working alone with his or her patient, usually in relative isolation from the organisational culture or community of practice around him or her.

The concept of safety culture includes the following dimensions: leadership commitment to safety; open communication founded on trust; organisational learning; a non-punitive approach to adverse event reporting and analysis; teamwork; and a shared understanding and belief in the importance of safety.(49)

The Manchester Patient Safety Framework is an excellent example of an intervention into the culture of a community of clinical practice. Developed in the UK, the tool is designed to increase staff awareness of patient safety within their organisation. All the team (doctors, nurses, receptionists, and others) individually score their perceptions of safety under nine different dimensions, a brief summary of which is listed in Box 11.6.(50)

BOX 11.6 MANCHESTER PATIENT SAFETY FRAMEWORK: DIMENSIONS

1. Overall commitment to quality
2. Priority given to patient safety
3. Perceptions of the causes of incidents
4. Investigating incidents
5. Learning following incident
6. Communication about safety issues
7. Staff management about safety issues
8. Staff education and training
9. Team working around safety issues

Adapted from Parker et al.(50)

Differences in attitudes and approaches to patient safety are illustrated by a set of criteria for each dimension. Table 11.1 outlines the criteria for Dimension 3 (Perceptions of causes of incidents). Once individuals have filled in their own scores, results are compared as a trigger for general discussion.

TABLE 11.1 MANCHESTER PATIENT SAFETY FRAMEWORK: DIMENSION 3

Perceptions of the causes of patient safety incidents and their identification *What sort of reporting systems are there? How are incidents viewed – as an opportunity to blame or improve?*	
A	Incidents are seen as bad luck, occurring as a result of staff errors or patient behaviour. Ad hoc reporting systems are in place but the practice is largely in blissful ignorance unless serious incidents occur or letters of complaint are received. There is a strong blame culture.
B	The practice sees itself as a victim of circumstances. Individuals are seen as the cause and the solution is retraining and punishment. There is an embryonic reporting system. Minimum data on the incidents is collected but not analysed. There is a blame culture, so staff are reluctant to report incidents.
C	There is a recognition that systems, not just individuals, contribute to incidents. A reporting system is in place. Attempts are made to encourage staff to report incidents (including those that did not lead to harm), though staff do not feel safe reporting the latter.
D	It is accepted that incidents are a combination of individual and system faults. Reporting of patient safety incidents is encouraged and they are seen as learning opportunities, although learning is not always disseminated. Accessible, staff-friendly electronic reporting methods are used. The practice has an open, fair and collaborative culture.
E	System failures are noted, although staff are also aware of their own professional accountability in relation to errors. It is second nature for staff to report patient safety incidents as they have confidence in the investigation process and understand the value of reporting. The practice has a high level of openness and trust.

Adapted from Parker(50)

Wallis and Dovey piloted a modified version of this intervention into general practices in New Zealand. Some practices made changes as a result, one group saying: 'We've started a patient called "Mr Patient Safety" and we've recorded a fair number of incidents … it's made us more aware.'(51) Participating staff reported that they became more proactive in their clinical practice after their individual scoring and group discussion.

Further research is needed to assess the long-term effect of this tool on each community of practice and to determine whether or not these interventions will impact on patient outcomes. There now appears to be a sufficient mandate to explore similar interventions into safety culture in both hospital practice and primary care.(52, 53)

Patient safety in medical education

Medical schools are beginning to include curricula on patient safety.(54) The World Health Organization is leading the way with its Patient Safety Curriculum Guide, published in 2009.(55) (Box 11.7)

BOX 11.7 WHO PATIENT SAFETY CURRICULUM GUIDE: TOPICS

1. What is patient safety?
2. What are 'human factors' and why are they important to patient safety?
3. Understanding systems and the impact of complexity on patient care
4. Being an effective team player
5. Understanding and learning from errors (types of errors, mistakes, violations)
6. Understanding and managing clinical risk
7. Introduction to quality improvement methods
8. Engaging with patients and carers
9. Minimizing infection through improved infection control
10. Patient safety and invasive procedures
11. Improving medication safety

Adapted from WHO Patient Safety Curriculum Guide for Medical Schools.*(55)*

This curriculum covers a comprehensive range of topics related to adverse outcomes and patient safety. The intention is that, compared with those practising today, future graduates will have a much better understanding of the risks to patients and of how to be more proactive in creating methods of prevention.

While the idea of patient safety curricula is laudable, many commentators have noticed the lag between innovations in clinical practice and what occurs in training: 'Medical education has yet to fully embrace patient safety concepts and principles into existing medical curricula. Universities are continuing to produce graduate doctors lacking in the patient safety knowledge, skills and behaviours thought necessary to deliver safe care.'(56)

Admittedly, there are significant barriers to implementation of such courses. Academic clinicians have differing ideas on when to introduce these subjects. Many do not want to 'damage' younger students' naïve enthusiasm about their choice of a medical career, or even tell them they will observe a number of serious adverse outcomes in the future.

Educationally, the design and implementation of new topics into an existing curriculum is difficult. Existing clinical rotations have their own agenda and newer subjects usually require an influential champion. Furthermore, current assessment is still largely based on knowledge-based recall, rather than on competence within clinical settings. If examinations drive learning, then patient safety has particular challenges in creating workplace-driven assessment. Ideally, though, students' capacity to recognise and prevent errors in the clinical setting needs to be assessed.

Additionally, comparing the evidence from medicine and aviation reveals that many doctors deny the existence of error and are unwilling to discuss it.(57) In other words, most current clinicians were not themselves trained in a patient safety model of practice and so feel diffident about introducing new subjects into their field of teaching.(54)

The main barriers to implementing curricula on patient safety, however, appear to be psychological. If academic staff are to demonstrate their understanding of these issues, they need to have worked through their own experiences of adverse events and be able to talk about them freely and openly with their students. They need to model reflective practice and be aware of the complex nature of change management within conservative institutions. They also need to be aware that discussing adverse outcomes can generate both individual and collective shame.

Our own experience of introducing modules on patient safety to both under- and postgraduate students is pertinent. In the undergraduate setting we introduced pre-clinical students to the concept of patient safety using Topic 1 of the WHO Patient Safety Curriculum and the WHO 'Learning from Error' video (which graphically illustrates the incorrect administration of vincristine). At first it was a challenge even to find teaching space in the absence of an overarching curricular consensus or approach to patient safety. Tutors delivering the course were largely supportive, but students were initially quite shocked by the video. Some mentioned a desire to give up medicine altogether. With further group discussion, however, feedback from students was supportive: 'Better to introduce these topics now so we are more prepared for the realities of clinical practice.'

We have also used the WHO video with several groups of mature GPs. The accompanying workshop materials suggest doing a 'fish-bone analysis' as a worked example of a systems approach to that particular event. However, many GPs were initially quite affected by the film. Instead of working through a cognitive analysis of contributing factors, the sessions were largely taken up with their own retrospective discussion of similar events. The video had triggered memories of traumatic clinical experiences, many of which had not been adequately processed, theorised, or used as vehicles for improvements in practice.

These experiences from both under- and postgraduate groups illustrate several of the themes in this chapter: differences between the expectations of clinical practice and reality; the expectation of perfection; overwhelming emotional responses to adverse outcomes and error which (initially at least) inhibit cognitive analysis; and the continued absence of systematic patient safety training.

While the principles of responding in more constructive ways to adverse outcomes can be introduced to students at undergraduate level, the real learning for such competence needs to occur within clinical settings, both in hospitals and in general practice. Role modelling by current staff is crucial in developing a more responsive culture surrounding these highly problematic situations. Lack of laudable role modelling remains a significant barrier to the profession's ongoing approach to adverse outcomes.(58)

Figure 11.4 summarises the approach to reducing the incidence of adverse outcomes in the future. Training for certitude has been replaced by specific training for patient safety, awareness of culture, and professional resilience.

FIGURE 11.4 REDUCING ERROR TRAPS AND ADVERSE OUTCOMES

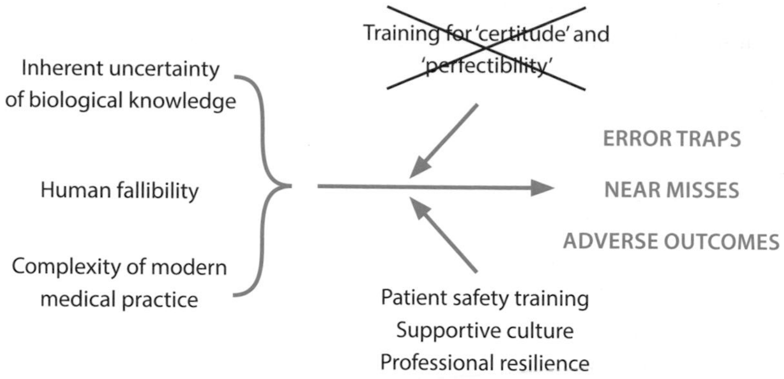

Training for 'certitude' and 'perfectibility'

Inherent uncertainty of biological knowledge

Human fallibility

Complexity of modern medical practice

ERROR TRAPS

NEAR MISSES

ADVERSE OUTCOMES

Patient safety training
Supportive culture
Professional resilience

Conclusion

The reactions of current doctors to complaints and adverse outcomes are often highly idiosyncratic and potentially unhelpful. Most practitioners have not been trained in a patient safety approach to clinical practice and may still be trying to practise 'perfect' medicine. Many doctors are suffering vicarious traumatisation from patient deaths or other adverse outcomes they have witnessed and/or feel partially responsible for. They may not have experienced a supportive environment in which they can openly discuss their reactions and fears. There is a defended fragility – vulnerable, without being open to discussion – which can make them very difficult to help.

Modern medical practice is increasingly complex. Given the combination of human fallibility and clinical uncertainty, error traps are omnipresent within medicine. Traditional goals of training for certitude and perfection have been ineffective in preventing adverse outcomes. Instead, students and graduates need to have much more specific and comprehensive training for patient safety. As this is now an overt agenda for undergraduate education, it seems likely that by 2020 every medical school will have a coherent and vertically integrated curriculum on patient safety, starting from day one. While there will be problems in implementation, graduating students need to be more realistic about the combination of uncertainty, medicine as a complex system, and human fallibility.

In brief, future students need to acknowledge and incorporate medicine's capacity to do harm, rather than learn to deny it. This means being trained to look for worst-case scenarios, to receive commendation for pointing out near misses, and to have training on how to respond to unintended consequences, both for the patient and for themselves. Embracing the capacity for doing harm means there is no longer a 'hidden shadow'. It has been precisely the denial of the shadow that has given it such power.

These long-term ideas require a significant change in medical culture, a change which is starting to take place, as Wallis and Dovey note: 'The current focus internationally is on the prospect of improving patient safety through cultural transformation.'(51)

Students also need more training for professional resilience and wellness. In brief, this requires:

- better understanding of emotional intelligence and how to respond to psychologically difficult situations, such as adverse outcomes;
- reflective practice as an overarching approach to the practice of medicine;
- a much more supportive culture within medicine itself – as Gawande suggests, a culture of trust, humility, and teamwork.(47)

In summary, medicine has traditionally been rather blind to its own predominant culture, which in the last 50 or so years has been dominated by an ever more narrowly focused biomedical science. The traditional approach of training for certitude and infallibility has failed. What is now required is training for patient safety, improving professional resilience, and creating a more supportive learning culture that re-envisages near-misses and adverse outcomes as learning opportunities, without shame or institutional recrimination. The end result will be better patient outcomes and more resilient doctors.

SUMMARY POINTS

- All doctors are involved in, or have been affected, by adverse outcomes.
- Adverse outcomes must be expected. They are due to (1) the inherent uncertainties within medical science, (2) human fallibility, (3) the complexity of modern medicine.
- Doctors are just as fallible as anyone else. Being in the act of doctoring does not obviate human fallibility.
- The profession has always known about adverse outcomes but has been slow to respond to them.
- The patient safety movement is gaining momentum now because of influences from outside the profession.
- The traditional training for certitude and infallibility in response to the inherent uncertainty of medical practice will not prevent error traps and adverse outcomes.
- Responses of doctors to complaints and adverse outcomes are often highly idiosyncratic and potentially unhelpful. Defensive medicine is an indication of maladaptive learning by doctors.
- Health care is littered with error traps, yet doctors have been given very little training in understanding, anticipating, detecting, preventing and responding to errors.
- Training in patient safety, improving professional resilience and creating a supportive learning culture is required if patient safety is to be improved.

References

1. Semmelweis IF, Carter KC. *The etiology, concept, and prophylaxis of childbed fever*. Madison: University of Wisconsin Press, 1983.
2. Kübler-Ross E, Wessler S, Avioli LV. On death and dying. *JAMA* 1972, 221(2):174–79.
3. Reason J. *The human contribution: unsafe acts, accidents and heroic recoveries*. Farnham: Ashgate, 2008.
4. Vincent C. *Patient safety*. Chichester: Wiley-Blackwell, 2010.
5. Emanuel L, Berwick D, Conway J, Combes J, Martin Hatlie JD, Leape L, et al. What exactly is patient safety? In: Henriksen K, Battles JB, Keyes MA, Grady ML, eds. *Advances in patient safety: New directions and alternative approaches. Vol. 4. Technology and Medication Safety*. AHRQ Publication No. 08-0034-4. Rockville, MD: Agency for Healthcare Research and Quality, 2008. pp. 19–36.
6. Cosby K. Developing taxonomies for adverse events in emergency medicine. In: Croskerry P, Cosby KS, Schenkel SM, Wears RL, eds. *Patient safety in emergency medicine*. Philadelphia: Lippincott Williams & Wilkins, 2009. pp. 8–11.
7. Reason J. *Managing the risks of organizational accidents*. Aldershot: Ashgate, 1997.
8. Elder NC, Dovey SM. Classification of medical errors and preventable adverse events in primary care: a synthesis of the literature. *J Fam Pract* 2002, 51(11):927–32.
9. Weingart S. Epidemiology of medical error. *BMJ* 2000, 320(7237):774–77.
10. Davis P, Lay-Yee R, Briant R, Ali W, Scott A, Schug S. Adverse events in New Zealand public hospitals I: occurrence and impact. *NZ Med J* 2002, 115(1167).
11. Hilfiker D. Facing our mistakes. *N Engl J Med* 1984, 310(2):118–22.
12. Young SR. Response to facing our mistakes. *N Engl J Med* 1984, 310(25):1676.
13. Wears RL, Vincent CA. The history of safety in health care. In: Croskerry P, Cosby KS, Schenkel SM, Wears RL, eds. *Patient safety in emergency medicine*. Philadelphia: Lippincott Williams & Wilkins, 2009. pp. 8–11.
14. Cooper JB, Newbower RS, Long CD, McPeek B. Preventable anesthesia mishaps: a study of human factors. *Anesth* 1978, 49(6):399–406.
15. Pierce Jr EC. The development of anesthesia guidelines and standards. *Qual Rev Bull* 1990, 16(2):61–64.
16. Reason J. *Human error*. Cambridge: Cambridge University Press, 1990.
17. Reason J. Human error: models and management. *BMJ* 2000, 320(7237):768.
18. Reason J. Beyond the organizational accident: the need for 'error wisdom' on the frontline. *Qual Saf Health Care* 2004, 13(suppl 2):ii28–ii33.
19. Noble DJ, Donaldson LJ. The quest to eliminate intrathecal vincristine errors: a 40-year journey. Qual Saf Health Care 2010, 19(4):323–26.
20. Ferner RE, McDowell SE. Doctors charged with manslaughter in the course of medical practice, 1795–2005: a literature review. *J Roy Soc Med* 2006, 99(6):309–14.
21. Kohn L, Corrigan J, Donaldson M. *To err is human: building a safer health system*. Washington, DC: National Academy Press, 1999.
22. Fox R. *Essays in medical sociology: journeys into the field*. New Brunswick: John Wiley & Sons, 1979.
23. Guenter D, Fowler N, Lee L. Clinical uncertainty: helping our learners. *Can Fam Phys* 2011, 57:120–23.
24. Esmail A. Clinical perspectives on patient safety. In: Walshe K, Boaden RJ, eds. *Patient safety: research into practice*. Maidenhead: Open University Press, 2006. pp. 9–18.
25. Smith R. Why are doctors so unhappy? *BMJ* 2001, 322(7294):1073.
26. Sinclair S. *Making doctors: an institutional apprenticeship*. New York: Berg Publishers, 1997.
27. Christensen JF, Levinson W, Dunn PM. The heart of darkness. *J Gen Int Med* 1992, 7(4):424–31.

28. Wu AW. Medical error: the second victim. *BMJ* 2000, 320(7237):726.

29. Near JP, Miceli MP. Retaliation against whistle blowers: predictors and effects. *J Appl Psychol* 1986, 71(1):137–45.

30. Wright T. The Stoke CNEP Saga: how it damaged all involved. *J Roy Soc Med* 2010, 103(7):277–79.

31. Bolsin S, Pal R, Wilmshurst P, Pena M. Whistleblowing and patient safety: the patient's or the profession's interests at stake? *J Roy Soc Med* 2011, 104:278–82.

32. Samuels A, Shorter B, Plaut F. *A critical dictionary of Jungian analysis*. London: Routledge & Kegan Paul, 1986.

33. Bismark MM, Brennan TA, Paterson RJ, Davis PB, Studdert DM. Relationship between complaints and quality of care in New Zealand: a descriptive analysis of complainants and non-complainants following adverse events. *Qual Saf Health Care* 2006, 15(1):17–22.

34. Murff HJ, France DJ, Blackford J, Grogan EL, Yu C, Speroff T, et al. Relationship between patient complaints and surgical complications. *Qual Saf Health Care* 2006, 15(1):13–16.

35. Wu AW, Folkman S, McPhee SJ, Lo B. Do house officers learn from their mistakes? *BMJ* 2003, 12(3):221–26.

36. Hershey N. The defensive practice of medicine: myth or reality. *Millbank Mem Fund Q* 1972, 50:69–97.

37. Nash LM, Walton MM, Daly MG, Kelly PJ, Walter G, Van Ekert EH et al. Perceived change in Australian doctors as a result of medicolegal concerns. *Med J Australian* 2012, 193(10):579–83.

38. Studdert DM, Mello MM, Sage WM, DesRoches CM, Peugh J, Zapert K, et al. Defensive medicine among high-risk specialist physicians in a volatile malpractice environment. *JAMA* 2005, 293(21):2609–17.

39. Cunningham W, Dovey S. Defensive changes in medical practice and the complaints process: a qualitative study of New Zealand doctors. *NZ Med J* 2006, 119:1244.

40. Cunningham W, Wilson HJ. Complaints, shame and defensive medicine. *BMJ Qual Saf* 2011, 20:449–52.

41. Lewis M. *Shame: The exposed self*. New York: The Free Press, 1995.

42. Jacoby M. *Shame and the origins of self-esteem*. London: Routledge, 1994.

43. Davidoff F. Shame: the elephant in the room. *Qual Saf Health Care* 2002, 11(1):2–3.

44. Cunningham W, Wilson HJ. Shame, guilt and the medical practitioner. *NZ Med J* 2003, 116(1183).

45. McManus IC, Gordon D, Winder BC. Duties of a doctor: UK doctors and good medical practice. *Qual Health Care* 2000, 9(1):14–22.

46. Cunningham W, Cookson T. Addressing stress related impairment in doctors: a survey of providers' and doctors' experience of a funded counselling service in New Zealand. *NZ Med J* 2009, 122(1300).

47. Gawande A. *Checklist manifesto: how to get things right*. London: Profile Books, 2010.

48. Haynes AB, Weiser TG, Berry WR, Lipsitz SR, Breizat AHS, Dellinger EP, et al. A surgical safety checklist to reduce morbidity and mortality in a global population. *N Engl J Med* 2009, 360(5):491–99.

49. Halligan M, Zecevic A. Safety culture in healthcare: a review of concepts, dimensions, measures and progress. *BMJ Qual Saf* 2011, 20:338–43.

50. Parker D, Lawrie M, Carthey J, Coultous M. The Manchester patient safety framework: sharing the learning. *Clinic Risk* 2008, 14(4):140–42.

51. Wallis K, Dovey SM. Assessing patient safety culture in New Zealand primary care: a pilot study using a modified Manchester patient safety framework in Dunedin general practices. *J Prim Health Care* 2011, 3(1):35–40.

52. Flin R. Measuring safety culture in healthcare: a case for accurate diagnosis. *Saf Sci* 2007,

45(6):653–67.

53. Robb G, Seddon M. Measuring the safety culture in a hospital setting: a concept whose time has come? *NZ Med J* 2010, 123(1313).

54. Mayer D, Klamen DL, Gunderson A, Barach P. Designing a patient safety undergraduate medical curriculum: the Telluride interdisciplinary roundtable experience. *Teach Learn Med* 2009, 21(1):52–58.

55. *WHO Patient Safety Curriculum Guide For Medical Schools*. New York: World Health Organization, 2009.

56. Walton M, Woodward H, Van Staalduinen S, Lemer C, Greaves F, Noble D, et al. The WHO patient safety curriculum guide for medical schools. *Qual Saf Health Care* 2010, 19(6):542–46.

57. Sexton J, Thomas E, Helmrich R. Error, stress, and teamwork in aviation and medicine. *BMJ* 2000, 320:745–49.

58. Runciman B, Merry A, Walton M. *Safety and ethics in healthcare: a guide to getting it right.* Aldershot: Ashgate, 2007.

Chapter 12

The Place of General Practice in Primary Health Care

CONTENTS

Introduction

While undergraduate medical students are often attracted to the *idea* of general practice, many are not quite sure what GPs actually do. Similarly, many hospital doctors feel quite intimidated by clinical practice in community settings, where patient problems are less well defined, there are no immediate laboratory or radiology facilities, and one is expected to know about a wide range of diseases and presentations. There is a shift in emphasis from a largely episodic, disease-based model to one of continuous, person-based care, where individual and social factors have a greater impact on disease. These factors might influence graduates to train in a particular specialty, where considerable depth of knowledge is gained, albeit within a narrower scope of practice.

Such concerns are understandable, given that most undergraduate training is based on treatment of acute disease within hospital settings. Some medical schools now provide general practice rotations where students work with GPs in primary care settings. More often, students are not provided with a systematic understanding of the role of the GP within the overall delivery of health care, or introduced to its history.

Given these factors, the transition from hospital training to general practice can be problematic. Working in primary care settings will provide other challenges. Do doctors known as general practitioners just diagnose and treat diseases within their particular community setting? Are they also charged with responsibility for identifying factors that might *cause* disease? If so, what factors do influence health and disease, and how might the GP identify these in a patient, the family, the community, or the environment? Furthermore, what are the divisions and relationships between primary and secondary care, and how should society allocate resources between them?

We start this chapter with a short history of general practice and primary health care. This leads to a discussion of determinants of health and circumstances of living. We then consider national health-care systems, noting that an overall primary care orientation provides better health and better equity, at a lower cost than those systems based on specialty care.(1) The discussion is intended to clarify both the scope and value of general practice or, in other words, to explore the place of the GP in modern society, as defined by relationships with patients, with communities and with society's health-care system.

The burden of illness

Before considering the origins of general practice and primary health care, it is useful to identify the usual range of health-related activities within each society. From an anthropological perspective, Kleinman identified three different sectors.(2) First, the **popular health-care sector** describes the initial responses of parents and families to illness. This healing role is often taken up by mothers and other women, who diagnose and treat using local handed-down knowledge.

The **folk sector** includes the traditional shaman or local healer. Folk healers often learn by apprenticeship, rather than by formal education. Two examples are the Peruvian curanderos and the traditional healer in Maori society called the tohunga.

Third, there is the **professional health-care sector**, where practitioners are trained in a standardised way to acquire an organised body of knowledge. Examples are traditional Chinese practitioners, Japanese herbal specialists and acupuncturists, ayurvedic practitioners in India, and biomedical doctors and nurses in Western countries.

Primary health care encompasses all these sectors, noting that the boundaries between them are always fluid and contested.(3) This chapter focuses on how the professional health-care sector in Western society is organised both to treat and to prevent illness.

Illness is very common. Within any given community, many people will be having symptoms, some will be getting treatment from various health providers, some will choose not to. The pattern of health-seeking behaviour varies from country to country. In a large study in 1996 in the US, about 800 people in 1000 were having physical or psychological symptoms of some kind.(4) About 330 of them were considering seeking medical help, 220 or so visited a doctor, but only half of those were in primary care. Sixty-five visited a complementary or alternative practitioner, 21 had a specialist outpatient appointment at a hospital, 14 were getting home health care of some kind, and 13 visited an emergency department. Eight were in hospital, but only one of those was being treated in a university teaching centre (Figure 12.1).

FIGURE 12.1 PREVALENCE OF ILLNESS IN THE COMMUNITY AND
SOURCES OF HEALTH CARE

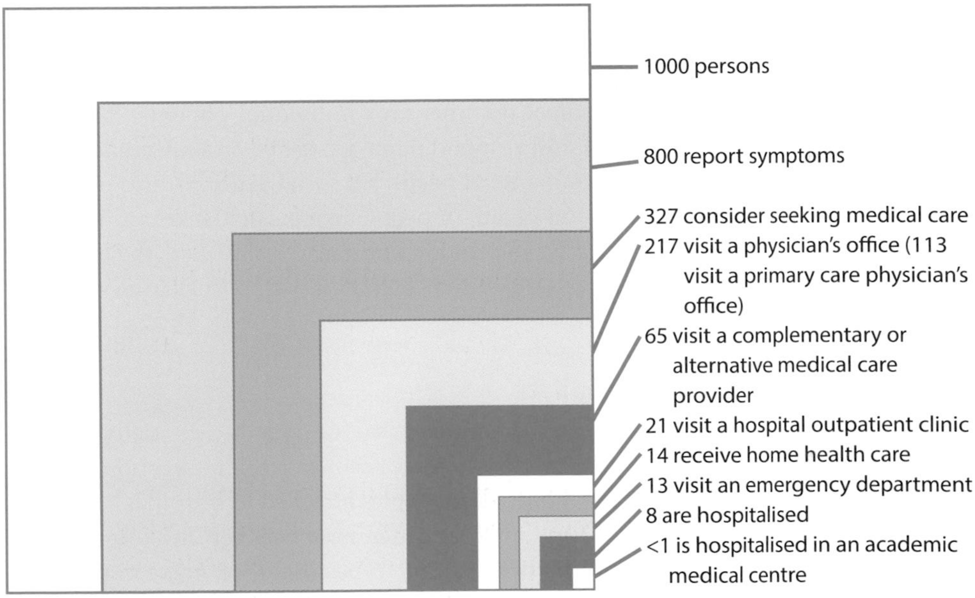

Numbers quoted are relative incidence only; groups are not 'nested'.
From Green et al.(4)

In Green's study, more than half the patients visiting a doctor were seeing a specialist, illustrating the specialist-led health-care system in place in the US. In most other countries, however, access to specialist care is restricted until *after* the patient has consulted their GP. Illness and disease are usually managed outside the hospital setting, with many people also choosing to visit practitioners *other* than doctors.

Of the 330 people receiving medical help, only a few are lying in a hospital bed. Most undergraduate medical training is based on this very small percentage of patients.

A brief history: general practice and primary health care

Until about 1800 in the UK, three different professions were learning about and practising biomedicine. The university-trained physician had expertise with internal disorders (cardiac and respiratory patients, and so on). The surgeon (or barber-surgeon) did operations, and the apothecary (pharmacist) gave out medicines prescribed by the physician. Between 1800 and 1840, a group of doctors started to develop expertise in all these areas, including midwifery. They became known as general practitioners. Their first organised group was the National Association of General Practitioners founded in 1844.(5)

For a hundred years or so, these early GPs practised largely by themselves. It was not until the 1950s that the Royal College of GPs in the UK was formally created and established. This national body was the start of more effective training worldwide for the specialty of general practice. Since then, the GP has become a central and effective figure in the delivery of health care in many countries.

The end of World War II saw the description 'primary health care' start to emerge as a unifying concept for health-care delivery. This was a wider concept than GPs simply providing medical treatment for individual patients. 'Primary health care' attempts to identify and respond in an accessible and affordable way to determinants of health. Determinants of health are social, cultural, and political factors that impact on the lives and health of people in a particular community or country. While generalists have always provided primary *medical* care, the modern GP has increasingly become more embedded or located within this larger context of primary health care.

The roles of GPs and specialists

General practitioners have quite different roles in health-care delivery in comparison with other doctors. On the whole, specialists work in secondary care hospitals, in private practice, or in outpatient clinics attached to hospitals.

Table 12.1 illustrates some fundamental differences between the orientation of specialists and that of generalists or GPs. Both types of doctor make important contributions to the health of individual patients: their different roles and responsibilities are synergistic and mutually cooperative. The GP treats disease in the context of the whole person and their supports. Specialist practitioners provide definitive biomedical interventions to patients where primary care practitioners do not have the skills or equipment to do so.

While GPs have a broad range of knowledge and skills in many areas, the specialist has greater depth of knowledge in one particular area. Working together, GPs and specialists provide both breadth and depth in medical care.

TABLE 12.1 GENERALISM AND SPECIALISM COMPARED

	GENERALISM	SPECIALISM
Knowledge	Breadth of knowledge	Depth of knowledge
	Multi-disciplinary, many organ systems	Single discipline, usually one organ system
	Undifferentiated disease	Differentiated
	Prevention, investigation, management, rehabilitation and chronic care	Investigation and management of specific disease
	Disease in the context of multiple systems and the whole person	Disease in the context of a single organ system
Site of work	Community- and hospital-based	Mostly hospital-based
Skills	Predominantly non-invasive approach	Often invasive techniques required
Attitudes	Whole person care, includes social background, supports and wider context	Uses reductionist principles to provide latest disease management.

Adapted from Starfield(6)

Knowing and appreciating these different roles can help to reduce the apparent competition between different specialties. Patients are frequently referred from GP to specialist and back again. The table above can help clarify the goals of such referrals, creating mutually cooperative relationships in the service of the patient. The role of the GP is further defined below, beginning with a review of the background to primary health care.

The Declaration of Alma-Ata

A turning point for the emerging concept of primary health care was the 1978 World Health Organization conference in Alma-Ata, USSR. This seminal conference re-envisaged primary health care as an international philosophy and policy for health-care delivery in both developed and developing countries. Speakers from many nations called on the world community to 'protect and promote the health of all the people of the world'.(7) Delegates proposed ideas that seem quite familiar in today's medical environment, including the idea that health is a fundamental human right: that it should be not merely the absence of disease, but 'a state of complete physical, mental and social wellbeing'. These statements provided direction and guidelines for governments around the world as they sought to improve the health of their people.

The major outcome of this conference was the Declaration of Alma-Ata. This contains both an overall political agenda and specific ideas for primary health care.

The broad agenda includes these principles: inequalities in health status between developed and developing countries (as well as between different socio-economic groups within countries) are unacceptable; health is linked to, and promotes, economic and social development in a reciprocal manner; people have a right to participate in their own health care; governments are responsible for the health of their people; governments should formulate strategies to launch and sustain primary health care; and the redistribution of resources from military conflict into social and economic development is essential for the promotion of health.(7)

According to the Declaration, primary health care 'reflects and evolves from the economic conditions and sociocultural and political characteristics of the country and its communities'. It should provide promotive, preventive, curative and rehabilitation services to address the main health problems in the community; be concerned with educative, treatment and preventive tasks relevant to those problems; involve national and community development, agriculture, industry, education, housing and public works; promote community and individual self-reliance and participation; be sustained by appropriate referral systems in order to provide comprehensive health care for all; and rely on health and community workers to work as a team, responsive to the health needs of the community.(7) The Declaration states that primary health care is the 'first level of contact with the national health system' and 'constitutes the first element of a continuing health process'.(7) GPs, therefore, play an important role as gatekeepers into the health system.(8)

While these ideals have been criticised as unrealistic,(9) primary health care is a system that is designed to respond to social and economic issues that impact on individual health. Poverty, for example, has long been known to be a major factor in the creation and spread of disease.(10) It is now measured through the 'deprivation index', and is the subject of considerable research.(11) We will now identify various social and economic factors that impact on health.

The social and economic determinants of health

In New Zealand in 1998, the National Health Committee released a major report addressing health inequalities. This report noted how social, cultural and economic factors are the main determinants of health.(12) While this discussion is set within the New Zealand context, the underlying issues are generic for all countries and societies (Figure 12.2).

FIGURE 12.2 SOCIAL AND ECONOMIC DETERMINANTS OF HEALTH

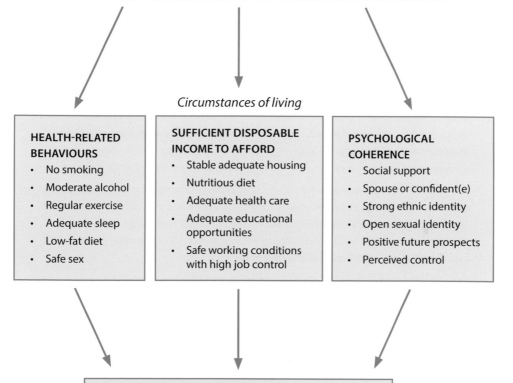

STRUCTURAL FEATURES OF SOCIETY, ECONOMY AND ENVIRONMENT
- Low unemployment
- Clean, healthy environment
- Safe working conditions with high job control
- Education and health services available
- Low disparities in income and wealth
- Low crime
- Favourable economic conditions
- All ethnic groups feel able to participate in society
- Negotiation between indigenous and immigrant groups

Circumstances of living

HEALTH-RELATED BEHAVIOURS
- No smoking
- Moderate alcohol
- Regular exercise
- Adequate sleep
- Low-fat diet
- Safe sex

SUFFICIENT DISPOSABLE INCOME TO AFFORD
- Stable adequate housing
- Nutritious diet
- Adequate health care
- Adequate educational opportunities
- Safe working conditions with high job control

PSYCHOLOGICAL COHERENCE
- Social support
- Spouse or confident(e)
- Strong ethnic identity
- Open sexual identity
- Positive future prospects
- Perceived control

HEALTHY INDIVIDUAL/FAMILY/'WHANAU'
HEALTHY COMMUNITY / STRONG SOCIAL CAPITAL

Adapted from Howden-Chapman and Tobias(12)

Structural features of a society that influence health include employment, working conditions, education and health services, and crime. These features link to concepts within the Declaration of Alma-Ata and impact on individual circumstances of living. These are:

- health-related behaviours such as smoking, alcohol and exercise;
- having sufficient disposable income to access adequate housing, diet, education, and health care;
- psychological coherence with respect to social and spousal supports, ethnic and sexual identity, a positive future and a sense of individual control.

While these concepts may appear quite theoretical, the following clinical story is an attempt to illustrate the complex issues and relationships involved.

VIGNETTE 12.1 ROBYN AND HER BABY

Robyn (30 years old) had recently shifted to my practice. Most of our consultations were initially about Joel, her one-year-old baby whose congenital heart defect had been surgically corrected. Robyn also had three other children, who had been removed from her care by welfare services. Two of these children were also in my practice, but were cared for by a foster family. Both illustrated the effects of disordered upbringing, with developmental delay and behavioural problems.

Robyn had lived with her mother and her mother's partner, but when this relationship became strained, she found her own place to live with Joel. Welfare services were often in contact with us about this at-risk baby, given Robyn's use of alcohol. Under pressure from welfare, Robyn agreed to start oral Antabuse (disulfiram). Her mother visited each day to ensure it was taken.

One day I took a call from welfare. Robyn's relationship with her mother had once again deteriorated and she was drinking heavily. I arranged to see her, pointing out that if she kept drinking, this child would also be removed by the state. I had always been pretty straight with her, and she took this to heart. We talked about how she could use the medication to stay off the alcohol and to keep her baby.

She was subsisting on a government benefit. While we charged her minimal fees, her payment was inconsistent. She acknowledged she was unreliable with her medication, so we agreed she could attend our practice three days a week, where the practice nurse would administer it. It would not have been unreasonable to charge for this service, but we did not, as the cost to us was low and the potential gain for Robyn and her child was high.

For about three months the system worked well. Robyn was settled, taking reasonable care of Joel. Then her mother's relationship with her partner broke down. The mother shifted away and Robyn lost her most significant (though inconsistent) social support. She moved away from the area and resumed drinking. We believe her child is now in welfare care.

This narrative illustrates some of the background social factors that contribute to individual patient health and their impact on medical work. Robyn's circumstances of living include her alcohol abuse, diet, lack of exercise, and sexual behaviour leading to unplanned pregnancies. She lacks sufficient disposable income to provide stable and adequate housing for herself and her baby. She cannot afford to pay for the health care that she needs. Her chances of becoming educated or trained sufficiently to escape her poverty cycle are poor and she is unlikely to reduce her reliance on social welfare. Her relationship with her main social support (her mother) is strained. She has separated from her former partner and lacks a strong sense of cultural identity and community. Her perceived control over her life varies as she grapples with alcoholism.

Some of the roles of general practice within primary health care become apparent in this narrative. The GP provides up-to-date and accessible medical care for both Robyn and her baby. The GP also attempts to keep track of other health professionals who are involved: social workers, nurses, pharmacists, paediatricians, alcohol counsellors, and so on. Understanding and working with this cluster of professionals who have input into Robyn's care is part of the GP's role.

The determinants of health will be outside the GP's control, but awareness of the impact of behaviour, income and psychological coherence allows careful consideration of how the doctor might intervene, or at least assist. This might involve contact with an employer of the patient if working conditions are poor, the local authorities if housing, sanitation or water supply is implicated, or the extended family or other social supports and networks if they are either part of the problem or the potential solution. In this diagnostic approach to circumstances of living and the role of the doctor, an analogy might be finding a rare dolphin entangled in a fisherman's net: doing so might stimulate thoughts about the relationships between food sources and commerce, conservation and politics.

Similarly, a child with delayed milestones (such as Joel) might trigger thoughts on the wider context, such as unemployment and poverty, disparities of income, the availability of street drugs and diversion of prescriptions, social services that provide unemployment and sickness benefits, and intergenerational aspects of unemployment. While the GP has responsibility for ensuring that the child receives adequate health care, other contributing factors need attention through social welfare, economics, and politics.

In summary, the GP is not responsible for solving complex social issues, but may have some responsibility for advocacy. Taking a patient's 'circumstances of living' into account enables shared responsibility between a wide range of parties.

We return now to primary health care systems and how they work.

Characteristics of primary health care

The Declaration of Alma-Ata can be translated into practical terms and activities. Systems of primary health care display the following characteristics: availability, accessibility, continuity, coordination, and comprehensiveness of care for all members of society. These terms are explained in more detail below.

Availability means that health care is readily available to all members of the community or society, regardless of their socio-economic group or background. This may require government subsidy of health-care services or special facilities for special groups such as cultural minorities, those with disability, and so on.

Accessibility or first contact care means that *all* new illnesses are seen in the primary care setting and that there are no structural barriers to access (lack of transport within the community, available hours, and so on).

Continuity of care or 'person-focused care over time' means that the focus is on the person, rather than on the disease. As most patients have many concurrent problems (co-morbidity), the place of treatment remains the same for that person.

Coordination of care means that the central locus of care remains within primary care, but that there is good coordination of services delivered by a multitude of other providers. Coordination of care between GPs, hospital services and specialists can have a significant impact on disease outcomes.

Comprehensiveness of care means that *all* health problems are cared for in that particular setting, except for those conditions that are too rare or require expertise or technology that cannot be provided by primary care teams.

Enrolment is how the characteristics above are put into practice. Patients in a particular community need to enrol or register with a general practice group or other locally based health provider. Identifying the demographics and health status of this enrolled population is a crucial first step, as otherwise the health-care team is unaware of that community's needs. On the other hand, if patients always see a new provider or use emergency departments for acute health needs, then there is no continuity of care, overview of disease trends, screening for disease, or attempts at health promotion. Primary health care thus requires considerable organisation, attempting to address the health inequalities of various socio-economic groups within each society.

This model of health care has made a significant impact in both developing and developed countries.

The impact of primary health care systems

Since 1979, the seminal Alma-Ata proposal for primary health care has been a helpful template as countries around the world attempt to address poverty-related mortality and morbidity. Taking just one example in Gambia in 1981, infant mortality dropped substantially after the introduction of primary health care. For various reasons this system weakened after 1994, and infant mortality rose again (Box 12.1).

BOX 12.1 INFANT MORTALITY IN GAMBIA

Over a 15-year period from 1981, 40 villages with and without primary health care (PHC) services were compared in terms of infant and child mortality. The 'PHC villages' were provided with a health nurse, a health worker and a trained birth attendant. Maternal and child health services with a vaccination program were also accessible to residents in both PHC and non-PHC villages. There were marked improvements in infant and child (<5 years) mortality in both PHC and non-PHC villages. Infant mortality dropped from 134/1000 in 1983 to 69/1000 in 1994 in the PHC villages and from 155/1000 to 91/1000 in the non-PHC villages over the same period.

Ongoing supervision of the PHC system weakened after 1994, and infant mortality rates in the PHC villages rose again to 89/1000 in 1994–96. Overall child mortality rates rose significantly when the PHC services weakened.

Adapted from Hill et al.(13) and Hall and Taylor(14)

While the above example is striking, the benefits of primary health care are just as applicable to more developed countries. Health outcomes of patients *within* a country depend on the local numbers of primary care physicians. For example, in the US an increase of three primary care doctors per 10,000 population increases life expectancy by about four years.(15)

These observations are even more apparent when comparing 'specialist' versus 'primary health care' systems in different countries around the world. Belgium, France, Germany and the US have health services that are **specialty** oriented. In these countries a high percentage of practising doctors are specialists. Patients have direct access to them as soon as they have symptoms. These countries have a lower primary health care score, as measured by various characteristics of the health system: financing, type of primary care practitioner, the percentage of active physicians who are specialists, professional earnings of primary care physicians relative to specialists, cost sharing for primary care services, patient enrolment, requirements for 24-hour coverage, and strength of academic departments of family medicine.(16, 17)

On the other hand, patients in **primary health care**-oriented countries are assessed and treated by generalist doctors or other primary health care professionals *before* they can access more expensive specialist services and treatment. Examples are Denmark, Finland, Netherlands, Spain, the UK, and New Zealand. In these countries, the bulk of disease management is provided by GPs, nurses, and other primary care providers. The overall health outcomes for these countries appear to be better than in countries where specialist doctors provide the greater part of care.(17)

Another observation is that countries vary enormously in terms of health expenditure per head of population. The US for example, spends almost twice as much on health care as many other countries.(18) However, because there is no primary health care system, many people have no access to basic health-care services. The overall outcome is that despite high health-care costs, there is no overall increase in life expectancy.(17).

The implication, then, is that spending more money does not necessarily improve health, unless the system is based on primary care. Specifically, primary care-oriented countries have fewer low-birthweight infants, lower infant mortality, fewer years of life lost due to suicide, and a higher life expectancy. The evidence arises from a wide variety of study types, including international comparisons, clinical studies and population studies within countries.(16, 17)

Why primary health care?

The feature that most distinguishes primary care-oriented countries from specialist ones is that of *comprehensiveness*. As defined above, this means that almost all health and medical needs are met within primary care, rather than from secondary care providers or disease specialists. These health needs describe the scope of practice of general practitioners and include: universal provision of health benefits for children such as vaccinations and development checks; medical care of the elderly, women and other adults; routine maternity care; mental health care at low cost; minor surgery; generic vaccinations and preventive care; treatment and follow-up of common diseases; minor technical procedures such as setting fractures, wart removal, assessment of acute eye injuries; contraceptive advice and cervical smears; and health education for various groups.(19)

Health care provided by specialists usually costs more than that provided by generalists. Although specialists usually have more in-depth knowledge of specific diseases, the generic outcomes of care (patient satisfaction, complications, referral to other services) are no better, and are often worse, than when general care is provided by primary care physicians.(20) This research finding might stem from the ready availability of invasive investigations and treatments within specialist health systems, where the benefit is marginal or even dubious.(21)

Starfield points out that comprehensiveness is 'a critical feature of primary care because it is responsible for avoiding unnecessary referrals to specialists and therefore avoiding unnecessary and inappropriate care and inappropriate expenditures'.(22) If primary care takes responsibility for the management of common diseases (even though their management can be complex and challenging), specialist resources are reserved for unusual or rare diseases, as well as for investigations and treatments that require particular expertise and technologies.

Co-morbidity

There is a further problem when a patient has more than one disease, also known as co-morbidity. If the patient sees a different specialist for each problem (rather than most of their health care being provided by one general practitioner), health-care costs rise exponentially and overall health outcomes turn out to be significantly worse. This is because diagnostic tests are used more, medication rates go up, and the possibility of drug interactions or other adverse outcomes increases. These issues illustrate a lack of continuity of care and the absence of an overall coordinator or director of referral and treatment decisions. In brief, the benefits of primary care are greatest for those patients who have high co-morbidity.(6, 21)

To summarise this chapter so far, the Declaration of Alma-Ata in 1978 was a turning point for health-care delivery around the world. Primary health care is now promoted as being a cost-effective and comprehensive method of providing health care, both for developed as well as for developing nations. Extensive research since then has confirmed that the Declaration was profoundly insightful: countries that have not followed these ideas spend more money on health care for less benefit. Recent commentaries have confirmed the continuing relevance of primary care.(23)

Responsibilities and relationships

As we have seen, there is more to the nature of primary health care than the treatment of disease. Primary care can also be defined by its underlying values and relationships. As noted, these include availability, accessibility, continuity, coordination, and comprehensiveness. The value that underpins these is commitment – not to a 'person with a disease', but to the person. As McWhinney explains: 'The commitment is open ended. The relationship is ended only by retirement, removal, death, or a decision by either party to end it.'(24)

The doctor's immediate task is to manage the illness, be aware of the compounding effects of co-morbidities, and engage secondary care when circumstances of experience, competence and resource dictate. However, the GP's role is the overall care of that patient, who is embedded in a particular community. The GP has a commitment to the community as well as to the patient. As noted above, identifying the health needs of the enrolled population for the practice allows GPs to become more proactive in relation to specific diseases, immunisations and health promotion. However, the GP cannot meet these commitments alone. Clear division of labour and tasks is required within each health-care team.

The organisation of general practice and teamwork

Organised general practice is a system in which groups of general practices are owned, funded and run so that they can take collective action to improve the quality of health care in a particular area. Quality primary care is dependent on how these health professionals relate to each other, as it is not possible for one person to perform the wide variety of tasks. If a general practice team is not functioning well, their practice population may not be well cared for. It is also essential that GPs are aware of the links between their own health and the quality of their clinical care, have a supportive work environment and use various methods of work review or reflection to continually improve their medical practice.

The concept of collaborative practice underpins the primary health care philosophy, even at a global level. Effective teamwork in general practice requires shared objectives, participative safety, and open communication.(25) However, collaborative practice can be undermined by structural and funding issues that make it difficult for team members to meet, share ideas and achieve common goals. Different types of funding streams can diminish the ability of the practice to effectively care for the needs of the practice population. In particular, fee-for-service and task- or intervention-based funding tend to encourage a focus on maximising income. Methods of payment can influence health-care outcomes.(25).

From hospital work to general practice

Many doctors in hospital or specialist training know little about primary care medicine, so to contemplate a move to general practice can feel like a leap of faith. One underlying problem is that modern medical training largely focuses on treatment of individual patients with one particular disease, especially in acute care settings. This training does not effectively prepare graduates for the approaches and tasks needed in general practice.

Furthermore, the professional and institutional *culture* of hospital and specialist medicine is vastly different from that of general practice, where hierarchical structures are much flatter, both within the profession and in relation to other professions. GPs are required to work independently across a wide spectrum of disease. Undifferentiated symptoms present considerable diagnostic difficulties and require the capacity to sit with uncertainty, especially as investigations take time. Responsibility for screening and health promotion is shared with other professionals. Shifting to clinical work in community settings requires awareness of these differences and their challenges.

Conclusion

This chapter has attempted to demystify the tasks of general practice and primary health care. It takes time to understand the different concepts, roles and tasks required, but those doctors who make a successful transition can be richly rewarded. Long-term relationships with patients and colleagues can contribute to a sense of job satisfaction that is unmatched in other specialties. Acknowledging circumstances of living, teamwork and relationships between primary and secondary care will provide clarity, determine responsibility and help to provide that unique sense of place that comes with being an effective and successful GP.

SUMMARY POINTS

- General practice is located within the wider concept of primary health care (PHC) as defined in the Declaration of Alma-Ata.
- Social and economic determinants of health can be identified and defined. PHC is a political strategy to address social determinants and health inequalities within countries.
- Primary health care systems provide better health outcomes for communities and society at lower cost and with greater equity than specialist-oriented systems.
- Having an enrolled population of patients in primary care (usually at a specific general practice) can lead to more accurate assessment of community health needs.
- Recognising determinants of health allows a diagnosis based on circumstances of living. This helps to determine responsibility for advocacy.
- A mutually respectful relationship between primary and specialist care, identifying and respecting different roles and strengths, is essential to sharing medical care.
- General practitioners meet a wide range of health needs in the community and are crucially important in the delivery of national health care.

References

1. Stange KC, Ferrer RL. The paradox of primary care. *Ann Fam Med* 2009, 7(4):293–99.
2. Kleinman A. *Patients and healers in the context of culture*. Berkeley: University of California, 1980.
3. Joralemon D. *Exploring medical anthropology*. Boston: Allyn and Bacon, 1999.
4. Green LA, Fryer Jr GE, Yawn BP, Lanier D, Dovey SM. The ecology of medical care revisited. *N Engl J Med* 2001, 344(26):2021–25.
5. Sturmberg J. *The foundations of primary care: daring to be different*. Seattle: Radcliffe, 2007.
6. Starfield B. Comprehensiveness of care: concept and importance. Keynote address. Wellington: Quality Symposium, Royal NZ College of General Practitioners, 2009.
7. Fendall N. Declaration of Alma-Ata. *Lancet* 1978, 312(8098):1040–41.
8. Glasgow N. The gatekeeper controversy: why it exists and how it can be resolved. *NZ Med J* 1996, 109(1021):168–70.
9. Navarro V. A critique of the ideological and political position of the Brandt Report and the Alma-Ata Declaration. *Internat J Health Serv* 1984, 14(2):159–72.
10. Boudreau F. The cost of sickness and the price of health. *Am J Pub Health Nation Health* 1952, 42(4):452.
11. Sundquist K, Malmström M, Johansson S. Neighbourhood deprivation and incidence of coronary heart disease: a multilevel study of 2.6 million women and men in Sweden. *J Epidemiol Comm Health* 2004, 58(1):71–77.
12. Howden-Chapman P, Tobias N. *Social inequalities in health: New Zealand 1999*. Wellington: Ministry of Health, 2000.
13. Hill AG, MacLeod WB, Joof D, Gomez P, Walraven G. Decline of mortality in children in rural Gambia: the influence of village-level primary health care. *Trop Med Internat Health* 2000, 5(2):107–18.
14. Hall J, Taylor R. Health for all beyond 2000: the demise of the Alma-Ata Declaration and primary health care in developing countries. *Med J Austral* 2003, 178(1):17–20.
15. Shi L, Macinko J, Starfield B, Wulu J, Regan J, Politzer R. The relationship between primary care, income inequality, and mortality in US States, 1980–1995. *J Am Board Fam Pract* 2003, 16(5):412–22.
16. Starfield B. *Primary care: balancing health needs, services, and technology*. New York: Oxford University Press, 1998.
17. Starfield B, Shi L, Macinko J. Contribution of primary care to health systems and health. *Milbank Quart* 2005, 83(3):457–502.
18. Starfield B, Shi L. Policy relevant determinants of health: an international perspective. *HealthPolicy* 2002, 60(3):201–18.
19. Boerma W, Van der Zee J, Fleming D. Service profiles of general practitioners in Europe: European GP task profile study. *Br J Gen Pract* 1997, 47(421):481–86.
20. Baicker K, Chandra A. The productivity of physician specialization: evidence from the Medicare program. *Am Econ Rev* 2004, 94(2):357–61.
21. Franks P, Clancy CM, Nutting PA. Gatekeeping revisited: protecting patients from overtreatment. *N Engl J Med* 1992, 327(6):424–29.
22. Starfield B. Primary care: an increasingly important contributor to effectiveness, equity, and efficiency of health services. SESPAS report. *Gac Sanit* 2012, 26(Supl.1):20–26.
23. Lawn JE, Rohde J, Rifkin S, Were M, Paul VK, Chopra M. Alma-Ata 30 years on: revolutionary, relevant, and time to revitalise. *Lancet* 2008, 372(9642):917–27.
24. McWhinney I. Primary care: changing values in a changing world. *BMJ* 1998, 316:1807–09.
25. Pullon S, McKinlay E, Dew K. Primary health care in New Zealand: the impact of organizational factors on teamwork. *Br J Gen Pract* 2009, 59(560):191–97.

Chapter 13

The Doctor of the Future

CONTENTS

This chapter starts with a short review of the main topics in this book, using a series of diagrams to illustrate links between key themes: the person of the patient, the person of the doctor, their relationship, difficulties encountered, and so on. We then briefly discuss how the training of doctors might be re-envisaged, better preparing them for the challenges of clinical practice in the twenty-first century. The doctor of the future needs both a coherent philosophy of medicine and an effective clinical model.

Chapter review

This book has covered a wide variety of topics. In Chapter 1, we asked if doctors considered medicine to be a 'healing' profession, or if doctors think of themselves as healers. Such questions are quite uncommon in our usual discourse, but they were designed to provoke thought about the goals of medicine and our role as physicians. As we noted in Chapter 2, illness can cause suffering; relieving that suffering is a legitimate goal of medicine. To achieve this goal, doctors need to understand the illness experience, how the health of the person is threatened and how to usefully respond. At its most simple, the interaction between doctor and patient is illustrated in Figure 13.1.

FIGURE 13.1 PATIENT AND DOCTOR

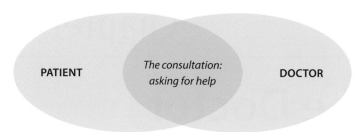

While this looks quite straightforward, the complex world of the patient is quite different from the modern understanding of what ails the human body. In Chapter 3, we reviewed the biomedical model. Without being dismissive of the advances in biological understanding and benefits this model has provided, we noted that its origin lay in the natural sciences of the seventeenth and eighteenth centuries. Applying the principles of science to the human body enabled the emergence of the 'disease model' of individual organ pathology. However, the model is also problematic, especially when patients are unwell, but no 'real disease' is found.

Borrowing from Kuhn,(1) we believe that even if medicine has not quite reached a paradigmatic crisis, somatisation and the meaning response (placebo effect) present a conceptual challenge to the rules or assumptions that underpin biomedical theory (Figure 13.2). Although biomedicine remains dominant, there is a degree of paradigmatic tension within current clinical practice.

FIGURE 13.2 THE WORLDS OF PATIENT AND DOCTOR

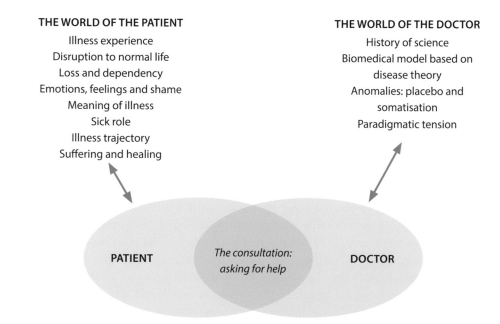

The one-to-one interpersonal interaction between doctor and patient is where these two worlds intersect, or even at times collide. We discussed the doctor–patient relationship in Chapter 4, noting the central importance of listening and the impact of the quality of the relationship on patient outcomes. We also noted that satisfactory doctor–patient relationships link to job satisfaction and professional meaning. Conversely, this relationship can at times be quite problematic, leading to a 'heartsink' experience for the doctor (Chapter 5). We highlighted the importance of self-awareness, emotional intelligence and transferences in the doctor–patient relationship.

Chapter 6 explored the consultation itself as the subject of considerable analysis and development. While various models are in use, none of the current ones adequately address the problem of illness without disease (Chapter 7). In our view, some revisions are required, not only to these consulting models, but also to the underlying conceptual basis of medicine that has arbitrarily (even if usefully at times) separated mind and body. Despite all the advances in medicine, many patients with somatisation in the twenty-first century are still waiting for their doctor to come up with a more helpful synthesis of their symptoms. This would go beyond simply saying 'Well, it is not disease X or Y.' Instead of the doctor increasing the tendency towards somatic fixation, patients need more effective suggestions for management (Figure 13.3).

FIGURE 13.3 PATIENT AND DOCTOR – THE MEETING OF TWO WORLDS

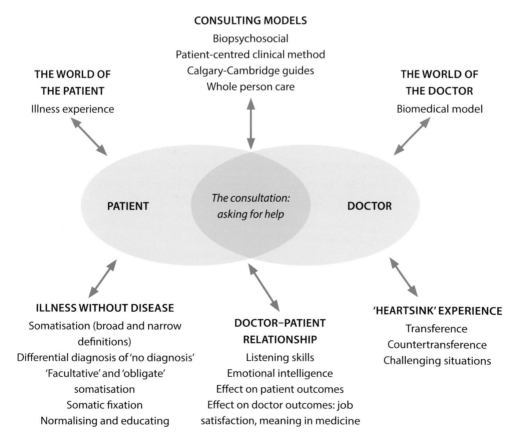

Chapters 1–7 were thus focused on doctors' interactions with patients and how that interaction might be conceptualised. In contrast, Chapter 8 (Doctors' Health and Wellness) focuses on the self of the doctor, set within the wider context of medical culture. Once again, there are some contradictions. Although doctors are highly trained and have considerable knowledge of the human body, some have problems with their own psychological health. From an occupational point of view, a medical career carries considerable rewards, but also some risks. Medical students need to learn how to look after themselves if they are to be resilient to the stresses of clinical practice. Fortunately, there are now well-identified methods to enhance wellness. These can lead to a greater sense of meaning and personal accomplishment for the doctor, as well as benefiting their patients.

Personal health and wellness are inextricably linked to the context and culture of medical practice. As we saw in Chapter 9, training is aimed at helping students to care for others, but the culture of training has often led to the blunting of emotional intelligence and a reduction in empathy. While the assumptions of modern medicine are remarkably homogeneous around the world, subcultures of clinical practice vary considerably, some being respectful and supportive of individual doctors, others being less so. We support the concept of reflective practice (Chapter 10), where doctors identify and critique their experiences of clinical work and medical culture, not only to learn from difficult situations, but also to reconnect with their original goals of doing medicine.

Such reflection is critical when a patient is harmed by health care. As we noted in Chapter 11, adverse outcomes have always been present, but their incidence has increased in the last few decades with the increasing complexity of clinical practice, pharmaceutical products and technological innovations. The discipline of patient safety is aimed at addressing this potential for harming patients, using insights on human fallibility, uncertainty and complex social systems. This revised approach to health care also results in a much greater understanding of how the doctor is embedded within the wider health-care team. Medical culture itself is crucial to patient safety. How the doctor reacts to both adverse outcomes and complaints from patients is also crucial. Defensive medicine is one possible outcome, but it can be prevented by attending to personal resilience, practising reflection and having a supportive culture.

Primary care is a model of health-care delivery that is applicable to both developing and developed countries. This model delivers greater benefits for more people at lower cost, largely through better access to, and comprehensiveness of, care by general practitioners and primary health care teams (Chapter 12). Figure 13.4 illustrates the links between all the chapters in this book.

FIGURE 13.4 THE WIDER CONTEXT OF DOCTORING

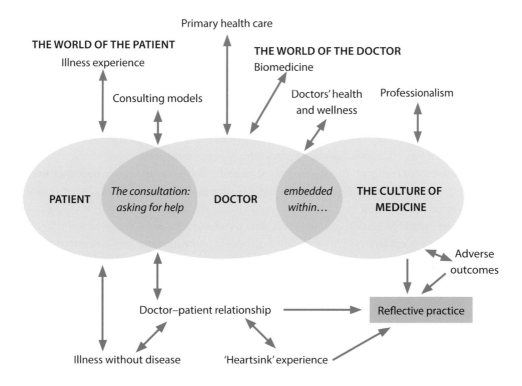

Figure 13.4 includes a number of arrows that point towards reflective practice. Reflection should be part of a systematic approach to clinical work, especially in relation to problematic situations such as a 'heartsink' experience, a patient without disease, an adverse outcome, issues in the doctor–patient relationship or even illness of one's own. As we noted in Chapter 10, deeper levels of reflection may help doctors to re-examine the hitherto taken-for-granted assumptions or premises that govern daily practice. Reflection can create a revised set of expectations about the role of the doctor and the goals of medicine: such outcomes are known as perspective transformation.

The remainder of this chapter looks to the future: the challenges ahead and the skill set of doctors that will be required.

Challenges in future practice

In the twenty-first century doctors are faced with considerable challenges. The demographics of disease and disability have changed significantly in the last hundred years. People in the Western world are living longer, increasing the elderly portion of the population. The incidence of chronic and multiple morbidities is rising. Inequities in health persist both between countries and within countries. Health care is now more costly and complex, yet fails to reach all patients. Globalisation and increased migration between countries will change the infectious, environmental and behavioural risks to personal and global health.(2) Global flows of doctors will also impact on the health resources of developing countries.(3)

Furthermore, there is considerable disquiet about the direction of health care towards more expensive interventions that offer only marginal benefit.(4) Elderly people are being given drugs in increasing quantities, the clinical efficacy of which is doubtful.(5) Inappropriate drug and narcotic use are increasingly complex and expensive problems.(6) As a result of these issues, many patients are becoming disillusioned with modern medicine: complementary and alternative practices are challenging the dominant paradigm.(7) Likewise, the influence of pharmaceutical companies on clinical practice is under scrutiny. There is considerable concern about methods of research, as well as about marketing strategies and their role in the creation of guidelines for patient management.(8) Finally, while evidence-based medicine initially promised to provide more rational use of science-based knowledge, it is now attracting criticism.(9,10)

In brief, while biomedicine has been effective in elucidating categories of disease and remains especially effective in acute illness and injury, the health issues of the twenty-first century demand a wider perspective. The question then arises: What sort of training might be required for future doctors to address these broader issues? The next section briefly recaps the history of medical education and indicates future directions.

Shifts in medical education

For most of the twentieth century, following the Flexner report of 1910,(11) undergraduate doctors have been trained in what is known as a 'traditional' model. The pre-clinical curriculum focused on basic medical sciences (pathology, biochemistry, physiology, anatomy), while in the clinical curriculum, students applied their knowledge to real patients, almost exclusively in hospital settings.

However, criticism of the Flexnerian model of training grew in the latter half of the twentieth century. Learning was considered to be too theoretical and the process too didactic (largely lectures away from the bedside). Cooke et al. criticised the 'older conceptualizations of learning [which] overemphasise the individual learner's acquisition of the knowledge and skills of medicine as the principal form of learning'. (12) Other studies also found that institutional learning was not adequately preparing students for the problem-solving nature of clinical practice, especially given the often harsh and overly critical learning environment.(13,14)

In response to these issues, 'problem-based learning' emerged as part of a second wave of educational reform. Problem-based curricula emphasise small group learning rather than didactic lectures. Learning is initiated by a particular clinical problem, rather than starting from the underlying pathology. Standardised patients are used to assess clinical competencies of students, while the context of learning is broadened to include community settings.(15,16) This shift was conceptually quite radical, as shown in Table 13.1.

TABLE 13.1 CONCEPTUAL SHIFTS IN UNDERGRADUATE TRAINING

Traditional medical education (Flexner, 1910)	Modern emphasis (late twentieth century)
Bioscience core	Problem-oriented learning
Didactic pedagogy	Integration of theory and practice
Factual overload	Patient-centred approach to patient care
Division of learning: preclinical/clinical	Population-based
Context of clinical learning: secondary care	Greater range of clinical settings for learning: primary care and community settings
Doctor-centred model of training and practice	Case presentations, early clinical skills
Focus on disease rather than on patient as an individual	Ethical and professional development
Learning by rote accumulation of facts	Preparation for independent lifelong learning
Learning by humiliation	Interprofessional learning

Adapted from Howe et al.(16)

The Flexnerian revolution set the scene for the dominant learning metaphor of the twentieth century, that of **knowledge acquisition**. In this understanding of learning, knowledge is provided to the student who learns, conceptualises, makes sense, shares with others, and so on.(17) It is not surprising that the metaphor became so dominant, given the vast number of facts required.

However, the list in the right column of Box 13.1 is now starting to illustrate a quite different metaphor of learning and of clinical practice: the **participation** metaphor. Instead of simply *having* knowledge, learning emerges through *doing*, especially within a particular context. The learner is viewed as 'a person interested in participation in certain kinds of activities rather than in accumulating private [knowledge].'(17) Learners gradually become embedded within particular 'communities of practice', learning to participate and contribute to the work of that group of professionals.(18) Clinical practice is considered to be knowledge-in-action.

Despite these conceptual shifts, Frenk et al. are particularly critical of the continued mismatch between the ethos of medical training and clinical practice:

Professional education has not kept pace with these challenges, largely because of fragmented, outdated, and static curricula that produce ill-equipped graduates. The problems are systemic: mismatch of competencies to patient and population needs; poor teamwork; persistent gender stratification of professional status; narrow technical focus without broader contextual understanding; episodic encounters rather than continuous care; predominant hospital orientation at the expense of primary care; quantitative and qualitative imbalances in the professional labour market; and weak leadership to improve health-system performance.(2)

Similarly, Cooke, Irby and O'Brien call for reform of medical school and residency training:

Clinical education involves far more than outfitting individual physicians with scientific knowledge and technical skills. The clinical work and the other professional activities of physicians are *social practices*, and physicians must be prepared to work in *relationships* with their patients and with other professionals and non professionals in clinics, medical centres and communities. Care of patients is an *interpersonal* endeavor, involving *transactions* between clinicians and patients, which even in a simple clinical situation involves many people, let alone in more *complex settings* where an array of specialists from a variety of fields are engaged.(12) [Our emphasis]

What sort of doctor is required for this quite different conception of clinical medicine? In answering this question, we first need to consider and review the theoretical understanding of what we understand by 'medical science' and the role of the doctor. In other words, is there a particular science that might best underpin future medical practice? Second, what sort of clinical approach or model might work best?

What sort of science?

The description of clinical practice above seems far removed from the doctor of the early twentieth century, who at worst was narrowly focused and largely uncontested in his knowledge and power. We contend that the underlying philosophical basis of clinical medicine also needs to be critiqued and revised, if clinical work as described above is to be well theorised. As an example, Engel proposed a philosophic review, arguing that medical practice was *inappropriately* based on the science of Newton and Descartes, 'where what is being studied exists external to and independent of the scientist, who discovers and characterizes its properties and behavior. This is the essence of the objectivity that is required if one is to be considered a scientist.'(19)

We have already outlined McWhinney's formulation of the biomedical model in Chapter 3.(20) Norton and Smith also captured the essence of biomedicine with a remarkably similar summary (Box 13.1). Both descriptions adhere quite closely to Engel's summary of a 'seventeenth-century understanding' of science.

BOX 13.1 BIOMEDICINE DEFINED

'The medical model of disease has long been the basic paradigm of medicine following the development of the germ theory of disease in the nineteenth century. It remains the principal form of explanation in scientific medicine. Its fundamental assumptions can be stated as follows. First, all disease is caused by a specific agent (the 'disease entity'), such as a virus, parasite or bacterium. Second, the patient is to be regarded as the passive target of medical intervention, since scientific medicine is concerned with the body as a sort of machine, rather than with a person in a complex social environment. Third, restoring health requires the use of medical technology and advanced scientific procedures. While being eclipsed, especially in primary care or preventive medicine, this view of disease continues to underpin much of medical practice and particularly so in hospital medicine.'

From Norton and Smith(21)

Alternative philosophical understandings

In contrast, Engel also described a 'twentieth-century science' based on Einstein and Heisenberg: 'What is being studied is inseparable from the scientist, who derives mental constructs of his/her experiences with it as a means of characterizing his/

her understanding of its properties and behavior.'(19) Heisenberg himself said that: 'Natural science does not simply describe and explain nature; it is part of the interplay between nature and ourselves; it describes nature as exposed to our method of questioning.'(22)

These descriptions of science are a closer match to the reality of medicine.(23) As we suggested above, the prevailing paradigm of medical practice is under tension, if not actually in paradigmatic crisis. The anomalies of somatisation, meaning response (placebo effect), and the effect of the doctor–patient relationship on health-care outcomes are observations that fail to fit within the prevailing theory of biomedicine.(24)

While clinical medicine is certainly evolving, we argue that the underlying assumptions have not in fact altered substantially. If they had, then the meaning response would be better understood and utilised as part of clinical practice (rather than being disregarded and avoided); doctors would more readily see their engagement with patients as part of treatment; and the somatising patient (illness without disease) would be diagnosed and managed in a more coherent, comprehensive way. Similarly, the health of the doctor would be considered important in the overall quality of health-care systems.

What sort of science, then, is a better match for modern medical practice? Several revised definitions have already been proposed, two of which are listed in Box 13.2.

BOX 13.2 PROPOSED PHILOSOPHIES OF MEDICINE

WILSON (2000)	ABRAHAM AND MEADOR (1976)
'Patients suffer from illnesses arising from a matrix of cultural beliefs and biological systems. A complex interaction occurs between patient and clinician, and behavioral outcomes are constructed from their negotiations and the doctor's physical interventions. Patients are accorded "sick" status according to social conventions unique to each sub-culture. Recovery from illness will depend on individual beliefs, cultural support systems for the patient, the influence and process of the doctor–patient relationship, and biological factors.'	'I do not believe in a single causation for most diseases. I believe the symptoms of disease arise in a highly complex mix of genetic weakness, psychosocial events and stresses, physicochemical abnormalities, and a host of other factors. I see patients as people with problems who may or may not also have a demonstrable physicochemical defect. If the defect is definable, I prescribe medication aimed at correcting the physicochemical abnormality or I recommend a surgical procedure. I also listen to the patient in a manner that will permit him to bring up whatever is bothering him. I am impressed with the frequency with which my patients can tell me what happened in their lives just before getting sick. I believe that man's mind and his body are highly interconnected and related, and that it is virtually impossible to have disease of one without disease or some dysfunction of the other.'
Wilson(25)	*Abraham and Meador(26)*

Both these descriptions are more consistent with a twentieth-century science, where the observer and what is observed are linked: each affects the other, in a reciprocal manner. The philosophical stance here could be identified as 'social constructivist':

the meaning of events, situations, and even knowledge, is created by participants in an iterative way.(27) This theoretical stance also underpins modern theories of learning and is widely used in education.(28)

In medicine, without discarding biological factors, this philosophy would legitimise various factors that influence the outcome of disease: the doctor–patient relationship; the context of care; and the social milieu in which the patient is held. It is also a better fit with the concept of communities of clinical practice, where professionals create meaning through shared participation.(18)

In our postgraduate courses, we put forward these various understandings of clinical practice to GPs. This usually triggers robust discussion on the nature of medicine, enabling them to consider and develop a philosophy that best matches their own goals and experience. Two approaches to clinical practice that appear to align closely with a social constructivist theory are those of narrative medicine (Chapter 2) and of whole person care (Chapter 6).

Narrative medicine

Narrative medicine is an emerging method of understanding the processes of clinical care.(29,30) It focuses on the story of illness and the relationship between the doctor and patient. It can also encompass the doctor's own relationship with herself, her relationship with peers and the profession of medicine, and the wider relationship between the profession and society.(31) Narrative medicine is closely linked with 'relationship-centred care', another emerging model.(32)

By way of illustration, we now return to Vignette 2.3, where one of our postgraduate students related the story of a patient with cancer who had been doing poorly. The patient was upset about the diagnosis, had difficulty communicating with her oncologist, and was generally struggling with life now her future was at risk. When her doctor asked 'What is it like for you to have cancer?' she burst into tears, not from fear or anxiety, but from being recognised as suffering. Despite her apparent difficulties, no health professional had ever asked such a question. She talked of her experiences in getting the diagnosis and difficulties in accepting chemotherapy, and left the room feeling much more at ease within herself. She subsequently engaged in treatment and coped quite well.

This patient's personal story or narrative is integral to her recovery from cancer. Narrative medicine looks at the patient's illness as a whole: in this case, a life story that felt broken. For this patient, the trajectory of illness was profoundly altered by the doctor's intervention, not through suggesting a better regime of chemotherapy or trying other treatments, but simply through acknowledging and validating her felt experience. It is only through careful listening that the patient's story may emerge: it may be impossible to say 'how it is' until someone listens. Patient and doctor work together to construct a new outcome. Charon asks that doctors have the 'courage and generosity to tolerate and to bear witness' to patients like the one above.(31)

Perhaps the doctor's intervention helped shift the narrative from 'chaos' (a painful lived expression of illness without meaning) to an early phase of 'restitution' (more accepting of cancer, engaging in treatment). As Brody suggests, the doctor can help the narrative back on track.(33) Many doctors can relate similar stories, where they manage to change the trajectory of illness.

Narrative medicine also has roots in the humanities, where stories of sickness and of doctoring are well-chronicled in literature, drama and film. Through studying these resources, doctors can resonate more with patients and with their own personal journey in medicine.(34) Shakespeare, for example, provides numerous clinical vignettes where characters faint, fit, or even die as a result of emotional upset.(35) Learning about somatisation can thus be grounded in history and culture.

Dr Rachel Remen's lifetime of work is another example. Her celebrated book of clinical stories illustrates the effectiveness of listening respectfully, searching the narrative for creativity and personal strengths.(36) The patient's story emerges and is further shaped through its telling. Similarly, her work in creating safe spaces for doctors to reflect on their work, looking for the *meaning* in being a doctor, has been a profound initiative in nurturing doctors for greater professional resilience and wellness.(37) Sharing stories about the challenges of doctoring with one's peers in a supportive environment is part of a narrative approach to clinical competence and contributes to doctors' well-being.

Whole person care

As we noted in Chapter 6, whole person care is an emerging model of training and clinical practice that builds on the strengths of previous suggestions such as patient-centred clinical method. This particular model is conceptually easy to understand, reminding doctors of their two traditional tasks: attending to the disease and attending to the person with that disease. As outlined in Chapter 7 on somatisation, we now suggest a third task (Figure 13.5).

FIGURE 13.5 THE THREE TASKS OF MEDICAL PRACTICE

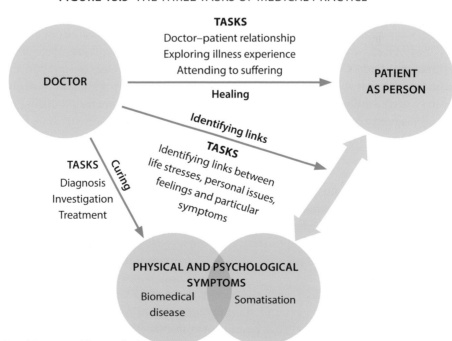

After Hutchinson and Brawer(38)

These three tasks require a diverse range of attitudes and skills. Competence with respect to disease uses knowledge and technical skills gained from biomedical research. Facilitating the journey toward healing requires interpersonal engagement, based on quite a different epistemology. Relationship skills include respect for the patient, an awareness of the doctor's role as a potential healing agent, and methods of reflective practice where skills can be further developed. The third arrow indicates the role of the doctor in somatisation, where the task is to help patients make links between their current life and their symptoms.

The doctor of the future

While we have explored medical theory and models of clinical practice in this book, we have also explored doctors as persons and as health professionals. As the authors, then, what sort of doctor would we like in the future when we develop serious disease and ask for help?

As noted in the Introduction, we assume that this doctor will have both adequate training and sufficient clinical competence: this means performing the usual biomedical tasks well, and if in doubt, having no reservations about asking others for advice. Acknowledging the tasks of medical practice, this doctor will also attempt to explore the nature of the illness, realising that such enquiry may be therapeutic in itself and may alter the illness trajectory. She will be fully aware that biomedicine is a very useful tool, but that her current knowledge may not be specific enough for each particular patient. She will be aware of the uncertainty in predicting the outcomes of disease, acknowledging how all her interventions carry a meaning response that can be either positive or negative. The patient's life factors and social supports may also contribute to the onset and future course of each illness. She will be aware that patients may or may not be 'adherent' to suggestions; she will also be aware that doctors can have trouble in *being* a patient and may require careful negotiation.

Further, the doctor will be aware that sometimes it is difficult to engage or connect with some patients. However, such situations will be a trigger for consultation analysis, wondering what is happening between them and being aware that both doctor and patient can contribute to such difficulties. She will be well practised in using a range of methods to explore her own discomfort, including discussion with others, writing, mentoring, or supervision. Over time, this reflection will help her become more relaxed when patients do not quite fit her expectations of practice, personal agency or clinical effectiveness.

Without becoming psychotherapists, all doctors will have more psychological understanding of common disorders such as anxiety, depression and grief and the impact of these on other illness. Similarly, they will be well accustomed to the somatising patient, accurately identifying those who respond readily to education about mind–body connections and those who require more delicate interventions over time.

Such doctors will feel well supported by their peers, meeting regularly for discussion aimed at both mutual support and clinical review. They will be aware that illness of their own is always possible, being conscious of the complex problems ahead for the doctor-as-patient. Likewise, their workplace will be aware of the links between doctor wellness and patient outcomes and the need for all health workers to feel valued and respected.

The culture of clinical practice will be quite proactive in identifying and preventing medical error, realising that modern health-care delivery depends on complex interacting systems. Doctors will work well with other health professionals, respecting their various contributions to teamwork and health outcomes. Mistakes and adverse events will be viewed as triggers for review, moving beyond the simplistic blaming of individual practitioners. Instead of complaints leading to shame, doctors will be more realistic about the inherent uncertainties within clinical practice, acknowledging that 'perfect' medicine is simply not possible. In this understanding of clinical practice, primary medical and health-care systems will provide the bulk of clinical management and disease prevention. GPs and hospital-based specialists will see their roles as complementary rather than competitive, working together in the service of the patient. Finally, undergraduate medical education will be based on a participatory, experiential style of learning, better preparing students for their role in the workplace environment.

Conclusion

In this chapter we have reviewed the various links made throughout this book, coming up with a model of medical practice based on a revised philosophy of medicine. While biomedicine has been a superb vehicle for the diagnosis and treatment of disease, it tends to disregard both the patient's suffering and the doctor's role in healing. Moving towards a stance of social constructivism, narrative-based medicine and whole person care can help to integrate the patient's treatment with the underlying objective of medical practice – the care of the patient.

Doctors need to be aware of the underlying framework of their practice, including the complex nuances of the doctor–patient relationship. A high level of clinical competence and performance is important. This demands self-care and reflective practice. Just as patients need 'whole person' care, the profession needs 'whole person' doctors.

References

1. Kuhn TS. *The structure of scientific revolutions*. Chicago: University of Chicago Press, 1962.
2. Frenk J, Chen L, Bhutta ZA, Cohen J, Crisp N, Evans T, et al. Health professionals for a new century: transforming education to strengthen health systems in an interdependent world. *Lancet* 2010, 376:1923–58.
3. Omaswa F. Human resources for global health: time for action is now. *Lancet* 2008, 371(9613):625–26.
4. Zucker MB, Zucker HD. *Medical futility and the evaluation of life-sustaining interventions*. Cambridge: Cambridge University Press, 1997.
5. Garfinkel D, Mangin D. Feasibility study of a systematic approach for discontinuation of multiple medications in older adults: addressing polypharmacy. *Arch Intern Med* 2010, 170(18):1648–54.

6. Manchikanti L, Singh A. Therapeutic opioids: a ten-year perspective on the complexities and complications of the escalating use, abuse, and nonmedical use of opioids. *Pain Phys* 2008, 11(2):S63–S88.

7. Eskinazi D. Factors that shape alternative medicine. *JAMA* 1998, 280(18):1621–23.

8. Brody H, Light DW. The inverse benefit law: how drug marketing undermines patient safety and public health. *Am J Public Health* 2011, 101:399–404.

9. Feinstein AR, Horwitz RI. Problems in the 'evidence' of 'evidence-based medicine'. *Am J Med* 1997, 103(6):529–35.

10. Cohen AM, Stavri PZ, Hersh WR. A categorization and analysis of the criticisms of evidence-based medicine. *Internat J Med Informatics* 2004, 73(1):35–43.

11. Flexner A. *Medical education in the United States and Canada: a report to the Carnegie Foundation for the advancement of teaching*. New York: The Carnegie Foundation for the Advancement of Teaching, 1910.

12. Cooke M, Irby DM, O'Brien BC. *Educating physicians: a call for reform of medical school and residency*. San Francisco: Jossey-Bass, 2010

13. Kassebaum DG, Cutler ER. On the culture of student abuse in medical school. *Acad Med* 1998, 73(11):1149.

14. Wilkinson TJ, Gill DJ, Fitzjohn J, Palmer CL, Mulder RT. The impact on students of adverse experiences during medical school. *Med Teach* 2006, 28(2):129–35.

15. Neville AJ. Problem-based learning and medical education forty years on. *Med Princ Pract* 2009, 18(1):1–9.

16. Howe A, Campion P, Searle J, Smith H. New perspectives: approaches to medical education at four new UK medical schools. *BMJ* 2004, 329(7461):327–31.

17. Sfard A. On two metaphors for learning and the dangers of choosing just one. *Educ Res* 1998, 27(2):4–13.

18. Wenger E. *Communities of practice: learning, meaning, and identity*. Cambridge: Cambridge University Press, 1999.

19. Engel GL. How much longer must medicine's science be bound by a seventeenth century world view? *Fam Syst Med* 1992, 10(3):333–46.

20. McWhinney I. Changing models: the impact of Kuhn's theory on medicine. *Fam Pract* 1984, 1(1):3–9.

21. Norton K, Smith S. *Problems with patients: managing complicated transactions*. Cambridge: Cambridge University Press, 1994. p.9.

22. Heisenberg W. *Physics and philosophy: the revolution in modern science*. New York: Harper, 1958. p.81.

23. Engel GL. The need for a new medical model: a challenge for biomedicine. *Science* 1977, 196(4286):129–36.

24. Wildes KW. The crisis of medicine: philosophy and the social construction of medicine. *Kennedy Inst Ethics J* 2001, 11(1):71–86.

25. Wilson H. The myth of objectivity: is medicine moving towards a social constructivist medical paradigm? *Fam Pract* 2000, 17(2):203–09.

26. Abraham HS, Meador C. *Basic psychiatry for the primary care physician*. Boston: Little, Brown and Company, 1976. p.9.

27. Kukla A. *Social constructivism and the philosophy of science*. New York: Routledge, 2000.

28. Bandura A. Social cognitive theory: an agentic perspective. *Ann Rev Psychol* 2001, 52(1):1–26.

29. Greenhalgh T. Narrative based medicine in an evidence based world. *BMJ* 1999, 318(7179):323.

30. Launer J. *Narrative-based primary care*. Abingdon: Radcliffe, 2002.

31. Charon R. Narrative medicine: a model for empathy, reflection, profession, and trust. *JAMA*

2001, 286(15):1897–902.

32. Suchman AL. A new theoretical foundation for relationship-centered care. *J Gen Int Med* 2006, 21(S1):S40–S44.

33. Brody H. *Stories of sickness*. New Haven: Yale University Press, 1987.

34. Helman C. *Suburban shaman*. Cape Town: Juta and Co, 2004.

35. Heaton K. Faints, fits and fatalities from emotion in Shakespeare's characters: survey of the canon. *BMJ* 2006, 333:1335–38.

36. Remen RN. *Kitchen table wisdom: stories that heal*. 10th edn. New York: Riverhead Books, 1997.

37. Remen RN. Recovering the soul of medicine. Interview by Gazella KA, Snyder S. *Altern Ther Health Med* 2006, 12(3):86–93.

38. Hutchinson T, Brawer J. The challenge of medical dichotomies and the congruent physician–patient relationship in medicine. In: Hutchinson T, ed. *Whole person care: a new paradigm for the 21st century*. New York: Springer, 2011. pp. 31–44.

Appendix

Balint groups: Reflecting on clinical work

CONTENTS

Introduction

A Balint group is a small group of health professionals who meet regularly to discuss clinical cases, the focus being on psychological aspects of practice, especially the doctor–patient relationship. The groups are named for Dr Michael Balint, a Hungarian-born psychiatrist and psychoanalyst who, together with his wife Enid, developed Balint groups in London in the 1950s and 1960s.(1) Their initial focus was on helping GPs to develop their skills in managing their therapeutic relationships,(2) although the method is now being used by psychotherapists as well.

Balint groups are primarily aimed at learning about the doctor–patient relationship and 'heartsink experiences' (Chapters 4, 5 and 7). Over time, the method increases doctors' self-awareness, contributing to general wellness and professional resilience (Chapter 8). It is also an excellent example of reflection-on-action (Chapter 10).

While Balint groups remain uncommon, Balint himself had an enormous influence. He was instrumental in the recognition of the importance of general practice and the establishment of the Royal College of General Practitioners in the

UK. The Balint method of exploring the illness experience and the doctor–patient relationship initiated the development of patient-centred medicine, consultation analysis, training programmes for GP registrars and the rise of peer groups as a method of support and training.

In the last 10 to 20 years, interest in the Balint method of group work has increased, especially in Europe, the US, the UK and Australia. The International Balint Federation has over 20 member countries and holds an international conference every two years. Each country runs workshops for health professionals, as well as 'intensives' to train future Balint leaders, who now undergo a formal accreditation process.

Method

Balint groups usually meet weekly or fortnightly for one to two hours to talk about their 'cases'. Groups are usually closed, consisting of 8 to 12 members, with one or two leaders. Cases are those where the doctor or therapist has found a patient 'difficult' in some way, or where they feel frustration, ambivalence or uncertainty in dealing with them. The presenter 'brings' the patient to the group, by giving a fairly detailed oral presentation without notes. After brief questions from the group (confined to facts only), the presenter draws back from the group and is silent while the others discuss the case, speculating on the background, the patient and their details, and what it has been like for the patient and for the doctor so far (Figure 1).

The general focus is on the doctor–patient (or client–therapist) relationship, rather than on technical details about diagnosis or treatment. The presenter is then invited back to the group and may or may not comment on the discussion, which continues until the end of the session, usually 45 minutes per case.

FIGURE 1 SCHEMATIC REPRESENTATION OF A BALINT GROUP

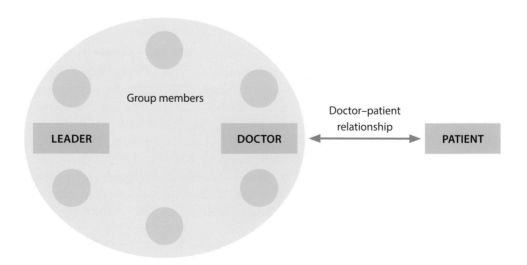

There are a number of features of this particular form of professional development that seem to be quite different from other methods in medicine.

Group process is the basis of training. The experience of group members is used to comment on the case and develop a collective wisdom that emerges from discussion. More specifically, this method could be characterised as 'action-research'. The aim is qualitative research on the doctor–patient relationship, acknowledging that such research will impact on participants' future work.

The task is **not diagnosis or solution focused**. It is generally assumed that the presenter is competent and that diagnosis and treatment is adequate. Usually the problem is not one of technical proficiency, as the cases are often those in which the presenter is troubled in some way and where biomedicine has no specific answers. Advice is not given to the presenter about how to manage the case, although the increased understanding of interpersonal issues will usually help them in their approach to the patient. Medical students or registrars can find this focus quite difficult, but they have many opportunities for technical advice or knowledge acquisition in other areas of training. It helps to be quite clear, at the start of new groups, about this particularly narrow focus, as clear direction will often pre-empt the reversion to more common methods of case discussion where advice is usually given.

Speculation and wondering are encouraged, even if ideas sound unusual or quite lateral. Saying 'the wrong thing' might be a clue to discussing what is missing or what is being avoided. In other words, one's contribution to the group is not necessarily about 'getting it right'. Intuition is encouraged.

Speculation in front of the presenter may at first appear to be quite contrived, using the third person ('he' or 'she') to talk about the presenter who remains in earshot. However, this is one of the gems of the Balint process. For a short time, the responsibility for the case is handed over to someone else. By hearing the discussion objectively, the presenter can bring a more dispassionate presence to the patient. Presenters develop a better capacity to 'sit with' the issues in the next consultation.

VIGNETTE 1 LUCY AND THE PATIENT'S RASH

This case is from Dr John Salinsky, a senior Balint trainer in the UK, where many GP registrars are now in a Balint group as part of their training. The case presentation and how the group responded is outlined below.(3)

Lucy is a GP registrar who was finding it difficult to manage a 27-year-old patient called Yvette, who had an extensive and non-responsive skin rash. The trouble for Lucy was that Yvette kept turning up during Saturday emergency clinics rather than during the week for her scheduled appointments. When Lucy raised this issue, Yvette became angry and defensive and swore at her. Lucy was 'shocked and hurt, but didn't retaliate'. She tried to retrieve the situation, but the consultation ended unsatisfactorily (at least for Lucy).

After this patient was presented, the group started to 'work on the case'. Salinsky reports how group members initially wanted to discuss the more general problem of how to discipline such patients in terms of their help-seeking behaviour. Salinsky then tried to get them back to the doctor–patient relationship by asking about the patient, Yvette: 'What sort of person was she?' The group then became rather critical of her: they also had difficulty in thinking how Yvette might have experienced that consultation herself. With further coaching, however ('What would you do if she was your sister?'), the group gradually started to wonder why this patient felt the need to be so provocative, and how the doctor might learn to 'sit with' this particular person.

Observations of this discussion are as follows. First, the doctor's goal was treatment of the skin condition, but she became sidetracked into a battle of wills about help-seeking behaviour. This became a barrier to a better connection with the patient. Instead of the patient becoming better known and understood by the doctor, she became more distant and estranged.

Second, the group initially found it difficult to focus on the relationship. It took some effort by the trainer to get the group to concentrate on the subjective experiences of both doctor and patient within that consultation. When they did so, however, the discussion was probably helpful, as Salinsky reports. On the next consultation, it seemed likely that Lucy would be a little less 'defensive' in her stance towards this patient, and perhaps more open to trying to figure out who her patient actually was. A deeper professional engagement might then result in better adherence to treatment and clinical outcomes.(3)

Three particular facets of Balint group work require further discussion. These are leadership, boundaries and parallel process.

Leadership

It is important for leaders to provide an adequate 'warm-up', setting the scene and ground rules for the work of the group. They need to be careful to maintain boundaries such as time management and the appropriate contributions from the group (avoiding technical details such as diagnosis or giving advice). They also need to help the group to manage the strong feelings and reactions arising in response to presented cases and issues.

Having two leaders seems to be more facilitative of group processes. This is because the leaders' task is to provide a bounded and safe space for the group to explore what are often difficult feelings and issues. The leaders must notice the broad issues arising from the presenter's story, then watch how the group grapples with three areas: the patient, the doctor and their relationship. Keeping track of the threads within the group discussion is not easy, especially as leaders can also become involved in the case, sometimes losing their objectivity about how the discussion is proceeding and/or what is missing.

The two leaders have a 'holding' function: they act as a 'mirror' for each other. This enables the group to 'play' with the material presented. This playful exploration allows creative ideas and possibilities to emerge. Such a potpourri of possibilities enables the presenter to mull over ideas about the patient that they may not have considered. Often it is reported that the patient is 'different' at the next consultation. The doctor's perception of the patient might be changed as an outcome of Balint discussion, which may cause subtle changes in the body language, attitudes, and even persona of the doctor in relation to this patient. Changes might also stem from an altered perception of the patient by the doctor.

Leaders make comments or 'interventions' into the discussion. These are usually aimed at deepening the understanding or empathy with respect to the three main areas of focus. Such interventions require considerable skill and leaders are trained to create a safe group, where intense issues can be discussed. Leaders-in-training require a focused debrief and review after each case if they are to learn quickly.

The close attention to boundaries, clear leadership, and the specific focus on the therapeutic relationship means that all members of the group can be welcomed and respected, regardless of experience or background. This usually enables a feeling of safety in the group, which then facilitates deep disclosure and a mature group process, where a wide range of ideas can be expressed without fear of saying something stupid or wrong.

Managing distress in the group

At times participants will be upset, angry, or sad, or will challenge other people, including the leaders: in short, they will demonstrate all the usual facets of significant relationships. It is helpful to see these behaviours as useful illustrations of the case and of the relationship between the presenter and the patient, instead of individual personal issues. Sometimes one person carries the emotional weight of the case for the group. The shared tension may coalesce into the response of that person. Observing this as it occurs helps members to be less judgemental of that participant and more understanding of the tensions within the case.

Being able to 'sit with' such strong emotions is an important part of Balint training. Acknowledging one's feelings, even distress, in an open and responsible way is one of the goals of Balint work. This helps to model back to the presenter how they might sit alongside similar feelings in the patient. The task is to learn how to *be with*, rather than to *act in response to*, certain patients. For example, an outcome of Balint training might be an increased capacity to stand steady with troubling feelings, rather than writing a prescription or referring to other providers.

Management of boundaries

Balint groups pay particularly close attention to the management of boundaries. This means the Balint group is a 'closed' group with stable membership. It is expected that there are no late arrivals or early departures and case discussion is kept strictly to time, regardless of how fascinating the discussion may be. Confidentiality means there is no discussion about the group or the case with outside persons and that there is no ongoing discussion of the case by members outside the group meeting. Participants usually disclose (and/or leave) if the case is someone they know personally or professionally.

Cases are based on the health professional relationship (doctor-to-patient, therapist-to-client). It may be tempting to discuss other health-related interactions, such as being asked for advice by family or others outside the formal consultation, but generally the focus is on the routine doctor–patient relationship. Some groups broaden the case to include supervisees or students who have significant and formal interactions with the presenter.

Parallel process

Parallel process occurs when the dynamic of the doctor–patient relationship is unconsciously replayed in another setting. This parallel process can occur between a registrar and their consultant when discussing a patient, in hospital presentations such as 'grand rounds', in fact in any situation where a significant relationship is presented to another person. In Balint groups, it is usually noticed and commented on.

Parallel process is where the group unconsciously acts out particular features of the patient or of their relationship with the doctor. For example, the group might start to experience some frustration with the presenter, parallel to the frustration the doctor feels with the patient. Or the group may avoid discussing issues around death and dying, in parallel to the doctor's avoidance of similar discussion with the patient.

Andrew Elder is an experienced GP and Balint leader. He describes parallel process as follows: 'After some initial responses, questions and comments [by the group], something rather mysterious happens: the doctor who has brought the case begins to behave a little bit like the patient to the rest of the doctors in the group, who themselves take on the role of the doctor … the group then begins to get a bit stuck with the doctor, just as the doctor had got stuck with the patient.'(4)

Initially at least, parallel process is unconscious. As group members become more aware of it, however, the underlying themes become more apparent. Observing and discussing parallel process is often the key to unresolved tensions in the case. Three relationships in question are illustrated in Figure 2.

FIGURE 2 PARALLEL PROCESS WITHIN GROUP DISCUSSION

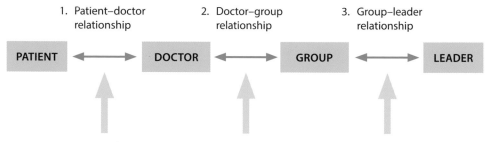

1. Patient–doctor relationship   2. Doctor–group relationship   3. Group–leader relationship

PATIENT ⟷ DOCTOR ⟷ GROUP ⟷ LEADER

The group's task: How is the doctor behaving towards this patient?

The leader's tasks: How is the group behaving towards this doctor? How am I behaving towards the group?

It is important that leaders are alert to the possibilities of these processes, which may not necessarily be disruptive to the group working on a case. Sometimes leaders notice and comment on them as an illustration of the difficulties for the doctor.

Here are two examples of parallel process where the doctor–patient relationship dynamic is played out in group discussion.[1] In Vignette 2, this occurs in the relationship between the *presenting GP* and the *Balint group*. It is also apparent in the relationship

---

1   Thanks to Dr John Barton for supplying the first example.

between the *Balint group* and the *leade*r. In Vignette 3, the father–son relationship is replicated by the group's passive response.

VIGNETTE 2 FEELING RESPONSIBLE

A 50-year-old male GP presented his patient to the group. This was a 42-year-old female patient with cancer of the tonsil who had refused radiotherapy (the treatment of choice). He knew her history of abuse by males in her life and had felt sympathy for her, not wanting to pressure her to change her mind. However, after she had died, he regretted his reticence, feeling quite guilty for '**breaking the rules** *of being a proper doctor'.*

During the discussion, the group wanted to engage more directly with the presenter than is usual and asked to go over time. They were sympathising with the GP when they did this. The leader also felt an urge to 'let the group get away with these requests'. In other words, all participants wanted to '**break the rules**' *of the usual Balint structure.*

The parallel process was that the group now felt responsible for trying to 'help' the doctor. Similarly, the leader felt the need to allow that dynamic in his relationship with the group.

VIGNETTE 3 THE SON, THE FATHER AND THE GROUP

A 45-year-old female GP presented her case to the group: a 24-year-old Greek man who had admitted to feeling suicidal. He was still living at home with his parents and he had a difficult relationship with his father. A highly respected banker, his father was critical of his son for not getting a job. The discussion focused mostly on the father and the effects of this parental relationship. When the presenter was invited back into the group, she provided more graphic details about the father's destructive attitude towards his son. The group then became very quiet and sombre and had difficulty in coming up with any ideas or speculations.

Parallel processes are quite subtle and intriguing, but as group members become more alert to the possibility that this is occurring, they start to see similar processes in their everyday work.

The outcomes of Balint work

There is international evidence that Balint work is very helpful for doctors.(5) However, there is a paradox. Balint has had an enormous influence on general practice and contributed to a deeper understanding of the generic nature of the doctor–patient relationship. Yet the number of health professionals who use the method as part of professional maintenance and development is relatively small.

The main reason for this paradox is the underlying assumptions of biomedicine, where there is more focus on diagnosis and treatment of disease (considered to be 'separate' from the person of the patient) than on interpersonal relationships. Another reason is that relationships are a difficult subject to focus on. By their very nature, relationships are subjective experiences. The Balint method helpfully uses the subjectivity of the group to explore complex health-care relationships.

With the increasing emphasis in medicine on accountability, patient safety, and self-care of the doctor,(6) Balint groups appear to offer considerable promise as a method of training, not only about significant relationships in medicine, but also about clinical reasoning.(7) The approach is applicable to postgraduate students and mature practitioners in medicine and in other health professional work. With the increased acknowledgement of burnout in health professionals,(8, 9) Balint work may become even more relevant.

Summary

A Balint case includes the patient, their problem, their interaction with their doctor and the doctor's responses. Balint groups are aimed at deepening the doctor's awareness of what was really going on in their presented case. Such deepening is achieved through group members wondering and speculating about all possible aspects of the case.

It is also helpful to say what Balint work is *not*. The aim is not to come up with better or different diagnoses, or better or different treatments. Group members put forward different ideas about the case, but it is also not a competition to be the most perceptive or accurate. The presenter does not award points at the end to the most prescient contribution.

At times the leaders may need to bring the group back to the task of speculation and wondering (instead, for example, of problem-solving or contesting someone else's point of view). These gentle corrections are made with the aim of canvassing all possible perspectives on the case, no matter how odd or 'left field'. Perspectives need to be offered and received without judgement: they are neither 'good' nor 'bad'.(10)

To achieve this, group members need to approach Balint work with an attitude of goodwill towards the presenter, the case, other group members and the leaders, whose interventions into the work may or may not be accurate or effective. All members of the group need to foster a spirit of enquiry. Overall, group members learn to listen to ideas from others with openness and curiosity, rather than with self-justification or defensiveness. This encourages a non-judgemental awareness, which in turn can lead to more intuition.

For many doctors just starting in Balint work, this overall orientation of goodwill and non-judgemental acceptance can feel quite different from the culture of medicine that involves intensively competitive training and strongly hierarchical relationships, both between doctors and with other health professionals. Balint work requires conscious readjustment of interpersonal culture. For new group members, this may take some time to filter in.

The task of the leader or leaders is to create a group in which a change in interpersonal culture might emerge. The more that leaders are clear about their tasks and attend to the boundaries around the work, the more group members can explore and play within it. Group members need to trust that such an extraordinarily different approach will eventually pay dividends.

Medicine is often a very serious enterprise: there are often better diagnoses and better treatments that might be used, and it is the responsibility of doctors to work hard at finding them. Play, speculation, and wondering are usually absent from these highly focused tasks. Balint work offers an alternative and enlivening approach to clinical competence and general well-being.

References

1. Balint M. *The doctor, his patient, and the illness*. London: Pitman, 1957.
2. Elder A, Samuel O, eds. *'While I'm here, doctor': a study of change in the doctor-patient relationship*. London: Tavistock, 1987.
3. Salinsky J. *Balint groups and the Balint method*. Balint Society of Australia and New Zealand, 2005.
4. Elder A. The role of the Balint group leader. *J Balint Soc* 2007, 35:15–7.
5. Kjelmand D. Balint training makes GPs thrive better in their job. *Pat Educ Couns* 2004, 55:230–35.
6. Benson J, Magraith K. Compassion fatigue and burnout: the role of Balint groups. *Austral Fam Phys* 2005, 34(6):497–98.
7. Lichtenstein A. Integrating intuition and reasoning: how Balint groups can help medical decision-making. *Austral Fam Phys* 2006, 35(12):987–89.
8. McCray LW, Cronholm PF, Bogner HR, Gallo JJ, Neill RA. Resident physician burnout: is there hope? *Fam Med* 2008, 40(9):626–32.
9. Paterson R, Adams J. Professional burnout – a regulatory perspective. *NZ Med J* 2011, 124:1333.
10. Barton J. *A beginner's guide to leading a Balint group*. Balint Society of Australia and New Zealand, 2011.

Index